Equine Behavior

A Guide for Veterinarians and Equine Scientists

Paul McGreevy BVSc PhD MRCVS

Senior Lecturer in Animal Behavior, Faculty of Veterinary Science,
University of Sydney, New South Wales, Australia

Foreword by

Professor Reuben Rose DVSc DipVetAn PhD FRCVS MACVSc

Dean, Faculty of Veterinary Science,
The University of Sydney, New South Wales, Australia
Vice-President, World Equine Veterinary Association

SAUNDERS

Edinburgh London New York Oxford Philadelphia St Louis Sydney Toronto 2004

SAUNDERS
An imprint of Elsevier Limited

First published 2004
    Reprinted 2005, 2006, 2008

ISBN 978 0 7020 2634 8

British Library Cataloguing in Publication Data
A catalogue record for this book is available from the British
Library

Library of Congress Cataloguing in Publication Data
A catalogue record for this book is available from the Library of
Congress

Notice
Veterinary medical knowledge is constantly changing. Standard
safety precautions must be followed, but as new research and
clinical experience broaden our knowledge, changes in treatment
and drug therapy may become necessary or appropriate. Readers
are advised to check the most current product information
provided by the manufacturer of each drug to be administered to
verify the recommended dose, the method and duration of
administration, and contraindications. It is the responsibility of
the practitioner, relying on experience and knowledge of the
patient, to determine dosages and the best treatment for each
individual patient. Neither the Publisher nor the authors assumes
any liability for any injuryand/or damage to persons or property
arising from this publication.
The Publisher

 ELSEVIER   your source for books,
journals and multimedia
in the health sciences
www.elsevierhealth.com

Working together to grow
libraries in developing countries
www.elsevier.com | www.bookaid.org | www.sabre.org
ELSEVIER BOOK AID International Sabre Foundation

The
publisher's
policy is to use
**paper manufactured
from sustainable forests**

Printed in China

Contents

Guest contributors

Chapter 3 was contributed by Dr Caroline Hahn and Chapter 13 was written jointly by Andrew McLean and Dr Paul McGreevy

Caroline Nora Hahn BS DVM MSc PhD MRCVS
Lecturer in Neuromuscular Disorders, Royal (Dick) School of Veterinary Studies, University of Edinburgh, UK

Andrew N McLean BSc DipEd
Director, Australian Equine Behaviour Centre, Victoria, Australia; PhD candidate

Foreword

The behavior of horses has intrigued horse-lovers, since ancient times. The domestication of the horse and subsequent modern use for recreational purposes has led to close observations of and fascination with horse behavior. Whether or not they realize it, those who get the best out of their horses are students of equine behavior. Many opinions exist in relation to what are regarded as normal and abnormal behaviors by horse owners and trainers. Most recently, this has culminated in a renaissance for the 'horse whisperer', who has supposedly mythical powers to commune with horses in their very souls. Undoubtedly, there are individuals who have rare gifts at an intuitive level, in understanding horses and their behavior. Popular interest in the skills of such individuals has accompanied demand for more humane training and handling techniques. Concurrently, the scientific study of equine behavior has been developing, and it is important to bring this to the attention of the horse industry.

For veterinarians and equine scientists, understanding the key aspects of horse behavior is critical to evaluation of health and welfare. It is only in relatively recent times that horse behavior has been subject to scientific study, and Dr Paul McGreevy has been one of a handful of veterinarians and scientists who have undertaken pioneering research in this field. This book is an important milestone in the progress towards better understanding of the effect of various equine management practices and their impact on horse performance and wellbeing. Dr McGreevy's book distills key scientific knowledge on horse behavior from over 1000 separate sources and covers the salient ethological characteristics of free-ranging horses, the impact of various management practices, as well as the significance of abnormal behaviors. In this latter area Dr McGreevy has undertaken groundbreaking research with Professor Christine Nicol on stereotypies, and this material will be of particular interest to those interested in applying equine science.

Dr McGreevy has provided an important guide for veterinarians and scientists and is to be congratulated for drawing together a veritable trove of scientific data on equine behavior that will be of benefit to the international horse industry.

Professor Reuben Rose

Preface

Equine Behavior: A Guide for Veterinarians and Equine Scientists has been an enlightening labor of love for me and I am honored to be commissioned to write it. Destiny may have had a hand in my selection, since legend has it that Ireland's McGreevy clan were keen horsemen and, indeed, were notorious for having stolen St Patrick's horses. For their alleged crime the Church forbade them to become priests. I doubt if that would have troubled them, as long as they had horses with which to work. For me the study of equine behavior is the most fascinating occupation in the world. Along with other enthusiasts, I delight in watching horses at work and play, and comparing notes on our observations. The aim of this book is to be a companion for all horse watchers.

Horse lovers are often tempted to conjure interpretations of how horses may process information and to imagine that horses share many of our value systems. On occasion, I have been criticized for failing to consider the rich emotional qualities horses may well possess. Suffice it to say that when we have a scientific way of measuring these qualities – and that time may not be too far away – I will be its strongest advocate, but until then I make no apology for confining myself to what we sometimes call the facts.

The past three decades have witnessed a terrific explosion in equine ethology – the science of horse behavior – so this is an exciting time for horse welfare. This book examines the truth behind modern trends and ancient traditions, by bringing together the latest cutting-edge research and best practice from around the world. The increased availability of data is matched by a growing sensitivity to what horses have been telling us for a very long time. The influence of science has helped to prompt fresh thinking about the relationship between horses and trainers. Science has also shown that horses learn in the same ways as other animals, in accordance with the principles of learning theory. This means that we are better placed to do the right thing by our horses and get the best out of them. This volume coins the term *equitation science* not as an attempt to undermine the art and skill of outstanding riders, but rather to demystify equitation and to allow more people to achieve better results and reduce wastage.

As a veterinarian and a qualified riding instructor I had two related audiences in mind: my colleagues in the veterinary profession and the veterinary students who will soon join us, and equine scientists and graduates in equine studies, who are assuming their place in the industry hierarchy. Veterinary professionals are uniquely placed to benefit from the book's scientific examination of those rare and poorly defined commodities, horse-sense and horsemanship. Owners naturally look to veterinarians for advice on the physical health of their horses, but this book is designed to empower veterinarians to become, also, a source of enlightened views on the mental health of their patients. Similarly, equine scientists can use the book to support scholarly approaches to enhance the management of horses. I hope this volume is written in a style that makes it accessible to a very wide audience and that it helps the industry as a whole to work with these two stakeholders in designing optimal scientific responses to behavior problems and in developing management and training systems that avoid their appearance.

Although this is a book that can be browsed, I strongly encourage you to digest some of its chapters in sequence. Specifically, the chapter on social behavior should be read before those on the behavior of the mare and stallion. Similarly, the chapter on learning contains material that facilitates understanding of the chapters on training, handling and miscellaneous problems.

The future for our relationship with horses seems bright. As we appreciate how to communicate with them sensitively and consistently, misunderstanding and misinterpretation by both parties will diminish. These advances are likely to be matched by greater sharing of knowledge among practitioners. Gone are the dark days when shamans locked themselves in stables to weave their magic on equine subjects and emerged with impressive results but no intention of divulging the techniques used. Information

technology means that, more than ever before, we can disseminate our observations, management innovations, and empirical findings and training successes through scientific abstracts, Internet discussion forums and email chat lists. Although horse enthusiasts are notoriously traditional and resistant to change, there is a pleasing uptake in these methods of exchanging information and an acceptance of new approaches.

I hope you enjoy *Equine Behavior: A Guide for Veterinarians and Equine Scientists* and that it improves your understanding of horses and inspires you to find out more. I warmly invite you to submit suggestions (through my website www.animalbehaviour.net) on how to improve future editions of this text. Finally, on behalf of my ancient and far-flung clan, I hope that St Patrick might regard my work as some kind of atonement.

Paul McGreevy
2004

Acknowledgments

Horses deserve the unique place they hold in the hearts and minds of humans, so it should be no surprise that horse behaviour as a research domain is populated by some extremely well-motivated and talented people, who have demonstrated their commitment to the species and their great kindness to me by providing invaluable feedback on various chapters of this book. They include Cheri Asa, Francis Burton, Hilary Clayton, Amy Coffman, Sharon Crowell-Davis, Nancy Diehl, Machteld van Dierendonck, Brian Farrow, Jane French, Debbie Goodwin, Caroline Hahn, Alison Harman, Kathe Houpt, Kevin Keay, Cecilia Lindberg, Andrew McLean, Finola McConaghy, Sue McDonnell, Christine Nicol, Kim Ng, Sarah Ralston, Ken Sedgers, Amanda Warren-Smith and Elaine Watson. One colleague, Daniel Mills, distinguished himself by going way beyond the call of duty and reading the entire draft manuscript. I am tremendously grateful to him for his advice and encouragement.

Other veterinary and academic colleagues who have provided helpful comments on specific topics include George Abrams, Ian Bidstrup, Heather Clegg, Sheila Crispin, Janet Eley, David Evans, Elsa Flint, Merran Govendir, Josie Hall, Lee Morris, Chris Murphy, Justine O'Brien, Trank Odberg, Mellisa Offord, Lesley Rogers, David Todd, Claire Weekes, Elsa Willis, Bonnie Williams and Carol Wyldes. Others who have helped me obtain particular illustrations include Victor Cabello, Natasha Ellis, Caroline Foote, Luke Henderson, Geoffrey Hutson, Peter Knight, Peter Read, Peter Thomson, and Clive Wynne and, most notably, John Conibear and Tracey Townsend-Sweeting from the University of Bristol. A number of undergraduate students studying both veterinary science and agricultural science made valuable contributions to early research for the book. They include Hilary Bugg, Russell Bush, Elvira Currie, Bradley Dong, Jayne Foster, Tanya Grassi, Lesley Hawson, Tammy Hunt, Kate Ireland, Lyndel Kruusamagi, Sally Leigo, Therese McGillion, Joe McGrath, Shawn McGrath, Sarah Mitchell, Kate Montgomery, Alex Nash, Katherine O'Toole, Claire Ruting, Denbigh Simond, Cathy Stimson and Joseph Toohey.

The staff at the University of Sydney Library have been characteristically helpful, efficient and professional in supplying research materials. In particular I would like to thank Joanne Bottcher, Ross Coleman, Su Hanfling and Alison Turner.

My extraordinary friends have been both supportive of my endeavours and tolerant of the extent to which writing has consumed my life over the past few years. Among the most helpful and supportive I wish to acknowledge Chris Coffey, Nick Copping, Lucy Hall, Claudia Jones, Emma Lawrence, Bryan McMahon, Alastair Paterson, Julia Perry, Jarther Taylor and Ben Scandrett-Smith. While Michael Jervis-Chaston gave the most refreshingly blunt advice on all the early chapters, Lynn Cole voluntarily cast an editorial eye over every last sentence and this has made the transition from manuscript to proofs smoother than any author deserves. I have learned a great deal in the process and will remain forever grateful. Meanwhile, Sandro Nocentini happily gave up an untold number of weekends to format illustrations and draw samples for the book.

Finally I would like to thank the outstanding horse riders, trainers and enthusiasts who have given their time and expertise to help with photography for the book. These include Terry Cooper, Valmai Furlong, Scott Glover, Brenna Harrison, Greg Hogan, Les Holmes, Portland Jones, Victoria Kendall-Hawk, John Leckie, Dave McConville, Deni McKenzie, Daniel Naprous, Gerard Naprous, Megan Roberts, Jo-Anne Rooker, Katie Rourke, Sigrid Schaerf, Daren Taylor and David Todd.

Special thanks to Richard Tibbitts of Antbits Illustration and Maggie Raynor for all their hard work in the illustration of this title.

1

Introduction

EVOLUTION AND CLASSIFICATION

Because the evolution of the horse has been dealt with many times elsewhere, I shall spare the reader detailed descriptions of three-toed forest-dwelling dog-like creatures. Suffice it to say that we have been left with a most remarkable animal that can exploit impoverished grazing niches by foraging on very poor fibrous material and digesting it quicker than ruminants. Various anatomical, physiological and behavioral features of the modern horse mean that it is useful to humans in many ways (Fig. 1.1).

EVOLUTIONARY BACKGROUND

A plains feeder that does not disperse and defend territories individually or in pairs as foragers of richer resources tend to, the horse has a long nose that allows it to graze while maintaining surveillance above the sward. As an animal without horns or antlers it relies largely on caution, speed and agility as its chief means of self-preservation. A social herbivore that capitalizes on companions for added safety, mutual comfort and enhanced detection of food, this is a creature that is likely to feel insecure when isolated.

To digest material ruminants generally discard, the horse needs a large fermentation chamber, the cecum. Obliged to carry such a voluminous digestive vat, the successful horse must therefore have tremendous muscular power to shift its necessary and considerable bulk from rest to top speed in the event of danger, so it has developed the ability

1

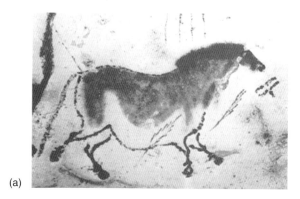

(a)

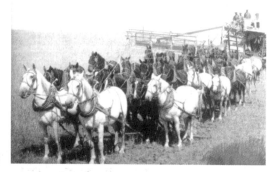

(b)

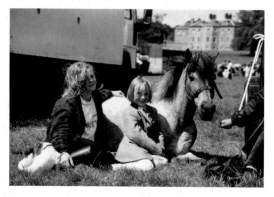

(c)

Figure 1.1 Humans and horses have had a long association. From depictions in cave paintings such as in Lascaux, France (a), we know that horses were originally hunted as a source of food, but since then the relationship has been developed through teamwork (b) and companionship (c). ((c) courtesy of Francis Burton.)

to use minimal physical effort to rest while standing. With its small stomach this 'trickle feeder' is obliged to forage frequently and has not evolved to eat and then ruminate in one spot. Instead it eats and moves and eats and moves. Restriction of movement and imposition of periods of fasting

are therefore likely to be more profound insults to equids than to members of many other species.

CLASSIFICATION OF EQUIDS

Prior to the beginning of domestication, in the late Pleistocene, long-term geographic isolation of equid populations occurred.[1] This led to the distinct species that exist today (Table 1.1). True horses (*Equus caballus*) occupied the Eurasian lowlands north of the great mountain ranges, while the asses occupied the arid zones of Asia. Crosses with asses, zebras and onagers are possible but the hybrids are normally sterile.

Order: perissodactyla (odd-toed ungulates)
Suborder: hippomorpha
Super-family: equoidea
Family: equidae

Despite their sometimes great morphological differences, all the breeds, groups and types of domestic horses belong to one species, *E. caballus*. Populations such as 'mustangs' and 'brumbies' found roaming in North America and Australia are feral representatives of this species. Within the *E. caballus* the occurrence of isolated environmental niches has given rise to the types we see among modern horses. Equine remains found in the Siberian permafrost suggest the presence of two distinct types of *E. caballus*: a small, heavily set type and a finer-boned 'Oriental' type of up to 14.3 hands (150 cm). The latter, less sturdy version was probably swifter and most likely the forebear of our modern 'hot-blooded' animals (so named because of their adapted suitability to hotter climes), the Arabians and Thoroughbreds. Reactivity and athleticism are the core characteristics of the hot-bloods that have led to their being favored as race, performance and sports horses. To respond rapidly to pivotal stimuli such as the opening of the starting stalls and the impact of the whip, racehorses have been selected for heightened reactivity to environmental changes. It seems likely that this is why they are over-represented in surveys of abnormal behaviors in stables, behaviors that are seen by many as responses to aversive

Table 1.1 Classification of equidae

Common name	Species	Diploid chromosome number
Prewalski's horse ([Mongolian] Wild Horse)	*Equus prewalskii*	66
Horse (domestic)	*Equus caballus*	64
African Wild Ass (and domestic donkey)	*Equus asinus*	62
Nubian Wild Ass	*Equus asinus africanus*	
Somali Wild Ass	*Equus asinus somalicus*	
Asian Ass	*Equus hemionus*	56
Mongolian Wild Ass	*Equus hemionus hemionus*	
Onager	*Equus hemionus onager*	
Indian Wild Ass	*Equus hemionus khur*	
Kiang	*Equus hemionus kiang*	
Grevy's zebra	*Equus grevyi*	46
Common zebra	*Equus burchelli*	44
Chapman's zebra	*Equus burchelli antiquorum*	
Grant's zebra	*Equus burchelli boehmi*	
Selous's zebra	*Equus burchelli selousi*	
Mountain zebra	*Equus zebra*	32
Cape Mountain zebra	*Equus zebra zebra*	
Hartman's zebra	*Equus zebra hartmannae*	

stimuli. The least reactive equids are the so-called 'cold-bloods', the heavy horses and solid ponies. In between the two groups are the 'warmbloods'. These can be described as crosses between hot and cold bloods and are exemplified by European performance horse breeds such as the Hannoverian.

Equus caballus and *Equus przewalskii*

Although mitochondrial deoxyribonucleic acid (DNA) studies suggest a divergence occurred as long ago as a quarter of a million years, it seems that the most likely link between modern horse (*E. caballus*) and its more numerous and diverse predecessors is the pony-shaped Mongolian Wild Horse, Przewalski's Horse (*E. przewalskii*). Apart from Caspian ponies that appear to be polymorphic in the diploid number (some having 64 chromosomes while others have 65),[2] *E. caballus* has 64 chromosomes. *Equus przewalskii*, on the other hand, has 66 chromosomes in the diploid state.

There is some debate as to how closely the first ancestors of *E. caballus* were related to *E. przewalskii*. Cross-breeding between *E. caballus* and *E. przewalskii* does produce fertile offspring, and there are similarities in their serum proteins and their blood groups. Geneticists explain that a

single fusion mutation in the haploid state (32) could have brought about their differences. They could be part of a single species exhibiting chromosomal dimorphism as occurs in the Asian ass *(Equus hemionus)*.[3] This then is the single-dichotomy theory that currently prevails over less-fashionable claims of multiple lineage.

Subsequent isolation of the two gene pools could perhaps have arisen because of capricious selectivity on the part of Caballus stallions (see Ch. 11) and the retreat of Przewalski herds into regions of the steppe uninhabited by humans.[4] While outnumbered by the similarities between the two species, the differences are fascinating. For example, the striking bistability of hock joints that allows a very rapid switch from one extreme position to the other is much more marked in domestic horses than in Przewalski horses and, for that matter, zebras.[5]

Przewalski horses became extinct in the wild in the 1950s.[6] However, from a nucleus of 11 foundation animals, they survive today in captivity and in successfully re-introduced wild populations, e.g. in Mongolia.[7,8] The survival story of the Przewalski horse is an extraordinary one, and we are indeed fortunate to be able to study them in a variety of contexts. It is fascinating that we now have data to refute the notion that Przewalski horses are socially more aggressive than domestic horses.[9] However, studies of their behavior should be treated with some caution since they have emerged from a shallow gene pool that has been filtered through 20 generations of captivity. Therefore before assuming that present-day Przewalski horses behave as true wild horses, we should bear in mind that some would regard them as survivors of the first stages of domestication.

In this text, I have selected examples of feral horse behavior rather than Przewalski horse behavior as benchmarks for what is normal. Discussions of such free-ranging behavior appear in each of the subsequent chapters.

CHANGING ROLES

Although initially horses found themselves in the human domain as a food source, their subsequent roles are nearly as varied as those of the other most domesticated species, the dog, and include the provision of power, leisure and companionship.

DOMESTICATION

French and Spanish cave paintings from around 15 000 years ago, depicting hunting for food and hides, represent the earliest record of human use of horses.[10]

While early horses would eventually provide their keepers with unprecedented mobility and power, the herding of horses probably had its origins in the consumption of horseflesh.[11] Hunters favor meat, such as that from horses, that has a high glycogen content. As a source of dietary sugar, this facilitates endurance, which is important for members of hunting cultures. Horses were regularly consumed in favor of other large herbivores. In the Palaeolithic, our ancestors hunted horses by driving them over cliffs and into traps and pitfalls. They continued to do so for thousands of years to the extent that they had a pivotal effect on population numbers.[12] It is thought that, along with climatic changes, this exploitation contributed to the extinction of wild horses in North and South America. Wild horse

remains elsewhere dating from periods since 9000 years ago are rare for this reason.[13]

Interestingly, it seems the 'true horse' (*E. caballus*) survived in Eurasia but with patchy distribution[14] despite, or perhaps even because of, this predation.

Archaeological evidence of horse domestication dates from 4000 BC (late Neolithic or Bronze Age) in the Eurasian Steppes of the Ukraine.[15] Ancient middens used as dumping grounds for the bony remains of human meals, most notably in a place called Dereivka on the steppes north of the Black Sea, have proved an especially rich source of domestication data. This is where river-valley agricultural economies evolved, relying on the use of stone enclosures to trap large numbers of game. The numbers involved in a draft often exceeded the immediate demand for consumption and prompted the maintenance of surviving herd members, to be slaughtered at a later stage.

From studies of the bone remains found in middens, the first pastoral species seems to have been bovine. A colder climatic shift that affected this region around 3500 BC is thought to have favored equids rather than other domestic or wild herbivores because, being large and long-legged, they were better able to forage in snow. The prevalence of horses in Ukrainian communities saw a dramatic rise at this time, with horse bones comprising 74% of animal bones at Dereivka.[16] Evidence of domestication at this site includes this dramatic rise and the predominance of colt skeletons. Analysis of the dental remains of horses in these sites suggests that humans consumed more males than females and that the age range of these animals did not show a normal distribution.

Some authors[12,17] maintain that the relatively high number of colts indicates domestication rather than hunting which would be more likely to harvest older animals, more often mares. Other workers suggest that the vast majority of horses at this time were hunted, by stalking (Fig. 1.2).[11] Perhaps the age distribution of horse teeth most closely matches what one would expect as remnants of such activity, but it is worth remembering that assessing age by dentition is an imprecise science.[18]

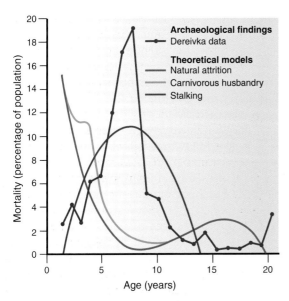

Figure 1.2 Graph of age distribution of remains of 151 horses found at Dereivka, Ukraine. In free-ranging horses death occurs most commonly in the very young and very old (natural attrition model). In populations raised for meat (carnivorous husbandry), the curve is skewed by preferential consumption of 2- to 3-year-olds. Meanwhile selective hunting of prime-age adults (stalking) produces a different pattern, with a sharp central peak. The age distribution of horse teeth found at Dereivka most closely matches the stalking model. (Reproduced by permission of Marsha Levine and Antiquity Publications Ltd, from Levine M, *The Problems of Horse Domestication in Antiquity* 64:727–740.)

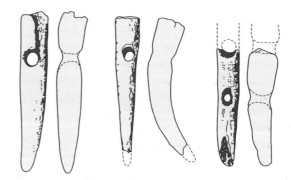

Figure 1.3 Artifact from what is believed to be an early bit fashioned from antlers.[19] The rope would have been held in place in the mouth by the cheek-pieces. (Reproduced by permission of David Anthony, Dorcas Brown and Antiquity Publications Ltd, from *The Origins of Horseback Riding in Antiquity* 65:22–38.)

The issue here seems to pivot on whether there is any reason for members of a domesticated population to be selected for consumption at 5–8 years of age. A more traditional farming approach would be to harvest the surplus while they were younger and their flesh was reasonably tender. Although one might also ask why hunters would target animals in a wild group that were undoubtedly in their prime and therefore most fleet of foot, it seems likely that they would be more abundant than adolescents or elderly horses.

The reported preponderance of what we regard as male type canine teeth seems to be crucial here. Could it be that small canines as found in many modern mares were erroneously identified as the teeth of stallions?

Horse remains at Dereivka have been characterized as being from large-headed, short and heavy-set animals,[15] a description strikingly reminiscent of the Przewalski horse. When the skull of a male equid was removed from a ritual burial site shared by two dogs and anthropomorphic figurines, it aroused considerable excitement in archaeological circles. Dating from the Copper Age, about 4300 BC, the ritualized nature of the burial was suggestive of profound domestication. Interestingly, in the same grave, excavations revealed antler tines that seemed to have been crafted into the cheek-pieces of a crude bit (Fig. 1.3). By facilitating the comparison of the teeth of modern domesticated and feral horses with those of the so-called Dereivka cult stallion, electronmicroscopic analysis of anterior premolar tooth wear has revealed bevels and fractures consistent with the use of a bit.[19] Even though the first bit was not as robust and therefore as damaging as modern hardware, the damage incurred was regarded as being consistent with 300 hours of bridled control. However, before making such comparisons, it is worth considering ways in which the evidence may have been skewed. Freshly domesticated horses may have been very headstrong and early equitation unrefined. Notwithstanding this minor point, the Dereivka stallion is regarded as the first ridden horse and is thought to have predated the invention of the wheel by at least 500 years.[20] The domestication of horses on the steppes may have been repeated in other places. Recent mitochondrial DNA evidence[21] indicates that a large number of founders was recruited over an extended time period. This 'multiple origins' scenario implies that horses may have been independently captured from diverse wild populations and then bred in captivity as the wild populations disappeared.[21] This suggests that what spread from that equine cradle was not necessarily the horses themselves but the innovation and technology of taming them.

Although it seems likely that meat production was the first reason for the domestication of horses, their prevailing impact was linked to their use in riding and haulage. When handling an orphan foal, early horse farmers would have appreciated the horse's ability to pull and the fact that control of the body depended on control of the head. A natural progression would have seen the development of harnesses for traction and headcollars for control. It may be that too much emphasis has been placed on the significance of bit wearing as the necessary step that took the use of horses beyond the dining table. It is implied that horses could not have been controlled from behind by anything less than a bit. This is something of a moot point since it precludes riding with bitless bridles. Equally, horses could have been used for non-riding purposes such as traction of non-wheeled haulage devices, or fallen prey for that matter.

Early farmers had to have some means of preventing the usual migratory dispersal of horses but men on foot, even if they were accompanied by trained dogs, would be no match for galloping horses.[22] Only when riding was attempted could the herding of horses become efficient. Furthermore, while using horses is a matter of taming the individuals as required, breeding them is far more technically demanding.[23] The difficulty of preventing domestic mares from dispersing in search of stallions whenever they were in estrus may have been the reason why domestication of the horse took such a long time. For these reasons, horses were domesticated after cattle, pigs, sheep and goats, which were all easier to herd and contain.

Although the horse was one of the last mammals to be domesticated, it has had more impact than most on humans, not least in terms of the dispersion of culture and language.[13,20] Beginning with the migration of humans across the deep steppes of the Ukraine that could not support large human populations prior to the emergence of riding, horses facilitated the spread of human genes. Because riders move two or three times faster and farther than pedestrians, exploitable territories expanded sixfold. At the same time grassland subsistence became more predictable, reliable and productive, and decisive military advantages were secured over more static neighbors.[20] As a consequence, human social groups grew tenfold, conflicts over resources escalated and patterns of trade and theft expanded in range and variety. While riding was established as the prime means of hunting, exploring and herding, the additional use of horses for milk and blood is likely to have peaked at the same time. One should not overlook the usefulness of horses in the haulage of fallen game, firewood, ploughs, produce and physically challenged members of the group. Such was the importance of the horse in the early dispersal of Copper Age humans that horses became one of the chief tradable items.

The emergence of equestrian cultures is also likely to have brought with it an increase in hit-and-run warfare (Fig. 1.4). This suggestion is borne out by the effective use of the horse by American Indians in the 1800s which resulted in the unprecedented rise in conflicts and accumulation of wealth leading to the tribal supremacy of the Sioux, Comanche and Apache.[24]

Interestingly it was not until approximately 2000 BC that horses arrived in the Middle East and displaced asses and ass-onager hybrids as the favored draft animals for battle carts from which arrows could be fired. A similar displacement took place in mid 19th century Africa when colonists' demand for the social status inferred by using apparently superior riding animals prompted the importation of often poorly adapted horses while the local equid, the quagga (*Equus quagga*), was hunted to extinction by English and Boer farmers.[25]

A new wave of horse-mediated military success emerged when the horse's speed and maneuverability was fully appreciated. In the first place,

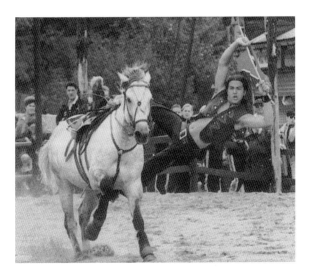

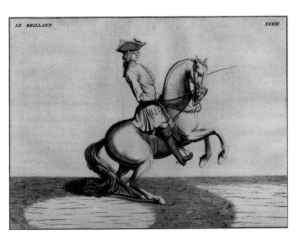

Figure 1.5 An etching showing the development of haute école training, as archived by Le Baron D'Eisenberg (from *L'Art de Monter a Cheval*, 1737).

Figure 1.4 Horse being ridden by stunt rider as a demonstration of use in combat. Equitation improved a warrior's usefulness and chances of survival. (Reproduced with permission of Gerard Naprous.)

chariots, as mobile platforms for archers, provided the means of delivering flanking blows to infantrymen,[26] then came the complete development of cavalry warfare. Many authors have discussed the introduction of modern equestrian techniques[27,28] and the development of the bits, saddles and stirrups[16,29,30] and the extent to which each lent a military advantage. The invention of the saddle that shifted the rider's weight bilaterally to the lumbar musculature and subsequently the stirrup that facilitated the use of weapons by mounted warriors are thought to have been major steps in the culture of mounted combat. With the increasing sophistication of equine-dependent power that led to the emergence of jousting tournaments and ultimately *haute école* dressage (Fig. 1.5), noblemen came to be judged by, among other things, the quality and quantity of horseflesh in their possession.[31] The role of the horse in colonial success was acknowledged by Cortes after the Spanish invasion of Mexico, when he noted that (next to God) he owed his victory to the horses.

The management of warhorses was often chronicled but the emphasis in these accounts seems to have been upon their training, nutrition[32,33] and medical care[34] rather than their housing. The use of horses by military and invading nations has been marked by considerable wastage. There is evidence that Roman equids in Britain sustained injuries consistent with poor living conditions and gross overwork.[35] Horses continued to serve in battle up until the end of the Second World War, when the Polish cavalry suffered horrific losses from the guns of Russian tanks.

CURRENT STATUS

Horses are regarded as a familiar part of many agricultural idylls but their role as farm animals is now in question. If we compare the life of a stabled riding horse to that of other farm species, some differences are obvious. Unlike most cows, pigs and sheep, horses are generally not kept with a view to productivity in terms of meat or milk and therefore are often on limited food rations. Because they cannot be regarded as production animals, horses are more often these days described as a 'companion animal species'. Unfortunately they do not fit terribly well into this category either, since they do not share living space with humans as do true companion animals such as cats, dogs and caged birds. Their contact with humans is largely restricted to being groomed, fed and ridden.

The key roles of the horse in human activity changed tremendously during the 20th century.

The overarching fields in which horses are now used include recreational and social purposes, breeding, sport and competition and to some extent meat production.[36] Huge reductions in the use of horses in military, agricultural and transportation activities have been matched, in developed countries, by increased equine numbers for sport and leisure.[37–39]

Prevalent modern breeds are often used in more than one activity (Table 1.2), and this may help to account for the retention of some diversity. Happily, horse breed societies have tended to avoid the sort of intense line-breeding that characterizes the bloodlines of many purebred

dogs, and very few populations are inbred. Notable exceptions are the horses of the Namib Desert, Namibia[40] and Blue Arabians from the USA.[41] In-hand showing as a sole means of selecting breeding animals removes many performance indicators from the selection process in breeding systems and is therefore short-sighted.

While donkeys are still used by the working classes in many parts of the world, the horse is now a status symbol in Western cultures, a luxury item or an emotional focus. Interestingly, this has done nothing to guarantee its welfare, since many owners of luxury items fail to budget for their maintenance. Despite the emergence of equine insurance

Table 1.2 Some generalizations about the attributes and uses of modern breeds and types

Horse use	Activities	Physical attributes	Behavioral attributes	Leading breeds
Show-jumping	Agility over fences and against the clock	• Tall yet built close to the ground[42] • Powerful hindquarters • Flat pelvis[43] • Forward-sloping femur[44] • Sloping, free-moving shoulders • Long humerus[43] • Large hock angles[43] • Agile • Deep-chested – thought to be associated with optimal lung and heart room	• Obedience • Boldness • Responsivensess • Tendency when jumping to tuck in the forelegs and kick back the hindlegs	• Thoroughbreds • Draft/TB crosses • Welsh Cob/TB crosses • Warmbloods, including Trakehners
Dressage	Controlled and yet demonstrably powerful execution of set maneuvers	• Classic good looks and impressive gaits help to keep the judge's eye on the horse • Powerful limbs • Forward-sloping femur[44] • Neck set on high • Short neck[42] • Long humerus[43] • Long upright phalanges[43] • Small hip angle[43] • Flexible and supple • >14.2 hands high (FEI height rule)	• Responsive • Calm • Classically correct, free, regular paces • Confident	• Draft/TB crosses • Warmbloods including Hannoverians, Dutch Warmbloods, Lipizzangers, Oldenburgs
Eventing	Combined demonstrations of stamina, agility and compliance in the dressage arena	• Generally athletic • Powerful limbs • Neck set on high • High withers • >14.2 hands high (FEI height rule 14 hands 2¼ inches high without shoes)	• Calm • Responsive	• Thoroughbreds • Draft/TB crosses • Australian Stock Horse • Warmbloods, including Trakehners • Warmblood crosses

(contd.)

Table 1.2   (Contd.)

Horse use	Activities	Physical attributes	Behavioral attributes	Leading breeds
Endurance	Long-distance riding and ride and tie events	• Stamina and resistance to dehydration • Short strong back • Strong legs • Hard hooves • A long stride and a floating action that helps to conserve energy	• Tendency to bond with humans[45] • Calm • Compliant • Drink readily	• Arabians • Arabian crosses • Paso Finos • Appaloosas • Walers • Australian Stock Horse
Children's sport	Junior versions of premier sports and team sports including vaulting and mounted games (gymkhana games) many of which have their origins in latter-day cavalrytraining e.g. tent-pegging	• Short backs (except for vaulting horses) • Short legs making turn about at speed easier • Agile • Fast over short distances • Athletic	• Tolerant • Calm • Unflappable • Fun-loving • Trainable • Responsive	• Arabian crosses • Ponies, especially Welsh
Racing	Racing: • Flat • Hurdles • Steeple chasing • Arab racing • Quarterhorse racing	• Croup high • Powerful hindquarters • Strong shoulders • Deep chests • Modest abdomens	• Reactive to stimuli • Desire to run • Perhaps a reluctance to be at the back of a group	• Thoroughbreds • Arabians • Quarterhorses
Trotting	Harness racing at the trot	• Tall withers[46] • Open angles at the shoulder and stifle joints[46] • Large girth circumference at the front of the thorax but narrow girth circumference at the lowest point of the back[43]	• Tolerant of harness and handling • Desire to run	• Standardbreds
Pacing	Harness racing at a pacing gait	• Elastic fetlock joints[47] • Long sloping shoulders[47] • Long muscular forearms[47]	• Tolerant of harness and handling • Desire to run	• Standardbreds
Ball sports	Polo and polocrosse	• Strong hindquarters that allow the horse to be light on the forehand and therefore easily accelerated • Athletic	• Reliable • Responsive • Hardworking • Agile • Swift to learn	• Polo ponies • Stock horses • Thoroughbreds (small) • Quarterhorses
Working horse competitions	Camp drafting Cutting	• Strong hindquarters	• 'Cow sense' • Reliable • Calm • Quick reaction times[42]	• Stockhorses • Quarterhorses • Draft crosses
Leisure	Recreational trail-riding/trekking/hacking Riding club activities including quadrilles and combined training	• Generally sound • Sloping pasterns	• Adaptable • Calm	• Any riding breed, especially Australian Stock Horse, American Saddlebred, Quarterhorses, Standardbreds, Arabian crosses, colored horses and pony breeds

(contd.)

Table 1.2 *(Contd.)*

Horse use	Activities	Physical attributes	Behavioral attributes	Leading breeds
Hormone, vaccine and anti-venin production	Regular removal of serum or urine for processing into human and animal medications	• Bulky	• Low reactivity	• Draft breeds, notably Percherons
Milk production	Milk production most notably in Russia where fermented mares' milk (koumiss) is a popular food for human infants	• Cup-shaped udders • Long lactation ($\geqslant$200 days)[48] • High yield $\geqslant$ 1600 kg/ lactation)[2] • Fast milk ejection rate ($\geqslant$28 ml/s)[48]	• Tolerant of daily separation from foal and machine milking	• Bashkir
Meat production	Slaughter for human consumption and pet food; notably: • Spent working animals • Poor young-stock specimens of all breeds • Some purpose-bred animals	Not applicable	Not applicable	• European heavy breeds • Small pony breeds • Feral horses
Draft	• Haulage of produce, wood and water in developing countries • Boutique tourism in developed countries • Ploughing matches	• Compact bodies • Strong, large feet • Strong neck and shoulders • Powerful hindquarters	• Low reactivity • Compliant • Phlegmatic temperament[49]	• Heavy horses including Shires, Clydesdales, Suffolk Punches and Percherons • Donkeys • Mules
Exhibition and production	• Showing • Breeding	• Conforming to written breed standard	• Impressive demeanour ('presence') in the show ring • Eye-catching gaits • Adaptable at stud	• Any registered purebreds and registered partbreds, color or types
Hunting and hunter trials	Cross-country riding over natural obstacles and terrain	• Strong hindquarters • Sloping 'jumper's' shoulders • Agility	• 'Bravery'	• Thoroughbreds • Draft/TB crosses • Cleveland Bays
Carriage driving	Dressage and cross-country driving of teams, pairs and singles	• Strong hind quarters • Relatively short, strong legs capable of scrambling, scurrying and turning	• Tough • Compliant • Tolerant of other horses in close proximity • Sure footed • Agile • High hock action	• Welsh ponies and Welsh cobs • Friesians • Gelderlanders • Cleveland Bays • Dales • Fells • Fjords • Shetland ponies • Standardbreds

FEI, Fédération Equestre Internationale; TB, thoroughbred.

policies that have helped to remedy the shortfall, many owners find themselves financially embarrassed when invoiced for colic surgery. Financial circumstances have considerable influence on the way horses are managed, as indeed does the value of the horse itself. Sometimes the value of a horse can prove an impediment to optimal welfare.[50]

Although many owners keep their horses in the best possible conditions that money allows,[39] sometimes it seems that when performance is less critical, management standards may drop and welfare may be affected. Ignorance and economies may combine to jeopardize the welfare of hobby-horses. This is not to suggest that high-performance animals always enjoy the best welfare, since, for example, intensive management of racehorses involves some of the greatest alterations in time budgets, some of which can reflect profoundly compromised welfare. It is interesting to contrast the management of a Thoroughbred stallion kept in a mahogany trimmed loosebox with brass fittings near Newmarket, on the one hand, with a child's pony tethered on common land in suburban Dublin. The relative absence of confinement of the latter may well enhance its welfare.

While private owners report increasingly emotional attachments to their horses,[51] large numbers of people work in the equine sector for little or no financial reward. With the shift of horse use from military and utilitarian services, the demographics of horse ownership changed, with women forming the majority.[52] It has been suggested that female horse owners are more affectionate than males.[53] There are interesting reports of an increasing proportion of male riders and an increasing number of older riders.[39]

Although there are no published data on the health benefits of horse ownership, there is convincing evidence that riding is a therapeutic activity.[54] Equine practitioners do well to consider the profundity of many human–horse bonds, especially at the time of euthanasia.[55] However, while some cultures have come to regard horses as companion animals, others have persisted in the pragmatism that leads them to consume young horses surplus to breeding requirements or those too old to be of use as breeders or as a means of conveyance.[36]

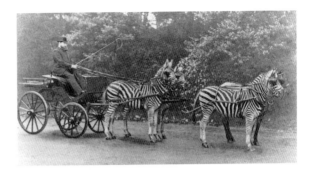

Figure 1.6 Lord Rothschild and his team of four zebras (*E. burchelli*), circa 1900. (Reproduced with permission of the Natural History Museum.)

Noting the human tendency to forget to appreciate horses for what they are, Rollin[56] highlights our 'unfortunate skill in putting square pegs into round holes'. Compared with close relatives such as zebras that have only very rarely been put to work (Fig. 1.6), horses can be manipulated to behave in many ways and persuaded to cope with a tremendous variety of uses and abuses. The behavioral flexibility of horses is fundamental to their utility in the domestic context. It allows them to tolerate negative reinforcement more than other domestic species but also explains why they are subject to tremendous abuse by clumsy and ignorant handlers (see Ch. 13).

The explosion in the popularity of riding for leisure and first-time horse ownership has led some veterinarians to bemoan the welfare of some present-day equids, e.g. inner city ponies. Ignorance is a considerable force to be reckoned with. I have encountered novice owners who believed their horses could thrive on remarkable diets, including rabbit food and, on one occasion, cat food.

THE HORSE'S FUTURE

Information technology should facilitate the education of horse owners and, one hopes, liberate their thinking. The impact of ethology on horse welfare has already been recognized,[57] and there is a growing demand for enlightened approaches to horse handling as evidenced by the success of the modern 'horse whisperers'.[58–61] Unfortunately, for some exponents the emphasis seems to be to placed on shows and the introduction of jargon rather than on education. It is hoped that ethologists will continue to demystify the language of showmen and shamans so that communication with horses can be enhanced wholesale.

The practice of identifying and logging the performance of non-racing sport horses has the potential to enhance the quality and, it is hoped, the depth of the gene pool. For that reason it is particularly sad to note the disappearance of the British Horse Database.

Similarly the introduction of novel reproductive technologies such as artificial insemination should allow horse breeders to capitalize on genetic material from overseas in the same way that shuttle stallions, flown in from the Northern hemisphere, have liberated Thoroughbred breeders in the Southern hemisphere.

Since we know that some unwelcome behaviors follow a familial pattern of inheritance, it may be that there will emerge a drive to breed from animals that can cope with the stressors of intensive management. Geneticists may also help to improve fertility, one of the most pressing problems in Thoroughbred circles. Globally, the annual reproduction rate for Thoroughbreds is approximately 50%.[37] This compares poorly with other single-offspring species such as cattle, in which 85% is normal.[37] This disturbing trend is certainly not helped by a rise in the rate of twinning, an unfit gene that is passed from one generation to the next almost exclusively by veterinary intervention.

It seems unlikely that, since it has been the single breeding objective for the past two centuries, speed on the track can undergo much improvement. Mirroring the current focus of human exercise physiologists, the role of lactic acid clearance as a limiting factor in racehorse performance continues to attract considerable attention.[62] It may be that selection of genotypes capable of accelerated lactic acid metabolism may reduce winning times in the longer classic races such as the St Leger and the Oaks.[63,37] Markers of speed may be identified by genome mapping studies but these are likely to combine a number of features,

including cardiac output and maximal oxygen consumption.

While there may be initiatives to identify the genes of horses that cope best with intensive management and do so without displaying stereotypies, it is hoped that the technology can be harnessed to improve horse welfare rather than simply to select for tolerance. The worldwide web seems an appropriate forum for information on the identification and treatment of common ailments and the showcasing of best practice in stable management.

Although grazing land will become harder to come by, stabling is likely to evolve to meet more closely the behavioral needs of horses. We may yet identify key elements of established management protocols that can have a deleterious effect on our horses.[64,65] Although these days it is common for owners and trainers to regard the risk of injury in sport horses as being great enough to outweigh the benefits of being turned out,[36] new evidence may emerge to fortify the case for increased opportunities for spontaneous exercise and social contact.

The welfare of riding-school horses is likely to improve as technological advances make it easier to detect those of a novice rider's signals that are particularly confusing and unhelpful. In France, an electronic riding machine has been developed with all of the paces of a horse (Fig. 1.7). Currently it has a predictable action that allows the rider to learn, for instance, how to rise at the trot and even jump a fence.[66] With sensors to detect and respond to the rider's signals, the simulator reduces the time required for novices to learn to ride.[67] It is not difficult to see how this technology may advance. It could be programmed to behave less predictably, to be more or less responsive or to demonstrate typical equine conflict behaviors in response to confusing commands.[68] One could even speculate that the welfare of those dependable riding-school horses that always carry novice riders will be of less concern in the future. Currently balance is acquired over weeks of crude education, for example, staying on board by pulling on the reins and therefore the mouth. The numbing effect this has on the horse's mouth reflects the discomfort it must endure. This

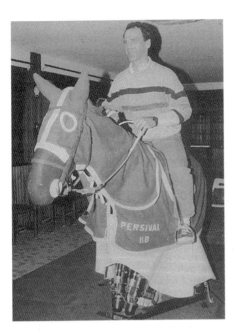

Figure 1.7 Persival, the Ecole Nationale d'Equitation's mechanical horse simulator.

inelegant and inhumane use of sentient beings in human education may disappear with the growing use of mechanical alternatives.

Digitization of the interaction of elite riders with their mounts may provide for a quantum improvement in the teaching of equitation. Measurement of tensions and pressures applied by the handler's hands, seat and legs can be correlated to observed behavior of the animal and provide an indication of the magnitude of stimulation required to be applied by the handler to modify the behavior of the animal. Logging devices of this sort will also provide teachers with some quantitative means of assessing the handling of an animal under the control of a student.

STABLE MANAGEMENT

Humans can control horses most effectively by stabling them. This imposes limits on the extent to which horses can meet their behavioral needs and can have profound effects on welfare. Equine behavior undergoes considerable modification when animals are removed from pastured (or feral) environments and placed in a stable.

TRADITIONAL STABLE MANAGEMENT

The horses sent over to the British Isles by the Roman conquerors would have included a variety of heavy, 'cold-blooded' and less weather-tolerant, 'hot blooded' animals. Archaeological evidence[69] suggests that they were small by modern standards. Evidence of how Roman horses were housed exists but is rather cryptic, with remnants often being limited to urine and manure staining on chalk beds and teeth in feeding channels. However, a site at Hod Hill in Dorset[70] appears to have been particularly well studied. Two types of stable division were noted, and the pattern of chalk-compression and the extent to which hooves had mixed chalk with manure gave the investigators an impression of how the animals were secured within the building. In one type of compartment, measuring 3.6 m × 3.3 m, three horses might have been tethered to the wall, their dung falling into a 2-meter channel to the rear. This channel also permitted access by grooms. The other compartment appeared to have accommodated six horses that again were tethered facing the wall. Measuring 3.6 m × 5.5 m, this house comprised a central dunging passage that was communal to both rows of horses.

Information regarding accommodation for military horses since that time is limited. Smith[71] indicates that the British Army billeted horses in lines and did not have stables until a program of building barracks and stables began in 1792. Of these stables little is known except that they were not ventilated and therefore precipitated considerable losses from glanders and other respiratory diseases.[71] Coach horses from the same era were confined to tie-stalls rather than individual boxes that were the reserve of saddle horses.

MODERN STABLE MANAGEMENT

Just as domestic horses are put to a number of uses, so they are housed for a number of reasons and in stables of varying design. The most common issues around the 'whys' and 'hows' of intensive horse management are considered below.

Reasons for stabling horses

Horse owners throughout the world house their animals for a number of reasons. Among these, the most important is often the need to spare limited grazing areas from damage underfoot, especially in regions of and in times of heavy precipitation. The danger of disease associated with exposure, such as 'rain-scald' and 'mud-fever', in these regions can be reduced by providing shelter and appropriate prophylaxis. Therefore, the economics of pasture management can prevail over horse welfare when owners consider stabling their horses for the winter.

By stabling their horses, owners eliminate food-stealing by dominant conspecifics and can have more control over food quality and intake. Food and water intakes are easier to monitor, with an eye toward early detection of disease, in the stable rather than the field. During the winter, time spent mucking-out and bedding a horse can be offset by the time saved by not having to groom a thick layer of mud off the horse prior to exercise. Clipping, made more feasible by the fact that the horse is sheltered, adds to this advantage since clipped horses sweat less in response to heavy work than their counterparts in a full winter coat and are therefore easier to clean.

Stabling may be favored by the owners of horses that are difficult to catch when at pasture. The limit on kinetic activity that is imposed by stabling is considered advantageous by trainers of performance horses since they can more easily control the amount of daily exercise taken by their charges.

Health advantages may accrue from stabling since injuries can be more effectively rested, worms can be better controlled and flies are less numerous than at pasture. Apparent advantages for the horses of being stabled include shelter (from sun, wind, rain and flies), freedom from bullying and a reduced physical requirement to work (e.g. forage) for food.

MANAGEMENT PRACTICES

The time of year and the seasonal nature of some sports such as hunting and eventing influence the way in which horses are managed. Traditionally during the summer, while gymkhana ponies undergo a peak in their use because children are on school holidays, hunters are 'let down' at grass.

Feeding

Horses are notoriously wasteful grazers (see Ch. 8). Many farmers remark that, in wet weather, when one considers the damage done by its unforgiving hooves, a horse is equivalent to the activity of five bovine mouths. The reluctance of owners to allow this damage means that time spent by horses at pasture in temperate climates is often limited during the winter months. While sparing the horses the pain of disorders such as mud fever and dermatophilosis, this intervention often has a deleterious impact on their behavior and nutrition.

Traditionally, horses are fed long fiber from a haynet or hayrack. This is intended to reduce wastage from contamination with urine or feces and possibly to decrease the likelihood of endo-parasite transmission. However, there is growing evidence that this unnatural foraging position can have a deleterious effect on the efficacy of the mucociliary escalator in clearing the upper airways of inhaled particles (Fig. 1.8), especially those inhaled from dried foodstuffs (which are to some extent unnatural in themselves).[72] Similarly, haynets reduce the space available in the stable, may increase the risk of the horse becoming snared (e.g. by trapping its hoof), and elevate the forage so increasing its potential as a source of ocular foreign bodies. It is also argued that feeding from a net or rack may adversely affect muscles and nerves in the neck.[73] Perhaps this is why, when financial considerations are almost insignificant relative to the value and maintenance of performance – for example, in the majority of racing yards[74] – horses are fed roughage, whether it be hay, haylage or silage, from the stable floor.

There are marked seasonal variations in feeding practices according to the weather and the

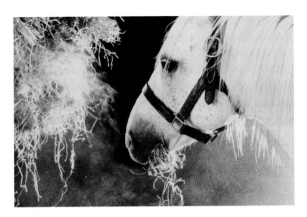

Figure 1.8 Dust plumes from a haynet as a horse forages. The position of the food and its contamination with fungal spores are unnatural. The harmful effects on respiratory health are well recognized. (Reproduced by permission of the University of Bristol, Department of Clinical Veterinary Science.)

availability of pasture. We do well to remember that the incidence of colic follows a similar pattern, with changes from fresh grass to a dried diet being associated with rises in various enteropathies, especially impactions. The use of concentrated feeds and the periods of fasting with which they are associated have been linked to unwelcome consequences, including increases in gastric acidity that can result in rapid ulceration.[75] Compared with those who ride mainly for competitive reasons, those who ride mainly for pleasure are less likely to feed cereal-based foods according to the manufacturer's recommendations during summer, when grass is available.[76]

Bedding

For a variety of reasons, including availability, ease of disposal and tradition, straw remains the favored bedding for horses,[76] with 65% of yards in a recent Irish study using straw only.[74] Although it raises concerns for some about the risk of impaction and chronic obstructive pulmonary disease (COPD), straw seems to have the added advantage of being the bedding preferred by horses themselves.[77] It may be worth noting that straw is regularly used as horse food in developing countries.

Depth of various bedding types that is needed to maximize their use has not been studied. However, it has been noted that horses lie down on deep litter bedding rather more than do horses at grass or on daily mucked-out beds.[78] The common practice of providing limited bedding to save money can affect choice by reducing the extent to which the horse can comfortably lie down. Houpt[79] notes that if bedding is present but inadequate, horses tend to lie down as soon as more bedding is supplied.

Whereas horses have evolved to be very sociable animals, many owners feel that their charges should be given solitary quarters to make bullying less likely. At pasture, horses choose their affiliates and will spend time interacting with them, for example, while playing, mutually grooming,[58] or settling reasonably minor disputes. On a stable yard, managers tend to dictate the distribution of horses with efficiency of service in mind rather than the associations established between pairs of horses at pasture. It is a shame that there are so few data on the effects of separating horses from preferred companions, or exposing them to agonistic approaches from neighbors whom they would normally avoid.

Watering

While some military horses are still communally watered on a three-times-daily basis, modern textbooks of stable management rarely commend the limited availability of water. However, the maxim that food should not be given before work and that water should not be offered after food probably represents a considerable limitation on the choice that stabled horses can exercise in terms of drinking behavior.[80]

Stable design

There are few publications on the design of stables, and these have been based largely on extrapolations of recommendations for shelter and ventilation of agricultural species. The Universities Federation for Animal Welfare (UFAW)[81] states that for a horse of average size – 500–600 kg body weight and 1.5–1.6 m (15–16 hands) – the loosebox should be at least 4 m × 4 m and preferably 4 m × 5 m. Ensminger[82] states that except for foaling mares and for stallions, there is no advantage in having box stalls larger than 3.6 m square. Evans et al[83] note that the popular size is 3.6 m × 3.6 m and that 3 m × 3 m is adequate for young horses but suggests that the more time the horse spends in the stall, the larger the stall should be. There are several differences between the housing of horses compared with that of other farm animals. Horses usually have individual living areas, and a much greater labor input per animal is present in stables than in farm-animal housing. A survey of racing stables in the Southwest of England found that floor space varied between 8.76 sq m and 21.8 sq m with a median of 12.1 sq m per horse.[84] This compares favorably with the floor space provided for other agricultural species per unit of body size.[85]

While box designs have been suggested by agricultural engineers and by horse-lore, there appear to be no recommendations in management texts about the amount of time that the occupants of these quarters should spend within them on a daily basis. There are a number of reasons for protracted confinement, including inclement weather, locomotory illness and isolation of contagious pathogens. Episodes of enforced confinement are popularly noted as being contemporaneous with the onset of stereotypies. Given that Evans[83] advocates the provision of more space for animals that are turned out less regularly, it could be argued that the design of all stables should meet the needs of the worst-case scenario that precipitates withdrawal of the daily turn-out period.

The traditional layout of a stable-yard includes the quadrangular enclosure of a central lawned area by boxes whose doors and windows face inwards. Walkways in many yards pass close to these portals and expose stabled horses to the unpredictable and arousing movement of humans, feed-buckets and conspecifics. Therefore, it has been suggested that regimented geometrical accommodation of this sort makes relaxation difficult for the occupants.[58]

Despite similar problems with the distracting effects of activity in the passageways and others to do with air hygiene, barn-style housing (in which horses are housed individually, under one roof, in pens made largely from bars and grilles), which facilitates communication between neighboring horses, is increasing in popularity. Studies on the effect of increasing visual contact with conspecifics on weaving[86,87] (see Ch. 5) suggest that whether a stable, rather than a tie-stall, is acceptable depends on its walls more than its size in that isolation is more of a problem than confinement.[79]

Modern stable management brings with it a number of disadvantages for both owners and horses. For the owner, the disadvantages of keeping their animals in stables rather than at grass revolve around time and money. Time commitments in stable management include bedding and feeding as well as having to exercise the confined horse on a more regular basis than its grazing equivalent in order to maintain a given level of fitness. The disadvantages of stabling from the horse's perspective are considered later.

BEHAVIOR

When practitioners are asked to comment on abnormal or unwelcome behaviors, they must first of all appreciate the range of normal behaviors.

NORMAL BEHAVIOR IN STABLED HORSES

Domestication affects behavior,[88] not least because it limits the amount of space in which stock is able to range. This limitation can be effective from day one of life, since many foals, especially valued Thoroughbreds, are born indoors.[89] Interestingly it has been suggested that myopia may be a consequence for horses that spend too much time in stables[90] (this is discussed further in Ch. 2).

The changes in equine behavior associated with confinement and limited choice merit particular consideration. From the horse's perspective, the ways in which stabling can compromise feeding, social and kinetic behavior and indeed health are considered below.

Feeding behavior

Because behavior is a response to an organism's environment, the more restrictive an environment is, the more limited are the choices available to the organism. It is possible that where choice is limited or eliminated, welfare may be compromised.[91] Choice allows animals to perform the behaviors that are important to them,[92] although the choices they make are not exclusively in the direction of their own welfare.[93] While the debate about the importance of environmental choice in the welfare of animals continues, there appears to be a number of ways in which modern stable management limits choice.

Choice is certainly reduced in feeding behavior when horses are stabled. Feeding behavior in stables seems to show the most marked difference from that at pasture since concentrated rations may be consumed more rapidly than a pure forage diet (Fig. 1.9a–e). While the feral or pastured horse may spend 70% of its day foraging, stabled horses on 'complete diets' may spend only 10% of their time feeding.[94] These diets for competition or maintenance can be eaten in less than 2 hours and have removed the feeding behavior of stabled horses even further from its evolutionary origins.

The time at which food is made available often adheres to a strict regime, which may have variable implications for gastrointestinal function. The designation of such feeding times may address the convenience of the operator rather than the needs of the horse. Horses have not been observed to fast voluntarily for more than 3–4 hours[95] but spells of this sort are imposed on many stabled animals.

It has been shown that after 2–3 weeks of continuous access to a single feed, ponies stabilize their bodyweights, consuming 2–3% of their bodyweight in dry matter in a 24-hour period.[96] Despite this finding in support of ad libitum feeding of housed equids, stable managers prefer to control intake, since it is known that to do otherwise is to risk temperamental volatility and metabolic disorders, e.g. laminitis.

There is considerable anecdotal evidence for the effects of diet on behavior in the horse,[1,97] but little has been done to determine the relative importance of factors such as energy, protein and fiber levels. (The relationship between diet and behavior is discussed in more detail in Ch. 8.)

It has been argued that the sleep pattern of a species can be used as an index of adaptation.[98] It is therefore interesting that, while drowsing accounts for 8% of the resting time of stabled horses, this figure has been shown to rise to 14% at pasture.[99] The concomitant dietary differences between intake at grass and in the stable may play a role in this phenomenon since a preliminary study in ponies has shown that, when oats replaced hay in the diet, total rest time increased.[100] This merits further scrutiny (see Ch. 10). Although the number of feeds per day can affect behavior via factors such as disturbances and arousal,[101] it could be that restlessness in horses peaks when stabled animals are fed small amounts of forage and after consuming them are left little to do in so-called vacuum periods.

Social behavior

The importance of social behavior to stabled horses has yet to be fully quantified with consumer demand studies. However, anecdotes that describe horses performing operant responses, such as undoing bolts with their lips to escape from the stable (Fig. 1.10) may indicate that housed individuals will perform work in order to return to their conspecifics.

It is known that frightened riding horses may bolt in a bid to return to their fieldmates, apparently because of an innate preference for the presence rather than the absence of equine company.[102] There are considerable data to suggest that isolation can be aversive.[103–106] When the choice of equine neighbors in a stable yard is dictated by the manager, bonded affiliates may be separated while individuals with mutually low tolerance may be housed next to one another. Disruption of an established social structure in this way may be associated with heightened aggression, especially at times of concentrated food delivery.[107]

Generally, the opportunities for social interaction with conspecifics, favored or otherwise, are

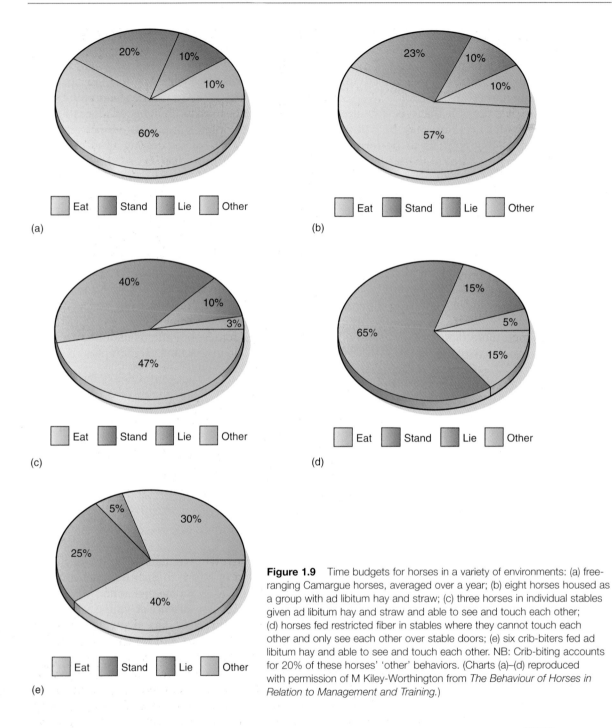

Figure 1.9 Time budgets for horses in a variety of environments: (a) free-ranging Camargue horses, averaged over a year; (b) eight horses housed as a group with ad libitum hay and straw; (c) three horses in individual stables given ad libitum hay and straw and able to see and touch each other; (d) horses fed restricted fiber in stables where they cannot touch each other and only see each other over stable doors; (e) six crib-biters fed ad libitum hay and able to see and touch each other. NB: Crib-biting accounts for 20% of these horses' 'other' behaviors. (Charts (a)–(d) reproduced with permission of M Kiley-Worthington from *The Behaviour of Horses in Relation to Management and Training*.)

minimized by the individual housing of horses. While olfactory, auditory and visual communication can often occur between stabled neighbors, tactile communication, which is of considerable importance in groups of horses,[108,109] is rarely possible in most stable designs.[84,101] Similarly, interactions such as mutual fly-swatting cannot be performed by isolated horses. These concerns

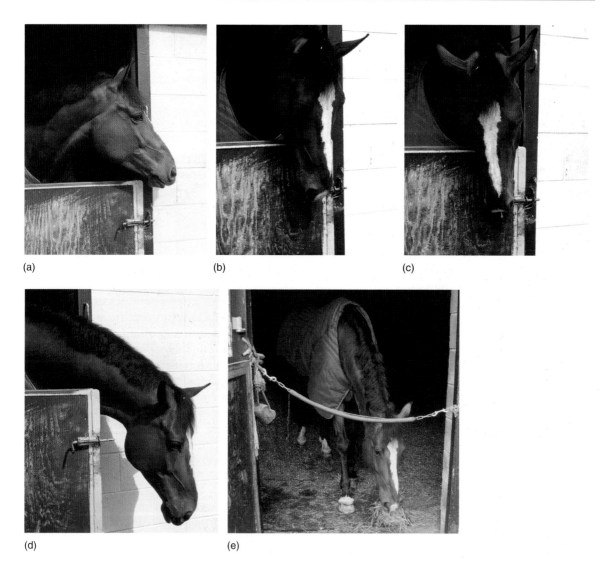

(a) (b) (c)

(d) (e)

Figure 1.10 a–d Irish Draft Horse undoing the bolt of his stable door. (e) After a chain was secured across the threshold to prevent his escape, he moved his hay so that he could watch activities on the yard while eating.

are of particular importance when tie-stalls are considered, with recent evidence to suggest that they do not sufficiently cater for horses' needs to perform social, recumbent resting and allogrooming behaviors.[110]

Stables of all sizes when designed for individual horses have the potential to conflict with many of their occupants' survival instincts.[10] While imposing the vulnerability of isolation and an unhelpful concentration of excretory products that may attract predation, they prevent detection of predators and

escape. Until we have costed out the value of resources or the absence of threats to safety and comfort, it behoves us to consider these impositions from the horses' perspective. For example, while stallions and occasionally geldings create stud-piles of feces in the stable, eliminative behavior in the stable differs markedly from that in the paddock, since the occupants cannot easily avoid contact with their urinary and fecal waste. Since fresh layers of bedding regularly prompt urination in male equids, some consider this a form of marking.[58] So, the extent to which bedding is managed to meet human rather than equine needs bears considerable merit but it is but one feature of the stabled horse's world that represents a removal of choice. In many ways horses attempt to meet their behavioral needs despite the shortcomings of intensive environments but may fail to do so because of management routines.

Kinetic behavior

Among the prevailing features that arise in intensively managed horses is restricted space. The physical limitations imposed on a horse by stabling mean that kinetic behavior is more difficult to perform than it is at pasture. For example, it has been estimated that an average sized horse needs a 6 m span to roll from one side to another, so many stabled horses are unable to perform this most basic of maintenance behaviors. The relative lack of space may either prevent the stabled horse from choosing to roll or precipitate casting. Confinement within looseboxes is common and is an important limitation on the amount of exercise that a horse can take through choice. After periods of confinement, horses show post-inhibitory rebound[111] that may explain why unwanted behaviors during training occur more frequently among stabled horses than those at pasture.[112]

It has been suggested[49] that voluntary kinesis indicates that, rather than being simply a substratum for most behavior, locomotory activity has a motivation of its own. However, the possibility of motivation for spontaneous locomotion is a contentious area because there is often difficulty in eliminating motivation to perform other behaviors for which locomotion is a prerequisite, e.g. intrinsic exploration.[113]

Although unacquainted horses from different yards may be mixed on a national and international scale for equestrian competition, isolation is often practiced when new horses arrive on a yard, in a bid to control the spread of pathogens. Should such animals perform an unwelcome behavior pattern, they will often remain in isolation, since stereotypies are traditionally regarded as contagious.

Space is certainly restricted when horses are housed, particularly in the case of tie-stalls. The extent to which stabled horses can see conspecifics is restricted. In a traditional loosebox, this can often be achieved only by looking over the stable door, while many tie-stalls restrict visibility further by having tall dividers between neighboring pens. This view is a contentious one. Marsden[114] maintains that the behavior of horses kept in tie-stalls is similar to that when they are kept at pasture. This was based on the fact that, in tie-stalls, horses showed no significant increase in the time they spent performing abnormal behavior. The proximity of neighboring horses was thought to facilitate social behavior more than is the case in individual looseboxes. It may be that the small sample size (n = 4) could have resulted in the inadvertent selection of horses that were especially unreactive and not predisposed to perform stereotypies. This work did, however, indicate that stalled horses spent significantly less time lying down and moving, with significantly more time standing in stalls than at pasture. Subsequent studies of pregnant mares in tie-stalls have shown their time budgets to be similar to those of free-range horses.[115] It would be interesting to see whether the mares' gravid state influenced this outcome.

Health

The continual proximity to feces and urine may be aversive to a stable's occupant and may also have an impact on health since humidity and airborne pathogen viability may rise, especially if air-changes per hour are insufficient.[84] An unnatural foraging posture, e.g. eating from a haynet for extended periods rather than from the ground, may compromise the function of the ciliary escalator in the respiratory tract[116] and precipitate pulmonary disease. Rhabdomyolysis[117] and chronic degenerative joint disease[118] are often exacerbated by the physical restriction that accompanies extended periods of stabling. A stable with insufficient or uncomfortable bedding may limit the willingness of its occupant to lie down.[119] This is thought to be associated with a foreshortening of the horse's working life.[120]

> **Box 1.1   The Five Freedoms**
>
> To analyze all the factors likely to influence the welfare of farm animals, consider whether the animal has:
>
> 1. *freedom from thirst, hunger and malnutrition* – by providing access to fresh water and a diet to maintain full health and vigor
> 2. *freedom from physical and thermal discomfort* – by providing a suitable environment including shelter and a comfortable resting area
> 3. *freedom from pain, injury and disease* – by prevention or rapid diagnosis and treatment
> 4. *freedom to express most patterns of normal behavior* – by providing sufficient space, proper facilities and company of the animal's own kind
> 5. *freedom from fear and distress* – by ensuring conditions which avoid mental suffering

Stabling has also been implicated as a predisposing cause of one of the most dreaded and frequently fatal equine disorders, colic.[121]

Conclusion

The five freedoms (Box 1.1) have been established as a means of judging the extent to which the needs of domestic and captive animals are met by human carers.[122,123]

If we apply this model of good animal welfare to horses, we can highlight areas in which wellbeing may be compromised. For example, we see many ways in which they are denied the freedom to express their normal behavior in a stable. When one considers the social nature of equids, one quickly appreciates the impediment that the isolation of single-horse housing represents to normal equine behavior. Therefore, while it has many advantages for the horse owner, the stable should be viewed not simply as a source of physical confinement but also as a limitation on behavioral choice.

ABNORMAL BEHAVIOR IN STABLED HORSES

Most changes in ingestive, eliminative and social behaviors that follow a horse's move from an extensive to an intensive management system are of little concern to the animal's owner. However, behavioral changes that are directly deleterious to the stable or the wellbeing, usefulness and value of its occupant are regarded as abnormal.

Tradition maintained that it was a form of disobedience when stabled horses did not behave as their owners required. Such miscreants were said to have 'vices' whether they ate their feces, bit their grooms or refused to lie down.[120] Far from elucidating the reasons for these unwelcome behaviors, this umbrella term tended to put the blame for them on the horses themselves, as if they had malicious intent.

In 1912, a Captain Moseley, writing in the *Veterinary Record*, described one such 'vice', crib-biting, as 'a form of mental masturbation'. However, while still saddled with a label that implied viciousness, the same behavior in 1959 was recognized by Summerhays[124] as being induced by confinement. Applied ethology has developed since then and serves to examine shortfalls in management that may have prompted the behaviors. Behaviors that have been described as vices[125] are now better categorized as either redirected behaviors, learned behaviors, physical problems, stereotypies or the consequence of inappropriate amounts of stimulation.[126]

Displacement and redirected behaviors

Displacement behaviors are regarded as responses that are inappropriate for the current situation. They are recognized in situations that involve behavioral conflict (see Ch. 13). For example, when a ridden horse is prevented from moving forward for longer than it can readily tolerate, it may start bending its neck laterally in an apparent attempt to groom its flank even though self-grooming is not the most appropriate response to restraint mediated through the bit. In the stabled horse, a similar self-grooming response as a result of frustration may be the kernel of stereotypic self-mutilation.

When a behavior (e.g. an act of aggression) is directed away from the primary target and toward another, less appropriate object, it is said to be redirected.[126] The term must be used with caution since it requires that the observer has correctly identified the primary target. For example, horses that eat their bedding material are thought by some to be performing a redirected behavior that meets their physiological needs for dietary fibre.[96] Others regard this as a form of coprophagia if the bedding is soiled, but since the remedies advocated involve increasing the provision of roughage (which redirects the behavior back to its evolutionary target), the distinction is descriptive rather than functional. Coprophagia is regarded as an adaptive behavior in foals[127–129] but as being an ethopathy in older individuals.[49]

Another common example of redirected behavior in equine husbandry systems is wood-chewing which is regarded as an ingestive behavior that would be more readily directed toward grass or other palatable fiber were it available.[96] However, it is known that horses at pasture will chew wood,[130–132] which implies that our understanding of the causes of this behavior is incomplete. It is possible that the ingestion of small quantities of bark may be adaptive as a means of acquiring micronutrients.[96]

Both redirected and displacement behaviors are subject to the rules of operant conditioning (see Ch. 4) and may be reinforced to become established unwelcome responses. For example, many horses paw at the ground or at the stable door prior to being fed. Although this may be a response that would be appropriate for a free-ranging horse that is being kept from its forage by a temporary barrier such as snow, some would see the targeting of the door as a redirection of the behavior. If the horse is fed during or shortly after pawing the door it will be more likely to paw the door in future.

Over-stimulation or under-stimulation of behavioral systems

While lack of stimulation is often cited as a cause of anomalous behavior,[46,133] including apathy, the opposite also merits consideration in the ontogeny of unusual behavioral strategies linked to housing. Kiley-Worthington[78] indicates that too much noise, excitement or exercise can cause over-stimulation, as can the presence of too many horses and humans to mix with socially. Raised levels of arousal in these horses may make them generally more reactive when being handled in the stable.[58] Similarly inappropriate levels of stimulation are thought to cause psychopathologies such as hyperphagia nervosa[49] and polydipsia nervosa.[134]

Learned behavior

Learning in companion animals is often not recognized and is therefore regularly misinterpreted. This often involves so-called superstitious learning whereby a response is acquired as a result of its accidental link with a reinforcer.[135] Misinterpretation arises because the handlers are unaware of the cues that their presence or actions represent to the animal. Chapter 4 is designed to allow readers to become conversant with learning theory and to understand why the term superstitious learning is virtually redundant, given that animals are learning all the time. Recognizing ways in which animals learn associations unanticipated by their handlers is a cornerstone of behavior therapy. A bizarre example is a case of psychogenic colic that was associated with a demand for human company.[136]

Another example is learned aggression to humans that can evolve as a result of inappropriate associations between agonistic posturing and the unwitting delivery of a food reward. Thus, arrival of the handler prompts hunger-motivated head-threatening behavior that is reinforced by the consequent acquisition of food as the human retreats. This agonistic behavior escalates when punished directly by the handler since his eventual retreat becomes a more valued goal.[137] Other learned responses, including conflict behaviors that arise during horse–human interactions, are considered in Chapter 13.

Physical problems

Problems that arise as a direct consequence of dimensions of the stable, such as 'refusal to lie down' have been blamed on some deficiency on the part of the occupants rather than the designers of the accommodation. Certainly, the area available influences resting behavior.[138] Other examples of physical problems include habitually getting cast, catching hips on the doorway (often exacerbated by learned fear that prompts faster, though not necessarily better judged, exits through doorways) and getting feet caught in haynets.

STEREOTYPIC BEHAVIORS

Stereotypic behavior is characterized by being repetitive, relatively invariant and apparently functionless.[139] Stereotypies are heterogeneous in their causes and their forms. Caged tigers that repeatedly pace up and down in their enclosures raise public concern about welfare in zoos. On a less exotic scale, similar behaviors are performed by horses and ponies. Historically known in horse-lore as 'stable vices' and given specific descriptive labels such as box-walking (stall-walking in the USA), weaving, wind-sucking and crib-biting, these seemingly irreversible behavior changes tended to cause more embarrassment than concern. Despite this, questions regarding 'stereotypies' (as these behaviors are more correctly described) have been fielded by behaviorists and vets for decades.

Most lay authors on the subject tend to use the blanket term 'boredom' to explain how these behaviors arise, and the remainder imply that it is the fault of the horses themselves. However, the days of dismissive attitudes to behavioral anomalies in horses and ponies would appear to be numbered. Therefore, while there are still those who regard the 'private life' of their stabled horses as being unimportant as long as it does not cause poor performance, others have begun to question the merits of traditional stable management that push the horse beyond its limits of adaptation.

Historical accounts of stereotypic behavior

Stereotypic behavior is not described in the earliest text on horsemanship and stable management[140] but archaeologists have used erosion on the incisors of equine skulls as an indicator of crib-biting and therefore domestication. Donkey teeth gathered from what are thought to be ancient sites of worship in Syria have shown signs of wear that have been likened to the erosion one finds in crib-biters.[141] The use of incisor wear to identify palaeolithic horses as crib-biters is not without its critics.[142] The current prevalence of crib-biting in donkeys is negligible and, while it is possible that crib-biting was more common in the past and has been selected out of the population to some extent, it seems strange that three of the five donkeys in this site had this stereotypy. The use of incisor erosion as a means of confirming that the bearer is or was a crib-biter remains controversial because pre-purchase evidence of erosion is cited in instances of litigation when the vendor fails to declare the behavior.

This link between crib-biting and domestication is made in the belief that stereotyped behavior occurs only in animals that have experienced captivity. Furthermore, the assumption that this wear is invariably the result of an oral stereotypy is not without hazards since sandy soils and particular species of grass may produce similar erosion of enamel on the labial surface and the tables of the incisors.

As well as crib-biting and a number of the other so-called stable vices, weaving is described in a number of antique texts on equine husbandry.[143–145]

Characteristics of stereotypic behaviors

Stereotypic behaviors are not recognized in free-living feral horses and are not purely a product of domestication since they are also reported in captive examples of wild equids such as the onager mountain zebra[146] and Przewalski horses.[147] In the horse, these behaviors have therefore been linked to a number of management practices.

A number of equine stereotypies have been identified,[78] including:

- chewing
- lip-licking
- licking environment
- wood-chewing
- crib-biting
- wind-sucking

- box-walking
- weaving
- pawing
- tail-swishing
- door-kicking (front feet)
- box-kicking (hind feet)
- rubbing self
- self-biting
- head-tossing
- head-circling
- head-shaking
- head-nodding
- head-extending, ears back and nodding
- kicking stall (hind feet).

This is an exhaustive list and includes a number of behaviors that are not morphologically invariant and therefore might be regarded as redirected behaviors by other authors. Other behaviors in the above list are difficult to define because changes in form may accompany aging of the stereotypy, e.g. weaving may change from a side-to-side pacing to a stationary head-swing.[148] More than one stereotypy may be performed by an individual horse, e.g. a box-walker may well be seen weaving on occasions.[149] Indeed if a horse has one stereotypy, it has a greater chance of having a second stereotypy than do normal horses.[150] The results of 13 studies into the prevalence of stereotypies and 6 into that of wood-chewing appear in Table 1.3.[151]

Since many stereotypies are popularly regarded as being transmissible by mimicry[119] and some are associated with health and performance problems, horses exhibiting them are often isolated. Some (such as box-walking, weaving and wind-sucking) must be declared at auction and tend to lower the value of affected animals. These are dealt with more thoroughly in subsequent chapters (see Chs 5 and 8).

The functional significance of stereotypies

There has been much recent debate about the functional significance of stereotypies performed by captive domestic animals.[152–154] One influential theory is that stereotypies enable animals to cope with stress.[155–158] However, experimental studies to examine the effects of preventing animals from performing stereotypies in order to assess the validity of the stress-coping hypothesis have produced equivocal results.[159–163] However, transient decreases in heart rates have been demonstrated in association with bouts of crib-biting (Fig. 1.11).[164,165] Furthermore, efforts to prevent the performance of equine stereotypies are linked to some increases in physiological stress parameters.[162,163] It has also been suggested that crib-biters may have higher basal sympathetic activity because they have been found to have higher overall mean heart rate.[165]

Stereotypies could help a horse cope with suboptimal environments or bring direct and immediate rewards that make the behaviors intrinsically gratifying. Endorphins have been implicated as a possible source of reinforcement for crib-biting[166] because opioid antagonists can reduce crib-biting by 84%, suggesting that at least one of the perceived benefits of crib-biting (from the horse's perspective) is mediated by opioid receptors at some point. However, because resting behavior in crib-biters was also significantly increased by opioid antagonists, it may be that the reduction in crib-biting was linked to a generalized sedative effect. The effects of opioid antagonists on weaving

Table 1.3   Reported prevalence (%) of stereotypies and wood-chewing from studies published between 1993 and 1998[151] (reproduced with permission)

	Mean	Standard deviation	Median	Minimum	Maximum
Crib-biting/wind-sucking (13 populations)	4.13	2.57	3.66	0	8.30
Weaving (13 populations)	3.25	3.23	1.98	0	9.5
Box-walking (13 populations)	2.20	2.33	3.50	0	7.32
Wood-chewing (6 populations)	11.78	6.12	12.00	5.00	20.00

are extremely variable, with reports of both decreases[167,168] and increases.[163] While it is possible that weaving may also be opioid mediated, further work with larger numbers of weavers would be required before there can be a clearer understanding of the mechanisms involved.[163]

A further suggestion is that a given stereotypy may retain a function within the motivational system from which it is derived.[78] Thus, an oral stereotypy such as crib-biting may provide a route to normal feeding and digestive activity within an environment that severely limits normal forage intake (e.g. an intensive training program characterized by the provision of high concentrate : minimal roughage diets).

Persevering with non-functional behaviors or previously trained but currently unrewarded responses is a characteristic of stereotypic animals.[169,170] Preliminary reports from a pilot study involving two stereotypic and two normal horses suggest that they may have developed a general

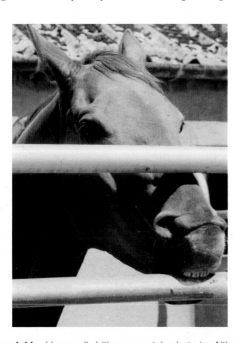

Figure 1.11 Horse crib-biting on metal substrate. Although horses prefer to grasp wood rather than metal (perhaps because it cushions their teeth), they will crib-bite on metal if no other substrate is available. This helps to demonstrate a considerable behavioral need to perform the stereotypy. (Reproduced by permission of the University of Bristol, Department of Clinical Veterinary Science.)

inability to suppress non-functional behavior (Daniel Mills, personal communication 2000). While this may have repercussions for the trainability of stereotypic horses, it should be borne in mind when equine scientists select subjects for studies of learning.

Management factors and abnormal behaviors in stabled horses

It is clear that the prevalence of crib-biting and weaving is greater in Thoroughbreds than in other breeds.[171,172] The prevalence of box-walking, wind-sucking/crib-biting and weaving in UK Thoroughbred populations has been estimated at 1.1%, 4.2% and 2.8%, respectively (n = 1033)[173] and in Italy at 2.5%, 2.4% and 2.5% (n = 1035).[174] Data from 4468 UK Thoroughbred horses in training showed the total prevalence of all three of these stereotypies to be 10.8%, similar to the prevalence of lameness.[175] Estimates of the combined prevalence of all stereotypies are more difficult; for example, when lip-licking, pawing, tail-swishing, head-tossing, head-nodding and box-kicking were included, the prevalence on some yards reached 26%.[78] However, it remains difficult to dissect the effects of management and breed because Thoroughbreds are generally raced and therefore managed intensively.

In other species, cage-design,[176] isolation-rearing[177] and food-deprivation[178] have been implicated as proximate causes of stereotypic behavior. Arousal, generated by frustrated motivation, is a possible shared underlying cause,[179] although others emphasize the possible heterogeneity of the cause and effect of different stereotypies.[139] Despite much work on farm and laboratory species, the proximate causes of stereotypic and redirected behavior in the horse have yet to be verified. However, the possible causal factors associated with oral and locomotory stereotypies are discussed in Chapters 8 and 5, respectively.

The role of genes and environment

Although they have failed to control for variability in management factors, studies into the role that heritability plays in stereotypy frequency have added weight to the view that certain family groups are more likely than others to demonstrate stereotypic behavior.[94,174,180] Meanwhile a growing branch of the literature identifies the importance of management factors that might frustrate motivation in the horse.[101,151] In horses bred for Flat racing, these include the amount and type of forage, the bedding type, the number of horses on the yard and the amount of communication that is possible between neighboring horses.[101] A parallel study in dressage and eventing horses demonstrated that the amount of time spent in the stable correlated with the likelihood of stereotypies being reported.[181]

Although feeding practices tend to have a greater effect than housing practices on the incidence of abnormal behavior,[114] a single causative factor is rarely to blame. For example, wood-chewing increased when high-protein rations were fed, because of a concomitant reduction in the total fiber content,[95] and when exercise was withdrawn.[131] Many authors have suggested other possible causes of anomalous behaviors,

including factors associated with weaning, social contact, crowding, feeding, housing and/or training practices.[78,182]

Some authors[120,149] emphasize the importance of mimicry rather than environmental deficits, believing that exposure to a stereotypic neighbor may increase the likelihood of stereotypy development or performance. Such social influences, known in voles,[183] may also affect stereotypy levels in horses,[184] despite no current indication that horses can learn by observation.[185–187] Even if observational learning is not involved, we should not rule out the possibility that having a stereotypic neighbor may increase the arousal of observing horses and therefore predispose them to developing stereotypic behavior.

An exhaustive study of abnormal behavior on Thoroughbred studs gathered data on more than 11 000 horses, which suggested that, as a result of emancipation, the prevalence of stereotypies tends to rise with age (Fig. 1.12).[175] Therefore, it seems likely that few horses are ever 'cured' of these behaviors. This implies that once these behavioral anomalies are established, they persist to an extent, despite attempts to improve any potentially causative deficiencies in the horse's management (Fig. 1.13). The continual reinforcement of stereotypic behaviors contributes to their resistance to therapy. Having said that, in one

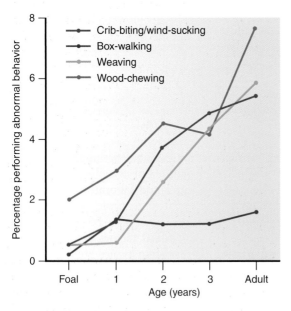

Figure 1.12 The percentage of Thoroughbreds reported as showing stereotypic and redirected behaviors from a sample population of 1023 foals, 746 yearlings, 1001 2-year-olds, 711 3-year-olds and 6250 adults.

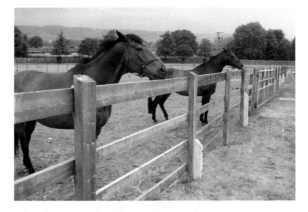

Figure 1.13 Two horses crib-biting at pasture. Since they have one another's company and optimal foraging opportunities they provide a useful example of emancipation. (Reproduced by permission of the University of Bristol, Department of Clinical Veterinary Science.)

study effective treatment of crib-biting was offered as a possible reason (along with euthanasia) for the largest percentage prevalence in crib-biting rates being found in foals.[188]

Fundamentally the possibility of emancipation means that it is better to implement environmental enrichment prophylactically rather than therapeutically. Notwithstanding its effects in maintaining normal behavior in youngstock,[189] it is also likely to increase learning ability[190] while at the same time promoting musculoskeletal health.[191]

The process of emancipation also means that stereotypic foals are better research subjects than mature stereotypers. Studies on cohorts of foals from neonates to 4-year-olds have yielded fascinating results. For example, time-related patterns for the development of oral behaviors differ from those of locomotory behaviors.[188] The results of these and other recent studies on oral and locomotory stereotypies are discussed in more detail in Chapters 8 and 5, respectively.

The future holds tremendous promise for sympathetic and productive understanding of equine stereotypies and the responsibility we must take for their emergence and effective management.

Management of stereotypies

Detailed therapeutic approaches to individual stereotypic behaviors will be considered in later parts of this book, but it is worth noting some overarching principles that apply to many of these ethopathies.

Of all of the anomalous behavior patterns in horses, stereotypies seem to have proved most insoluble to horse owners. Work on other species by different groups[154,159,192–194] often appears contradictory and has highlighted heterogeneity in stereotypies.[152] Since the study of equine stereotypies is in its infancy and because information from other species can be applied only with caution, it is perhaps not surprising that hippologists have found vices so mysterious and frustrating and have met with so little success when attempting to modify these behaviors.[120]

As the data demonstrating increasing prevalence with age suggest, stereotypic behaviors can become emancipated from their initiating causes.[195] Therefore, while stereotypies may arise in response to adverse management, they may persist in more enriched environments. Despite this, owners of stereotypic horses often feel responsible for their charges' behavioral anomalies. The behaviors are therefore unwelcome not least because they are a potential source of embarrassment to owners.

Stereotypic horses are considered undesirable for many reasons. Generally diminished performance in stereotypers has been identified by some authors,[78,196] while health problems associated with these behaviors have been highlighted by others.[102,119,197–199] Furthermore, it has been suggested that stereotypic horses in tie-stalls spend less time interacting with neighboring horses.[115] Prevention of crib-biting, involving physical or surgical approaches, is commonly attempted,[1,119,200–204] with considerable variation in rates of success. Certainly surgery is falling out of favor as the causes of stereotypies become better understood.

Although there is no empirical evidence that observational learning can occur in horses, the belief that behaviors can be learnt or copied affects the management of stereotypic horses. Physical prevention of the behaviors is the prevalent response, while isolation of affected horses from other horses is also common (Table 1.4). If these behaviors are not as functionless as assumed, e.g. they constitute a coping response to a suboptimal environment, the common practice of preventing stereotypic behavior may be of welfare significance. Conversely, managing stereotypic animals so that they are subjected to minimal frustration, e.g. by feeding and exercising before other horses on the yard, is very helpful.

The need to prevent stereotypies for aesthetic and occasional health reasons has prompted searches for permanent cures. A remedy that is effective for every crib-biter remains elusive (but readers are directed to Ch. 8 for a discussion of current humane approaches). The resourcefulness of horses in satisfying their motivation to perform this behavior seems to overwhelm humans' ability to physically prevent established forms of the behavior.

Table 1.4 Attitudes among professional horse owners to stereotypic behaviors[a]

	Racing stables	Riding schools	Competition establishments
Source of concern about stereotypic behaviors			
They reduce the performance of the animal	31	30	27
They have adverse clinical effects on the horse	52	55	56
They reduce the monetary value of the animal	45	59	31
Responses			
Remove causal factors	35	43	36
Physical prevention	77	67	79
Isolation	39	30	48

[a] The results of a telephone survey conducted with the owners of 100 racing stables, 100 riding schools and 100 competition establishments (n = 8427 horses).[205]

Environmental enrichment, often mentioned in the context of captive exotic species, is no less important in the horse. Turning stabled horses out to pasture offers a dramatic illustration of the effects of enrichment. However, for some owners this is not an option. While many owners reach for the blanket term 'boredom' to describe the problems faced by the stabled horse, some are beginning to explore ways to increase complexity of stables.[206] For example, using a chain in place of the stable door is a surprisingly effective means of increasing the visual stimuli that enter at stable (see Fig. 1.10e). The key with any environmental enrichment is to ensure that the intervention is relevant and unlikely to provide a focus for simple redirection of abnormal behaviors, an outcome that is quite unsatisfactory. By studying this book, and most notably Chapters 5 and 8, readers will be well placed to design enrichment strategies that are likely to meet the behavioral needs of all horses, especially those that exhibit under-stimulation and frustrated motivation.

INTRODUCTION TO EVALUATING BEHAVIOR PROBLEMS

Many behaviors labeled abnormal are simply normal but unwelcome. It is the veterinarian's job to distinguish normal and learned behaviors from those with organic origins. Owners and grooms generally know their horses better than the consulting clinician and therefore it is important to keep one's counsel until a thorough case history has been taken.

Care should be taken to translate horsey jargon when taking a history. Various terms may be used to describe the same behavior; for example, depending on the observer, a horse may be variously described as sharp, keen, fizzy or flighty.[8,207] A survey of horses described by their owners as 'head-shakers' identified some that were simply nodding their heads.[208] Having said that, there is evidence that even among a large group of amateurs the use of a human personality inventory achieves high inter-correlations in the ranking of horses, with especially strong agreement being achieved for neuroticism and extraversion.[209] The reliability of these assessments increases the legitimacy of everyday use of psychological terms to describe animal behavior.[209] Additionally it is encouraging to note that when confined to the use of objective descriptive definitions, riders score horses' temperaments with significant agreement and that their scores correlate significantly with objective measures from temperament tests.[210]

Although clients tend to be impressed by shortcuts in history-taking, experience shows this tempting path to be more hazardous than worthwhile. Acquiring only half the salient facts means one is half as likely to emerge with a correct diagnosis and successful therapy.

More than dog and cat owners, horse owners tend to seek advice from each other before calling out the veterinarian, so it is often the case that horse-lore has been applied unsuccessfully in the past. At the end of a complete case history, one should have all the benefit of hindsight and therefore make intelligent suggestions based on what is known of previous attempts to remedy the problem.

How to take a case history

Behavioral consultations can be considered under two main headings: the background and management details, which constitute a behavioral profile, and the unwanted behavior. Although entirely a matter for personal preference, it seems good practice to establish details of the horse's management before exploring the details of the unwanted behavior. This is because, having acquired a picture of the way the horse sees its world, one can better understand the motivation it may have to deploy unwelcome counter strategies. Box 1.2 gives an example of factors constituting a typical behavioral profile.

Because such potentially dangerous behaviors as bucking and rearing can be both expressions of joie de vivre and evasions from pain, veterinarians undertaking behavioral consultations should begin by performing physical examinations to eliminate somatic causes before embarking on a program of behavior therapy. This book explores the normal behavior of horses in considerable depth so that practitioners are equipped to consider the adaptive significance of many signs that present as behavioral problems. Horses that shy provide a useful example in that they should undergo ophthalmological examinations that are complemented by information regarding the frequency and variability of shying, and the spatial relationships of objects at which they tend to shy.

Problem behaviors, especially those under saddle, can be learned through unfortunate experiences but may also reflect ongoing pain. To some extent it is a shame that the veterinary profession is called upon only as a last resort when a horse starts refusing jumps it is capable of clearing. As a result, lower limb pain is probably under-diagnosed as a cause of such problems.[211] The application of various gadgets and escalated coercion often come before a full clinical examination.

Recognition of pain ranks as an extremely important feature of the examination in a clinical case with behavioral manifestations. Houpt[212]

Box 1.2   Behavioral profile

Name
Family includes
Address
Tel no
Animal's name
Breed
Age
Sex
If gelded, age at castration
Other surgical and medical history

Early history and education
Origin?
Was dam's behavior observed?
Since what age has horse been in present ownership?
Why was the horse obtained?
Is it still used for this purpose?
If there has been a change, why?
Previous owners and trainers?
Any 'imprint' training?
Circumstances at early rearing (numbers, ages and gender of companions, housing, exposure to humans)?
Age at and method of weaning?
Methods of training? (primarily operant vs classical)[a]
Do related horses have similar problems?
Do other horses that were raised or trained at the same yard have similar problems?

Environment
Type of housing (loosebox, pasture, run-out shed)?
Exercise?
a. Hours per week ridden or driven?
b. Hours per week in pasture or paddock? Size of enclosure?
c. Hours per week lunged?
d. Other?
Other horses in environment and its relationship with them (any recent changes)?
Other animals in the environment and its relationship with them?
Persons involved with the horse and its relationship with them?

About the horse's day
When fed?
What fed?
Where fed?
Who feeds?
Who feeds titbits?
Who can take food away from the horse?
Does he/she like to be groomed?
Is the horse head-shy?
Who grooms?
Where?
How often is the horse turned out?
What is the horse's response to being caught when at pasture?

---

[a]See Chapter 13.

suggests that a visual appraisal may help to indicate chronic pain, with the affected horse typically having a loose lip but clenched masseter muscles. Meanwhile, there may be a facial expression suggestive of 'concern', with decreased mobility of the eyes, puckering of the eyelids, backward inclination of the ears[211] and dilation of the nostrils.[49] As social herbivores, horses might not be expected to demonstrate signs of pain more overt than teeth-grinding, since to do so may single them out for predation. However, it is proposed that when vocalization accompanies pain, it generally takes the form of a squeal if the pain is of somatic origin and a grunt if visceral.[211] While reduced locomotion and postural attempts to shift weight away from the seat of pain can be spotted from a distance, guarding of muscle groups may be appreciated during palpation.

Although the role of neuropathic pain is now recognized in the etiology of head-shaking (see Ch. 3),[213] it remains unclear why some horses head-shake most when being ridden in certain ways, e.g. with a flexed poll. Sometimes the role of pain in emergent unwelcome behavior is not revealed without analgesics. While one horse that is slow to leave from and quick to return to its yard may have become overly bonded to a companion, another may refuse to leave the yard until placed on a course of anti-inflammatory drugs. The latter would be one of those horses that have learned that being ridden, especially on resilient surfaces, is reliably painful and therefore should be avoided.

In behavioral terms, donkeys are not small horses. Behavioral peculiarities in the donkey are sometimes of clinical significance. Compared with horses, donkeys give fewer overt signs of pain, tending instead to lie down or stand still with their heads lowered. Sweating and hyperpnoea are more common responses to abdominal pain than rolling and flank-kicking (Jane French, personal communication). Even during intestinal strangulation or rupture, donkeys rarely lie down and roll but instead show little more than inappetance, a mildly elevated heart rate and a vague reluctance to move.[214]

Because behavior modification relies on being able to redirect motivation that has prompted

unwanted behaviors, it pays to clarify the specifics of any behavior that seems to have departed from the norm. For example, if the animal is described as aggressive, considerably more information is necessary before the motivation to demonstrate agonistic behaviors can be understood. One should establish whether the horse is aggressive to other horses, other domestic species, humans or all of the above. Aggression toward specific targets merits further questioning. For example, aggression toward humans can be investigated further with questions such as:

- Under what circumstances is the horse aggressive?
- Does the horse avoid personnel or is it actively aggressive?
- Does the horse target particular individuals or types of people (male, female, large, small) or all people?

The unwanted behavior and the way it has evolved to its current form need to be clearly defined (Box 1.3). Given the apparent inconsistencies in the terminology and interpretation of equine behavior,[215] practitioners are commended to equine ethograms designed to establish standard nomenclature for equid behavior.[216] Because of the possibility of inconsistent labeling of behaviors,[175,213] direct observation or video material is certainly preferable to an oral account of the behavior. Problems in the ridden horse can be fully appreciated only if the patient is ridden saddled and unsaddled, preferably on more than one occasion by different riders.

Box 1.3   The unwanted behavior

- Description of what specifically happens
- Where does the behavior occur?
- When does the behavior occur?
- When was it first detected?
- What was the owner's reaction?
- What advice has the owner received to date?
- What problems has the owner encountered with any attempts at correction?
- Has there been any change in the frequency or appearance of the problem?
- What will be done with the horse if its behavior does not improve?

With a clear picture of the ontogeny and motivation of the unwelcome behavior, the development of an effective, tailored strategy to remove the reinforcement of the behavior and redirect the horse's motivation is likely to emerge.[217–220] This is behavior modification. Although a number of case studies are presented in this book, readers may find more exhaustive accounts of behavior modification elsewhere (for a series of 60 cases, see *Why does my horse…?*[50]). If applied with consistency, the results of behavior modification programs are rarely immediate in the horse, because of its innate resistance to extinction[78] but they are usually impressive. There have often been years of inconsistent and inappropriate handling which leave habits that must be surmounted before the slate is clean enough for fresh lessons to be learned. It is therefore worth reminding owners that, because horses have excellent memories, 'quick fixes' are generally a rarity in equine behavior therapy. Some apparently expeditious solutions may mask pain, so they should be used with tremendous caution and only after the role of discomfort has been assessed.

In the following chapters, we will explore the variety of innate and learned behaviors seen in horses. Given this information, the success of behavior therapy depends largely on the versatility of the practitioner and the compliance of the owner.

REFERENCES

1. Waring GH. Horse behaviour: the behavioural traits and adaptations of domestic and wild horses including ponies. Park Ridge, NJ: Noyes; 1983.
2. Hatami-Monagazah H, Pandit RV. A cytogenetic study of the Caspian pony. Journal of Reproduction and Fertility 1979; 57:331–333.
3. Ryder OA. The chromosomes of a rare equine: Equus hemionus kulan. Zoonooz 1977; 50:15.
4. Budiansky S. The nature of horses – exploring equine evolution, intelligence and behavior. New York: Free Press; 1997.
5. Alexander RMcN, Trestik CL. Bistable properties of the hock joint of horses. J Zool 1989; 218:383–391.
6. Mohr E. The Asiatic wild horse. London: Allen; 1971.
7. Boyd L, Bandi N. Reintroduction of Takhi, Equus ferus przewalskii, to Hustai National Park, Mongolia: time budget and synchrony of activity pre- and post-release, Appl Anim Behav Sci 2002; 78(2–4):87–102.
8. King SRB. Home range and habitat use of free-ranging Przewalski horses at Hustai National Park, Mongolia. Appl Anim Behav Sci 2002; 78(2–4):103–113.
9. Christensen JW, Zharkikh T, Ladewig J, Yasinetskaya N. Social behaviour in stallion groups (Equus przewalskii and Equus caballus) kept under natural and domestic conditions. Appl Anim Behav Sci 2002; 76(1):11–20.
10. Goodwin D. The importance of ethology in understanding the behaviour of the horse. The role of the horse in Europe. Equine Vet J Suppl 1999; 15–19.
11. Levine MA. Social evolution and horse domestication. 1993; Oxbow Monograph 33:135–141.
12. Bokonyi S. Evolution of domesticated animals. London: Longman; 1984.
13. Clutton-Brock J. Horse power: a history of the horse and donkey in human societies. Cambridge, MA: Harvard University Press; 1992.
14. Forsten A. Horse diversity through the ages. Biol Rev 1989; 64:279–304.
15. Bibikova VI. Studies on ancient domestic horses in Eastern Europe. Bjulleten Moscovskogo Obshchestva Ispytatelei Prirody, Otdel Biologicheskii 1967; 22:106–118.
16. Telegin DY, ed. Dereivka: a settlement and cemetery of Copper Age horse keepers on the middle Dneiper [Russian]. Pyatkovsky VK, transl; Mallory JP, ed. Oxford: British Archaeological Reports International Series; 287; 1986.
17. Bibikova VI. A study of the earliest domestic horses of Eastern Europe, parts 1 and 2, reprinted in 'Dereivka: a settlement and cemetery of Copper Age horse keepers on the middle Dneiper'. Ed: Telegin DY. 1986. Oxford: British Archaeological Reports International Series 1986; 287:135–162.
18. Richardson JD, Cripps PJ, Hillyer MH, et al. An evaluation of the accuracy of ageing horses by their dentition: a matter of experience. Vet Rec 1995; 137(4):88–90.
19. Anthony DW, Brown DR. The origins of horseback riding. Antiquity 1991; 65:22–38.
20. Anthony D, Telegin DY, Brown D. The origin of horseback riding. Scientific American 1991; 12:44–48.
21. Vila C, Leonard JA, Gotherstrom A, et al. Widespread origins of domestic horse lineages. Science 2001; 291(5503):412.
22. Anthony DW. The domestication of the horse. In: Meadow RH, Oerpmann HP, eds. Equids in the ancient world, vol II. Wiesbaden: Rechart Verlag; 1991: 250–277.
23. Levine MA. Domestication, breed diversification and early history of the horse. Havemeyer Workshop on Horse Behavior and Welfare, Holar, Iceland 2002; 64–69.
24. Ewers JC. The horse in Blackfoot Indian culture. Bureau of American Ethnology Bulletin 1955; 159.
25. Lawrence EA. Horses in society: In: Rowan AN, ed. Animals and people sharing the world. Hanover, NH: University Press of New England; 1988:95–115.
26. McMiken DF. Ancient origins of horsemanship. Equine Vet J 1990; 22:73–78.
27. Schulman AR. Egyptian representations of horsemen and riding in the new kingdom. J Near East Studies 1957; 16:263–271.

28. Moorey PRS. Pictorial evidence for the history of horse riding in Iraq before the Kassite period. Iraq 1970; 32:36–50.
29. Hancar F. Das pferd in prähistorisches and frühen historisches Zeit. Weiner Beitrage zur Kulturgeschichte and Linguistik, 11. Vienna: Harold; 1955.
30. Azzaroli A. An early history of horsemanship. Leiden: EJ Brill; 1985.
31. Cohen E. Animals in medieval perceptions, the image of ubiquitous other. In: Manning A, Serpell J, eds. Animals and human society, changing perspectives. London: Routledge; 1994.
32. Probst GF. The Kikkuli text on the training of horses (ca. 1350 BC). Lexington: University of Kentucky, King Library Press; 1977.
33. Anderson JK. Ancient Greek horsemanship. Berkeley: University of California Press; 1961.
34. Cohen C, Sivan D. The Ugaritic hippiaric texts: a critical edition. New Haven, CT: American Oriental Society; 1983.
35. Hyland A. Equus, the horse in the Roman world. London: Batsford; 1990.
36. Endenburg N. Perceptions and attitudes toward horses in European societies. The role of the horse in Europe. Equine Vet J Suppl 1999; 28:38–41.
37. Cunningham P. The genetics of Thoroughbred horses. Scientific American 1991; 5:56–62.
38. Mellor DJ, Love S, Reeves MJ, et al. A demographic approach to equine disease in the northern UK through a sentinel practice network. Epidemiol Sante Anim 1997; 31–32.
39. Robinson IH. The human-horse relationship: how much do we know? The role of the horse in Europe. Equine Vet J Suppl 1999; 28:42–45.
40. Goergen R. Life on the edge. New Scientist 2001; 2305:30–33.
41. Cothran EG, van Dyk E, van der Merwe FJ. Genetic variation in the feral horses of the Namib Desert, Namibia. J S Afr Vet Med Assoc 2001; 72(1):18–22.
42. Clayton HM. Performance in equestrian sports. In: Back W, Clayton HM, eds. Equine locomotion. London: WB Saunders; 2001.
43. Holstrom M, Magnusson LE, Philipsson J. Variation in conformation of Swedish warmblood horses and conformational characteristics of elite sport horses. Equine Vet J 1990; 22:186–193.
44. Holstrom M. The effects of conformation. In: Back W, Clayton HM, eds. Equine Locomotion. London: WB Saunders; 2001.
45. Hayes KN. Temperament tip-offs. Horse and Rider 1998; 37:46–51.
46. Magnusson LE. Studies on the conformation and the related traits of standardbred trotters in Sweden. PhD thesis, Swedish University of Agricultural Sciences, Skara, 1985.
47. Sellet LC, Albert WW, Groppel JL. Forelimb kinematics of the Standardbred pacing gait. Proc Equine Nutr Physiol 1981; 210–215.
48. Akhatova IA. A system for breeding horses for dairy purposes. Zootekhniya 1995; 10:13–15.
49. Fraser AF. The behaviour of the horse. London: CAB International; 1992.
50. McGreevy PD. Why does my horse ...? London: Souvenir Press; 1996.
51. Lagoni L, Butler C, Hetts S. The human–animal bond and grief. Philadelphia: WB Saunders; 1994.
52. Digard J-P. Research in the social science of horses: why? And how? The role of the horse in Europe. Equine Vet J Suppl 1999; 28:56–57.
53. Brown D. Personality and gender influences on human relationships with horses and dogs. In: Anderson RK, Hart BL, Hart LA, eds. The pet connection: its influence on our health and quality of life. Minneapolis: Center to Study Human–Animal Relationships and Environments, University of Minnesota; 1984:216–223.
54. Burch MR, Bustad LK, Duncan SL. The role of pets in therapeutic programmes. In: Robinson IH, ed. The Waltham book of human–animal interaction: benefits and responsibilities of pet ownership. Oxford: Pergamon/Elsevier; 1995:55–69.
55. Brackenridge SS, Shoemaker RS. The human-horse bond and client bereavement in equine practice. Equine Practice 1996; 18:19–22.
56. Rollin BE. Equine welfare and emerging social ethics. Animal Welfare Forum: Equine Welfare. J Am Vet Med Assoc 2000; 216(8):1234–1237.
57. Ewbank R. Contribution of ethology to clinical interpretation of the horse's welfare. Equine Vet J 1985; 17:1, 2–3.
58. Rees L. The horse's mind. London: Stanley Paul; 1984.
59. Dorrance T. True unity. Tuscarora, NB: Give-it-a-go Enterprises; 1987.
60. Parelli P. Natural horsemanship. Colorado Springs, CO: Western Horseman; 1995.
61. Hunt R. Think Harmony with Horses. Fresno, CA: Pioneer; 1995.
62. Fregin GF, Thomas DP. Cardiovascular response to exercise: a review. In: Snow DH, Persson SGB, Rose RJ, eds. Equine exercise physiology. Cambridge: Burlington; 1983.
63. Gaffney B, Cunningham PE. Estimation of genetic trend in racing performance of Thoroughbred horses. Nature 1988; 322(6166):722–724.
64. Gable AA. Metabolic bone disease: problems of terminology. Equine Vet J 1988; 20:4–6.
65. Jeffcott LB. Osteochondroses in the horse – searching for the key to pathogeneses. Equine Vet J 1991; 23:331–338.
66. Galloux P, Richard N, Dronka T, et al. Analysis of equine gait using three dimensional accelerometers fixed on the saddle. Equine Vet J Suppl 1994; 17:44–47.
67. Arabian AK, Clayton HM. Modeling of locomotion. In: Back W, Clayton HM, eds. Equine locomotion. London: WB Saunders; 2001: 365–371.
68. Herr HM, McMahon TA. A galloping horse model. Int J Robotics Res 2001; 20(1):26–37.
69. Walker RE. Roman veterinary medicine. In: Animals in Roman life and art. London: Thames & Hudson; 1973.
70. Toynbee J. Animals in Roman life and art, p 343. London: Thames & Hudson; 1973.
71. Smith F. The early history of veterinary literature, vol 3, p 17. Reprinted London: JA Allen; 1976.
72. Holcombe SF, Jackson C, Gerber V, et al. Stabling is associated with airway inflammation in young Arabian horses. Equine Vet J 2001; 33(3):244–249.
73. Hintz HF. Hay racks vs feeding hay on the stall floor. Equine Practice 1997; 19:5–6.

74. Townson J, Dodd VA, Brophy PO. A survey and assessment of racehorse stables in Ireland. Irish Vet J 1995; 48:364–372.

75. Murray MJ, Eichorn ES. Effects of intermittent feed deprivation, intermittent feed deprivation with ranitidine administration, and stall confinement with ad libitum access to hay on gastric ulceration in horses. Am J Vet Res 1996; 11:1599–1603.

76. Harris PA. Review of equine feeding and stable management practices in the UK concentrating on the last decade of the 20th century. The role of the horse in Europe. Equine Vet J Suppl 1999; 46–54.

77. Mills DS, Eckley S, Cooper JJ. Thoroughbred bedding preferences, associated behaviour differences and their implications for equine welfare. Anim Sci 2000; 70(1):95–106.

78. Kiley-Worthington M. The behaviour of horses: in relation to management and training. London: JA Allen; 1987.

79. Houpt KA. Equine welfare. In: Recent advances in companion animal behavior problems. Ithaca, NY: International Veterinary Information Services; 2001. A0810. 1201.

80. Hinton MH. On the watering of horses – a review. Equine Vet J 1978; 10:27–31.

81. UFAW (Scott WN, ed). The care and management of farm animals. London: Baillière Tindall; 1978.

82. Ensminger ME. Horses and horsemanship. Danville, IL: Interstate; 1969.

83. Evans JW, Borton A, Hintz HF, van Vleck LD. The horse. San Francisco: WH Freeman; 1969.

84. Jones RD, McGreevy PD, Robertson A, et al. Survey of the designs of racehorse stables in the South-west of England. Equine Vet J 1987; 19:454–457.

85. Sainsbury DWB, Sainsbury P. Livestock health and housing, 2nd edn. London: Baillière Tindall; 1979.

86. Cooper JJ, McDonald L, Mills DS. The effect of increasing visual horizons on stereotypic weaving: implications for the social housing of stabled horses. Appl Anim Behav Sci 2000; 69:67–83.

87. Mills DS, Davenport K. The effect of a neighbouring conspecific versus the use of a mirror for the control of stereotypic weaving behaviour in the stabled horse. Anim Sci 2002; 74:95–101.

88. Ratner SC, Boice R. Effects of domestication on behaviour. In: Hafez ESE, ed. The behaviour of domestic animals. London: Baillière Tindall; 1975:3–19.

89. Rossdale PD. Modern stud management in relation to the oestrus cycle and fertility of Thoroughbred mares. Equine Vet J 1968; 2:65–72.

90. Harman AM, Moore S, Hoskins R, Keller P. Horse vision and an explanation of the visual behaviour originally explained by the 'ramp retina'. Equine Vet J 1999; 31(5):384–390.

91. Wiepkema PR. Umwelt and animal welfare. In: Baxter SH, Baxter MR, MacCormack JAC, eds. Farm animal housing and welfare. The Hague: Martinus Nijhoff; 1983:45–51.

92. Dawkins MS. The current status of preference tests in the assessment of animal welfare. In: Baxter SH, Baxter MR, MacCormack JAC, eds. Farm animal housing and welfare. The Hague: Martinus Nijhoff; 1983: 20–26.

93. Duncan IJH. An ethological approach to the welfare of farm animals. In: Proceedings 19th International Ethological Conference, Toulouse, France, 1985:295–305.

94. Marsden MD. An investigation of the heredity of susceptibility of stereotypic behaviour pattern – stable vices—in the horse. Equine Vet J 1995; 27(6):415.

95. Ralston SL, van den Brock G, Baile CA. Feed intake patterns and associated blood glucose free fatty acid and insulin changes in ponies. J Anim Sci 1979; 49:838–845.

96. Ralston SL. Feeding behaviour. Vet Clin North Am Equine Pract: Behav 1986; 2:609–621.

97. McBane S. Behaviour problems in horses, p 304. London: David & Charles; 1987.

98. Ruckebusch Y. The hypnogram as an index of adaptation of farm animals to changes in their environment. Appl Anim Ethol 1975; 2:3–8.

99. Dallaire A. Rest behaviour. Vet Clin North Am Equine Pract: Behav 1986; 2:591–607.

100. Dallaire A, Ruckebusch Y. Sleep and wakefulness in the housed pony under different dietary conditions. Can J Compar Med 1974; 38:65–71.

101. McGreevy PD, Cripps PJ, French NP, et al. Management factors associated with stereotypic and redirected behaviour in the Thoroughbred horse. Equine Vet J 1995; 27:86–91.

102. Summerhays RS. The problem horse, p 93. London: JA Allen; 1975.

103. Houpt KA, Hintz HF, Pagan JD. The responses of mares and their foals to brief separation. J Anim Sci 1981; 53:129.

104. Houpt KA, Hintz HF, Butler WR. A preliminary study of two methods of weaning foals. Appl Anim Behav Sci 1984; 12:177–1881.

105. McCall CA, Potter GD, Kreider JL. Locomotor, vocal and other behavioural responses to varying methods of weaning foals. Appl Anim Behav Sci 1985; 14:27–35.

106. Mal ME, Friend TH, Lay DC, et al. Physiological responses of mares to short-term confinement and isolation. J Equine Vet Sci 1991; 11:96–102.

107. Keiper RR. Social structure. Vet Clin North Am Equine Pract: Behav 1986; 2:465–484.

108. Feh C, de Mazieres J. Grooming at a preferred site reduces heart rate in horses. Anim Behav 1993; 46:1191–1194.

109. Dougherty DM, Lewis P. Generalization of a tactile stimulus in horses. J Exp Anal Behav 1993; 59:521–528.

110. Zeitler-Feicht MH, Buschmann S. [Are standing stalls for horses acceptable today with regard to animal welfare?] [German] Pferdeheilkunde 2002; 18(5):431.

111. Houpt K, Houpt TR, Johnson JL, et al. The effect of exercise deprivation on the behaviour and physiology of straight-stall confined pregnant mares. Anim Welfare 2001; 10(3):257–267.

112. Rivera E, Benjamin S, Nielsen B, et al. Behavioral and physiological responses of horses to initial training: the comparison between pastured versus stalled horses. Appl Anim Behav Sci 2002; 78(2–4):235–252.

113. Nicol CJ. Behavioural responses of laying hens following a period of spatial restriction. Anim Behav 1987; 35:1709–1719.

114. Marsden MD. Feeding practices have greater effect than housing practices on the behaviour and welfare of the horse. Livestock Environment IV, 4th International Symposium of the American Society of Agricultural Engineers, University of Warwick, Coventry, 1993:314–318.

115. Flannigan G, Stookey JM. Day-time time budgets of pregnant mares housed in tie stalls: a comparison of draft versus light mares. Appl Anim Behav Sci 2002; 78(2–4):125–143.

116. Racklyeft DJ, Love DN. Influence of head posture on the respiratory tract of healthy horses. Aust Vet J 1990; 67:402–405.

117. Rose RJ. The TG Hungerford Vade Mecum series for domestic animals. Number 1: Horses, p 24. Sydney, Australia: Post-graduate Committee in Veterinary Science; 1983.

118. Richardson DW. Degenerative joint disease. In: Robinson NE, ed. Current therapy in equine medicine, Philadelphia: WB Saunders; 1992:137–140.

119. Schramm U. The trouble with horses, p 124. Bury St Edmunds, Suffolk: JA Allen; 1988.

120. Hayes MH. Veterinary notes for horse-owners. London: Stanley Paul; 1968.

121. Fraser A, Manolson F. Fraser's horse book. London: Pan; 1979.

122. Farm Animal Welfare Council second report on priorities for research and development in farm animal welfare. MAFF, Tolworth; 1993.

123. Webster AJF. Animal welfare: a cool eye towards Eden. London: Blackwell Science; 1994.

124. Summerhays RS. The problem horse. London: JA Allen, 1959.

125. Hamilton S. The vice squad: conquering your horse's behavioural quirks. Equus 1980; 32:68–71.

126. Fraser AF, Broom DM. Farm animal behaviour and welfare. London: Baillière Tindall, 1990.

127. Francis-Smith K, Wood-Gush DGM. Coprophagia as seen in Thoroughbred foals. Equine Vet J 1977; 9:155–157.

128. Crowell-Davis SL, Houpt KA. Coprophagia by foals: effects of age and possible functions. Equine Vet J 1985; 17:17–19.

129. Crowell-Davis SL, Caudle AB. Coprophagy by foals: recognition of maternal faeces. Appl Anim Behav Sci 1989; 24:267–272.

130. Crowell-Davis SL, Houpt KA, Carnevale JM. Feeding and drinking behaviour of mares and foals with free access to pasture and water. J Anim Sci 1985; 60:883–889.

131. Krzak WE, Gonyou HW, Lawrence LM. Wood-chewing by stabled horses: diurnal pattern and effects of exercise. J Anim Sci (USA) 1991; 69:1053–1058.

132. McCall CA. Wood-chewing by horses. Equine Practice 1993; 15:35–36.

133. Bush K. The problem horse – an owner's guide, p 160. Marlborough, Wilts, UK: Crowood Press; 1992.

134. Buntain BJ, Coffmann JR. Polyuria and polydipsia in a horse induced by psychogenic salt consumption. Equine Vet J 1981; 13:266–268.

135. Lieberman DA. Learning: behavior and cognition. Pacific Grove, CA: Brooks/Cole; 1993.

136. Murray MJ, Crowell-Davis S. Psychogenic colic in a horse. J Am Vet Med Assoc 1985; 186:381–383.

137. Beaver B. Aggressive behaviour problems. Vet Clin North Am Equine Pract: Behav 1986; 2:609–621.

138. Zeitler-Feicht MH, Prantner V. Recumbence resting behaviour of horses in loose housing systems with open yards. Arch Tierzucht 2000; 43(4):327–335.

139. Mason GJ. Stereotypies: a critical review. Anim Behav 1991; 41:1015–1037.

140. Xenopohon. The art of horsemanship (400 BC). Morgan MH, transl. London: JA Allen; 1999.

141. Clutton-Brock J, Davies S. More donkeys from Tell Brak. Iraq 1993; 55:209–221.

142. Bahn PG. Crib-biting: tethered horses in the Palaeolithic? World Archaeology 1980; 12: 212–217.

143. Lawson A. The modern farrier, p 47. London: Newcastle, Mackenzie & Dent; 1828.

144. Youatt W. The horse, p 448–451. London: Charles Knight; 1846.

145. Lupton JI. Evils of modern stables. In: Mayhew's illustrated horse management. London: WH Allen; 1884.

146. Holzapfel M. Uber Bewegungssterotypien bei gehalten Sangetieren; 2. Mitteilung: das Weben der pferde. Z Tierpsychol 1939; 60–72.

147. Boyd LE. Behaviour problems of equids in zoos. Vet Clin North Am Equine Pract: Behav 1986; 2:653–664.

148. Meyer-Holzapfel M. Abnormal behavior in zoo animals. In: Fox MW, eds. Abnormal behavior in animals. Philadelphia: WB Saunders; 1968: 476–503.

149. Sambraus HH, Rappold D. Crib-biting and wind-sucking in horses. Pferdeheilkunde 1991; 7:211–216.

150. Mills DS, Alston RD, Rogers V, Longford NT. Factors associated with the prevalence of stereotypic behaviour amongst thoroughbred horses passing through auctioneer sales. Appl Anim Behav Sci 2002; 78 (2–4):115–124.

151. Nicol CJ. Stereotypies and their relation to management. In: Harris PA, Gomarsall GM, Davidson HPB, Green RE, eds. Proceedings of the BEVA specialist days on behaviour and nutrition, 1999:11–14.

152. Mason GJ. Forms of stereotypic behaviour. In: Lawrence AB, Rushen J, eds. Stereotypic animal behaviour: fundamentals and applications to welfare. London: CAB International; 1993.

153. Broom DM. Animal welfare: concepts and measurements. J Anim Sci 1991; 69:4167–4175.

154. Cooper JJ, Nicol CJ. Stereotypic behaviour affects environmental preference in bank voles, Clethrionomys glareolus. Anim Behav 1991; 41:971–977.

155. Fentress JC. Dynamic boundaries of patterned behaviour: interaction and self-organization. In: Bateson PPG, Hinde RA, eds. Growing points in ethology. Cambridge: Cambridge University Press; 1976:135–167.

156. Levine MA, Weinberg J, Ursin H. Definition of the coping process and statement of the problem.

In: Ursin H, Baade E, Levine S, eds. Psychobiology of stress: a study of coping men. New York: Academic Press; 1978:3–21.

157. McBride G. Adaptation and welfare at the man–animal interface. In: Wodzickka M, Edey TN, Lynch JJ, eds. Reviews in rural science IV. Armidale, NSW: University of New England; 1980.

158. Wood-Gush DGM, Stolba A, Miller C. Exploration in farm animals and animal husbandry. In: Archer J, Birke LIA, eds. Exploration in animals and humans. London: Van Nostrand Reinhold; 1983:198–209.

159. Kennes D, de Rycke PH. Influences of performance of stereotypies on plasma corticosterone and leucocyte levels in the bank vole (Clethrionomys glareolus). In: Proceedings of the International Congress on Applied Ethology in Farm Animals, 1988:238–240.

160. Terlouw EMC, Lawrence AB, Ladewig J, et al. Relationship between plasma cortisol and stereotypic activities in pigs. Behav Processes 1991; 25:133–153.

161. Würbel H, Stauffacher M. Prevention of stereotypy in laboratory mice: effects on stress physiology and behaviour. Physiol Behav 1996; 59(6):1163–1170.

162. McGreevy PD, Nicol CJ. Behavioural and physiological consequences associated with the short-term prevention of crib-biting in horses. Physiol Behav 1998; 65(1):15–23.

163. McBride SD, Cuddeford D. The putative welfare-reducing effects of preventing equine stereotypic behaviour. Anim Welfare 2001; 10(2):173–189.

164. Lebelt D, Zanella AJ, Unshelm J. Physiological correlates associated with cribbing behaviour in horses: changes in thermal threshold, heart rate, plasma beta-endorphin and serotonin. Equine Vet J Suppl 1998; 27:21–27.

165. Minero M, Canali E, Ferrante V, Verga M, Ödberg FO. Heart rate and behavioural responses of crib-biting horses to two acute stressors. Vet Rec 1999; 145(15):430–433.

166. Gillham SR, Dodman NH, Shuster L, et al. The effect of diet on cribbing behaviour and plasma ß-endorphin in horses. Appl Anim Behav Sci 1994; 41:147–153.

167. Dodman NH, Shuster L, Court MH, Dixon R. Investigation into the use of narcotic antagonists in the treatment of a stereotypic behavior pattern (crib-biting) in the horse. Am J Vet Res 1987; 48:2,311–319.

168. McBride S. A comparison of physical and pharmacological treatments for stereotypic behaviour in the horse. In: Duncan IJH, Widowski TM, Haley DB, eds. Proceedings of the 30th International Congress for the International Society of Applied Ethology. Guelph, Canada: CSAW;1996.

169. Garner JP, Mason GJ, Broadbent H. Cage stereotypy in Blue tits (Parus caeruleus) and Marsh tits (Parus palustris) is associated with a deficit in the inhibition of non-functional behaviour. In: Veissier I, Boissy A, eds. Proceedings of the 32nd International Congress of the ISAE. Clermont-Ferrand, France: INRA; 1998:56.

170. Garner JP, Meehan CL, Mench JA. Stereotypic parrots fail the same psychiatric task as stereotypic autists and schizophrenics. In: Garner JP, Mench JA, Heekin S, eds. Proceedings of the 35th International Congress of the ISAE. Davis, CA: Center For Animal Welfare, University of California at Davis; 2001.

171. Luescher UA, McKeown DB, Dean H. A cross-sectional study on compulsive behaviour (stable vices) in horses. Equine Vet J Suppl 1998; 27:14–18.

172. Redbo I, Redbo-Tortensson P, Ödberg FO, et al. Factors affecting behavioural disturbances in race-horses. Anim Sci 1998; 66:475-481.

173. Prince D. Stable vices. In: McBane S, ed. Behaviour problems in horses. London: David & Charles; 1987.

174. Vecchiotti G, Galanti R. Evidence of heredity of cribbing, weaving and stall-walking in Thoroughbred horses. Livestock Production Sci 1986; 14:91–95.

175. McGreevy PD. The functional significance of stereotypies in the stabled horse. PhD thesis, University of Bristol, UK; 1995.

176. Ödberg FO. The jumping stereotypy in the bank vole (Clethrionomys glareolus). Biol Behav 1986; 11:130–143.

177. Morgan MJ. Effects of post-weaning environment on learning in the rat. Anim Behav 1973; 21:429–442.

178. Appleby MC, Lawrence AB. Food restriction as a cause of stereotypic behaviour in tethered gilts. J Anim Production 1987; 45:103–110.

179. Duncan IJH, Rushen J, Lawrence AB. Conclusions and implications for animal welfare. In: Lawrence AB, Rushen J, eds. Stereotypic animal behaviour: fundamentals and applications to welfare. London: CAB International; 1993.

180. Hosoda T. On the heritability of susceptibility to windsucking in horses. Jpn J Zootechnical Sci 1950; 21:25–28.

181. McGreevy PD, French NP, Nicol CJ. The prevalence of abnormal behaviours in dressage, eventing and endurance horses in relation to stabling. Vet Rec 1995; 137:36–37.

182. Luescher UA, McKeown DB, Halip J. Reviewing the causes of obsessive-compulsive disorders in horses. Equine Pract Vet Med 1991; 5(91):527–530.

183. Cooper JJ, Nicol CJ. Neighbour effects on the development of locomotor stereotypies in bank voles Clethrionomys glareolus. Anim Behav 1994; 47: 214–216.

184. Houpt KA, McDonnell SM. Equine stereotypies. The Compendium of Continuing Education for the Practicing Veterinarian 1993; 15:1265–1272.

185. Baer KL, Potter GD, Friend TH, Beaver BV. Observation effects on learning in horses. Appl Anim Ethol 1983; 11:123–129.

186. Baker AEM, Crawford BH. Observational learning in horses. Appl Anim Behav Sci 1986; 15:7–13.

187. Clarke J, Nicol CJ, Jones R, McGreevy PD. Effects of observational learning on food selection in horses. Appl Anim Behav Sci 1996; 50:177–184.

188. Waters AJ, Nicol CJ, French NP. Factors influencing the development of stereotypic and redirected behaviours in young horses: findings of a four year prospective epidemiological study. Equine Vet J 2002; 34(6):572–579.

189. Heleski CR, Shelle AC, Nielsen BD, Zanella AJ. Influence of housing on weanling horse behavior and subsequent welfare. Appl Anim Behav Sci 2002; 78(2–4):297–308.

190. Rosenzweig MR, Bennett EL. Psychobiology of plasticity: effects of training and experience on brain and behaviour. Behav Brain Res 1996; 78:57–65.

191. Bell RA, Nielsen BD, Waite K, et al. Daily access to pasture turnout prevents loss of mineral in the third metacarpus of Arabian weanlings. J Anim Sci 2001; 79(5):1142–1150.

192. Keiper RR. Causal factors of stereotypies in caged birds. Anim Behav 1969; 17:114–117.

193. Dantzer R, Mormede P. De-arousal properties of stereotypic behaviour: evidence from pituitary-adrenal correlates in pigs. Appl Anim Ethol 1983; 10:233–244.

194. Cronin GM, Wiepkema PR, Van Ree JM. Endogenous opioids are involved in abnormal stereotyped behaviour in tethered sows. Neuropeptides 1985; 6:527.

195. Cooper JJ, Ödberg FO. The emancipation of stereotypies with age. In: Appleby MC, Horrell RI, Petherick JC, Rutter SM, eds. Applied Animal behaviour: past, present and future. Hertfordshire: UFAW; 1991:142.

196. Straiton EC. The TV vet horse book, p 193. Suffolk: Farming Press; 1973.

197. Steele DG. El Cribbing (pica) y la aerofagia en los pura sangre. Ganaderia 1960; 18:74–78.

198. Karlander S, Mansson J, Tufvesson G. Buccostomy as a method of treatment for aerophagia (wind-sucking) in the horse. Nordisk Veterinär Medicin 1965; 17:455–458.

199. Hachten W. Cribbing treatment. The Equine Athlete 1995; 8:20–21.

200. Baker GJ, Kear-Colwell J. Aerophagia (windsucking) and aversion therapy in the horse. Proc Am Assoc Equine Practitioners 1974; 20:127–130.

201. Hamm D. A new surgical procedure to control crib-biting. Proc Am Assoc Equine Practitioners 1977; 23:301–302.

202. Firth EC. Bilateral ventral accessory neurectomy in windsucking horses. Vet Rec 1980; 106:30–32.

203. Hakansson A, Franzen P, Petersson H. Comparison of two surgical methods for treatment of crib-biting in horses. Equine Vet J 1992; 24:494–496.

204. Broom DM, Kennnedy MJ. Stereotypies in horses: their relation to welfare and causation. Equine Vet Ed 1993; 5:151–154.

205. McBride SD, Long L. Management of horses showing stereotypic behaviour, owner perception and the implications for welfare. Vet Rec 2001; 148(26):799–802.

206. Goodwin D, Davidson HPB, Harris P. Foraging enrichment for stabled horses: effects on behaviour and selection. Equine Vet J 2002; 34(7):686–691.

207. Mills DS. Personality and individual differences in the horse, their significance, use and measurement. Equine Vet J Suppl 1998; 27:10–13.

208. Taylor K, Cook S, Mills DS. A case-controlled study investigating health, management and behavioural features of horses commonly described as headshakers. Havemeyer Workshop on Horse Behavior and Welfare, 2002: 16–20.

209. Morris PH, Gale A, Duffy K. Can judges agree on the personality of horses? Personality and Individual Differences 2002; 33(1):67–81.

210. Visser EK, van Reenen CG, Rundgren M, et al. Responses of horses in behavioural tests correlate with temperament assessed by riders. Equine Vet J 2003; 35(2):176–183.

211. Casey R. Recognising the importance of pain in the diagnosis of equine behaviour problems. In: Harris PA, Gomarsall GM, Davidson HPB, Green RE, eds. Proceedings of the BEVA Specialist Days on Behaviour and Nutrition, 1999:1.

212. Houpt KA. Domestic animal behaviour for veterinarians and animal scientists, 3rd edn. London: Manson; 1998.

213. Taylor KD, Cook S, Mills DS. A case-controlled study investigating health, management and behavioural features of horses commonly described as head-shakers. Ippologia 2001; 12:29–37.

214. Taylor TS, Matthews NS. Mammoth asses – selected behavioural considerations for the veterinarian. Appl Anim Behav Sci 1998. 60(2–3):283–289.

215. Houpt KA, Rudman R. Foreword to special issue on equine behaviour. Appl Anim Behav Sci 2002;78(2–4):83–85.

216. McDonnell SM. The equid ethogram: a practical field guide to horse behavior. Lexington, KY: The Blood Horse; 2003.

217. McCall CA. A review of learning behavior in horses and its application in horse training. J Anim Sci 1990; 68:75–81.

218. Mills DS. Applying learning theory to the management of the horse: the difference between getting it right and getting it wrong. Equine Vet J Suppl 1998; 27:44–48.

219. Cooper JJ. Comparative learning theory and its application in the training of horses. Equine Vet J Suppl 1998; 27:39–43.

220. Barakat C, McGreevy PD. How cribbing takes hold. Equus 2002; 297:34–43.

2

Perception

Horses have been described as being among the most perceptive of animals.[1] By studying the sensory perception of horses, we gain valuable insights into their behavior. The differences between human and equine perceptions of the external environment can be explained by the differences in their sensory structures. The horse's adept perception has allowed it to be constantly aware of changes occurring in its surroundings and has played a pivotal role in the success of this species. An appreciation and understanding of the horse's well-developed sensory system are valuable tools, particularly when attempting to understand distinctive aspects of equine behavior.

VISION

The equine eye is among the largest, and held by some to be the largest, in terms of absolute dimensions, of any terrestrial mammal.[2,3] Leaving aside the aesthetic appeal this gives the horse, it suggests that the horse relies heavily on visual information about its environment. With large retinae and a relative image magnification that is 50% greater than that of humans,[4] the horse's eyes allow it to visualize a wide panorama of the horizon and also the area ahead where feet will be placed and fodder will be selected. As a herbivorous flight animal, the horse has good distance vision, allowing it to scan widely for danger and, despite being relatively poor at accommodation, with a vertical field of 178°,[4] is able to visualize the ground immediately ahead while grazing.

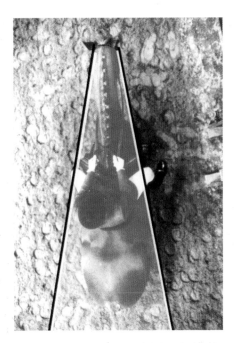

Figure 2.1 Aerial view of a horse showing the blind spot to its rear. The width of the blind spot is influenced by the horse's head carriage. (Adapted, with permission, from photograph 6.1a in *Equestrian Technique* by Tris Roberts, London: JA Allen; 1992.)

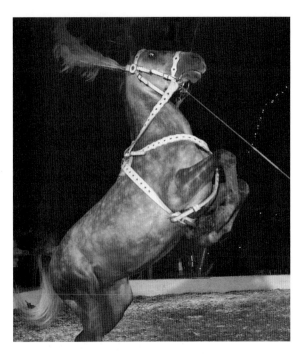

Figure 2.2 Rearing horse showing the white of its eye. (Reproduced with permission of the Captive Animals Protection Society.)

Horse eyes occupy a lateral position towards the back of the head, affording a panoramic view in front and on both sides, with only a narrow blind area to the rear (Fig. 2.1).

The narrow blind zone at the back of the horse of approximately 20° for each eye,[5] can be unveiled by a slight turn of the head. For example, when kicking with its hindlegs, a horse may turn its head to ensure that its target is no longer in the blind area. The width of the blind zone is determined by the level at which the head is carried. As most practitioners appreciate, the blind zone can be effectively increased by cupping one hand around the lateral canthus, an intervention which pacifies many horses that have learned to anticipate aversive stimuli as part of veterinary intervention (see Ch. 14).[5]

The price horses pay for having laterally placed eyes is that the muzzle gets in the way of forward vision. Depending on the carriage of the head, the particular breed and the setting of the eyes, there is a blind zone extending almost 2 meters directly in front of the horse. When the head is down the horse's binocular field is located down the nose in the direction of grass. Therefore horses can see where they eat especially well. This is why, if they do want to see directly in front rather than down the nose, horses have to lift up the nose and point it at the object of interest.

The exposition of more sclera is often noted in anxious animals (Fig. 2.2) because the eyes are opened wider to take in more visual information that may help them resolve the situation, while a fixed eye may be associated with reasonably chronic distress. It is widely believed that the extent of oscillation of eye movements and the amount of sclera shown can be helpful in assessing the disposition of horses,[6] but, if the horse has a relatively small iris, that may detract from the reliability of this effect.

ACUITY

There are a number of aspects of vision that can be measured. Visual acuity describes the ability

Figure 2.3 A system of vertical lines can be presented progressively closer to one another to measure visual acuity. (Reproduced with permission of Alison Harman.)

to distinguish the fine details of an object. Clearly, the nearer an object is to the eye, the finer the detail that can be distinguished. Horses' eyes are geared to be focused largely on more distant features and, like many mammal species, appear to have limited accommodation, i.e. the ability to focus on very close objects less than about 1 meter away. Animals that have been trained to discriminate between panels painted gray and those bearing black and white stripes can expose their species' acuity. As panels with ever finer stripes are presented to the observer, the discrimination task becomes more difficult (Fig. 2.3). The point at which the lines blur together and appear to be gray (the limit of acuity) is marked by a failure to discriminate. Most birds that have been tested excel at this task. They can distinguish extremely narrow stripes that occupy as little as 1/100th of a degree of their visual field. Horses can perceive stripes that fill about 1/20th of a degree.

An interesting way of expressing the horse's acuity is in comparison with normal human vision, as 20/33. This indicates that a horse can only discern at 20 meters what a human can at 33 meters,[7] and this compares favorably with the dog (20/50) and the cat (20/100).[7] Horses' eyes are extremely sensitive to movement in all areas of their visual field, but human peripheral vision is considered a good approximation of the visual detail horses can appreciate.[8]

The visual field is affected by the corpora nigra, which are found on the upper margin of the pupillary aperture, possibly as an anti-glare device.[9] The corpora nigra contain an intricate network of blood vessels, which suggests that they might also be used to oxygenate the anterior chamber of the eye (Alison Harman, personal communication 2002). For horses to see through their narrow pupils, they adjust their head position up and down or side to side. Best frontal vision of the ground in front is achieved when the horse flexes slightly at the poll. Horses commonly hold their heads in this position when they are moving in slower gaits. This was thought to improve focus and enhance images of the ground ahead.[6] However, when over-flexed so that the nose is behind the vertical, the horse cannot see the space in front of it and so, when being ridden, may occasionally collide with objects, people and other horses if not directed (Fig 2.4a & b).

A functionally important blind spot is created when a horse is ridden 'on the bit'. The blind spot is formed to the front of the horse, and is believed to be as wide as the body. Thus, when a horse is being ridden in such a fashion it cannot see directly in front of itself. Horses on the bit are said to be showing signs of submission and 'listening to their riders', but it is possible that compromising a horse in this way makes it more reliant on the rider for avoidance of obstacles and so more biddable. Before using physical constraints such as tie-downs and standing martingales to keep the head down or overchecks to keep it up, one should consider the effect of these restraints on the horse's ability to convey itself safely over rough terrain and most especially over jumps.

The horse has mostly monocular vision; that is each eye sees a completely different field of view. However, horses have a small binocular field at the front of the monocular fields. Therefore, the horse can adjust its view to overlap the visual fields of both eyes and achieve a binocular view (Fig. 2.5). This binocular field of view allows the horse to observe the ground in front with both eyes.

To see objects at a greater distance, the horse rotates its nose upwards because its binocular overlap is oriented down the nose (Fig. 2.6). It is believed that when focusing on objects to the fore, horses may momentarily lose the ability to observe from the rear and to the sides.[7] Having said that, when taking off for a jump, horses sometimes tilt their head sideways, using their

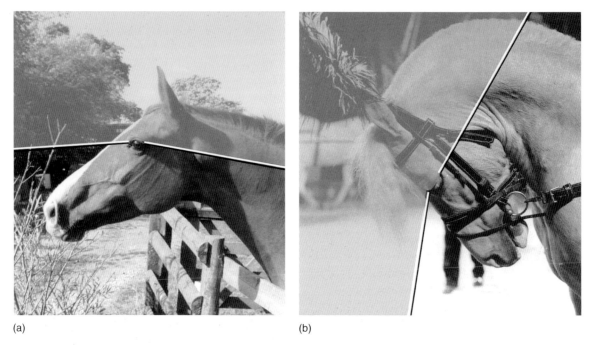

(a)   (b)

Figure 2.4 (a) The visual field in front of a horse when allowed to carry its head naturally. (b) The blind area in front of a horse when over-bent. ((b) Reproduced with permission of the Captive Animals Protection Society.)

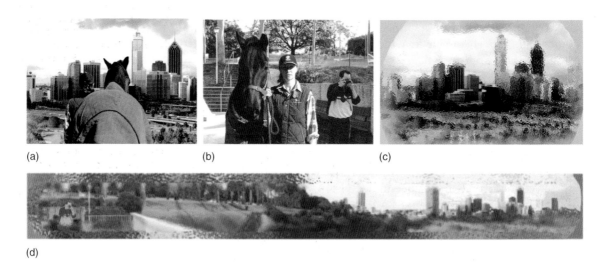

(a)   (b)   (c)

(d)

Figure 2.5 The visual field of one eye of a horse. Horse and human – (a) rear view, (b) front view – are standing looking out over Perth from a viewpoint in Kings Park. So in front of them they see Perth and to the back of them is a man taking a photo of Perth. The human view (c) is of Perth itself and not much more, since our vision is so frontal. Also we see just the very middle in high acuity. The horse (d) by contrast, sees Perth and everything else simultaneously right back to the man taking the photograph. (Reproduced with permission of Alison Harman.)

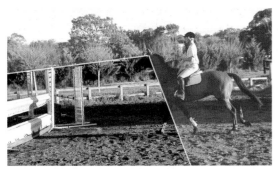

(a)

Figure 2.6a,b Show jumper approaching a jump with the horse's head either (a) up or (b) down. Visual field is indicated. (Reproduced with permission of Alison Harman.)

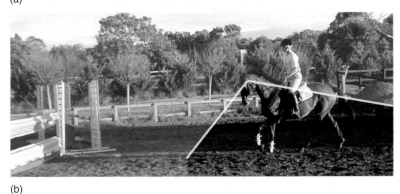

(b)

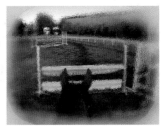

(c)

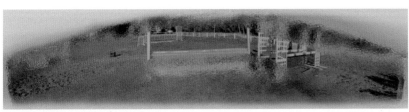

(d)

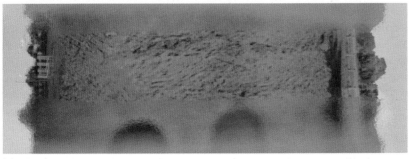

(e)

Figure 2.6c–e A view of what a horse sees when approaching a jump with head (d) up or (e) down. (d) shows that the horse sees the jump and also a lot of other things out to the side. (e) shows that if you hold the head down it sees its foot and knee and a bit of the world out to the side. Perhaps this is why a horse may be more compliant when its head is held down, since it is unlikely to make much sense of the visual world. (c) Shows what a human sees over the jump (remember we only really see the middle of our visual field in high acuity). (Reproduced with permission of Alison Harman.)

lateral vision to get a better look at jumps as they get up close. Perhaps this is why blinkers have found little favor in show-jumping circles, the traditional source of a multiplicity of gadgets. Blinkers are most effective in preventing shying and have been favored by carriage drivers because they make the horses less likely to attempt to turn in the shafts or bolt. It is also suggested that blinkers can render a horse more responsive to voice commands used to increase speed because they prevent it from seeing when the driver is not carrying or about to use a whip (Les Holmes, personal communication 2002). Blinkers on racing animals bring rather different benefits – especially, it seems, when used for the first time. It has been suggested that, if it is a generally low-ranking animal, a racehorse that sees another horse approaching from behind is more likely to defer to the challenger if not wearing blinkers. This assumes that more dominant horses are more motivated to assume the lead in a galloping herd, a hypothesis that has yet to be tested.

DEPTH PERCEPTION

It was long believed that animals with laterally placed eyes and extensive monocular visual fields did not have stereopsis – the ability to see in stereo and perceive depth. However, recent studies[10] have demonstrated that the horse's binocular field is an arc of approximately 60° in front of the head, affording good stereopsis and thresholds of depth detection comparable to those of cats and pigeons. These findings indicate that larger interocular distances, as found in the horse, may provide useful depth judgment. This may have arisen because the horse has evolved to make judgments over a range of several meters, whereas ground-feeding birds such as pigeons, with an extremely small interocular distance, have to focus at a distance of only a few centimeters. Horses also use monocular depth cues to judge distance.[4] This makes sense because they spend so much of their day with their heads to the ground, a position that makes stereopsis redundant.

Harman et al[11] suggest that when a horse lifts its head the binocular area of vision is directed at the horizon, enabling scanning and depth perception. In this position monocular lateral vision is compromised. However, when the head is lowered and the binocular vision is directed at the area directly in front of the head, the lateral monocular fields afford good lateral horizon vision.

Effective use of the binocular field is required when a horse attempts to discern an object that is close and low. The horse is best able to use its binocular field of view by arching the neck and rotating the head. It can focus on the object by simultaneous rotation of the eye downward to optimize orientation of the visual streak (see p. 43).

STIMULUS VISIBILITY

Factors that affect the visibility of a stimulus for a horse include size of the object, contrast and environmental illumination. When a moving horse spots something underfoot, it not only looks at the stimulus, but is also likely to change speed.[12] The level of arousal plays a part in the recognition of stimuli, an outcome that may be influenced by the horse's age and training because recognition of distant stimuli on the ground is facilitated by carrying the head at a lower angle. Saslow[12] found that younger animals tend to carry their heads higher and therefore may not notice stimuli as readily as older horses, especially those that have been trained not to carry their neck straight and head high.

Saslow[12] also found that horses were able to discern stimuli better in overcast rather than bright sunny conditions. This suggests that the equine rod-dominated eye may not find bright conditions as favorable as dull conditions. The high proportion of rods to cones (generally 20:1)[13] gives the horse excellent night vision but insufficient to make horses innately fearless of areas that are poorly lit. As we will see in Chapter 4, horses will work to keep a stable illuminated, and this helps to explain some of the aversiveness of small dark spaces, including trailers (floats in the USA) (Fig. 2.7). A reflective layer of cells behind the retina, the tapetum, enhances this. Acting like a mirror, the tapetum reflects light back on to the retina, enabling further light to be gathered. The downside of this arrangement is that the image is

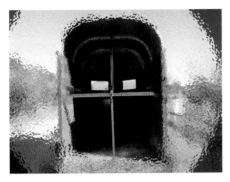

(a)

Figure 2.7 (a) human and (b) horse visual fields when looking into a trailer (float in the USA). (Reproduced with permission of Alison Harman.)

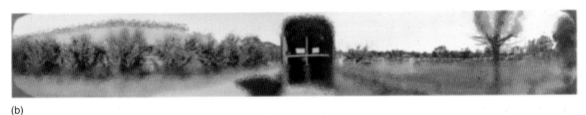

(b)

somewhat compromised. Because several receptors may be stimulated by incoming light, the image can become fuzzy and acuity reduced. This effect has been likened to the pixelation of a low-resolution digital image.[4]

ACCOMMODATION

Horses have a small degree of ciliary accommodation,[14] which relies on the contraction of ciliary muscles and contractile fibers that extend into the corpora nigra. However, despite weak lens muscles, horses' optics allow them to see between about 1 meter away and infinity on the whole, with little need to vary the lens. Accommodation is required if there is a need to see even closer than that with high acuity. Horses rarely need to do that; indeed because the eye's proximity to objects is generally limited by the length of the nose,[15] things very close are felt via the skin and vibrissae of the muzzle, and therefore highly focused vision is not essential.

According to what was originally referred to as the 'ramp retina' theory, it was believed that the distance from the nodal point of the eye to the retina varied so that the dorsal retina was farther away than the more central and ventral regions.

The idea was that the horse could move its head so that near objects would be focused on the back of the retina while far objects would be more easily focused on the dorsal part of the retina. This theory was supported by the observation that horses are likely to exhibit characteristic head-moving behavior when looking at things. For example, the head may be raised unusually high and the nose pointed forward when observing an object of interest to the fore. The horse may arch its neck sideways (cock its head) to look at an object of unusual interest beside it (Fig. 2.8).

First refuted by Sivak & Allen,[16] the ramp retina theory has fallen out of favor. By demonstrating that, except for the far dorsal and far ventral retina, the distance between the retina and lens was the same at all points on the retina, Harman et al[11] confirmed the absence of any ramp. Therefore, because movement of the head would not alter the focus of the image on the retina, they inferred that the horse has dynamic accommodation ability.

It has been shown that the horse's eye has a visual streak (Fig. 2.9). This linear retinal region contains high concentrations of ganglion cells, while low concentrations appear in the peripheral regions. Concentrations in the visual streak reach 6100 cells/mm^2, with the peripheral regions object with the visual streak. Movement of the head may bring into focus images that originally fell onto the regions of low acuity, in the same way that we may see movement in our peripheral visual field and turn towards it to see, with our high-acuity retinal region, what is the cause of the movement. The horse sees a movement in the peripheral visual field and reacts defensively. This may explain why a horse will suddenly raise its head and shy away from an object that has suddenly entered its field of view.

Accommodation in the horse appears to be no more than one diopter (light-bending power) in either direction.[11] In optical terms, horses are emmetropic with limited accommodation, which means they can see everything well but cannot focus close up. The normal horse's eye appears to be correctly focused with a tendency to long-sightedness (hyperopia) when older. It has been suggested, though, that domestication, inbreeding and constant stabling may lead to horses becoming myopic.[11] Though yet to be tested, the hypothesis (derived from work in human infants exposed to night lights while asleep) is that if a young horse has limited possibilities to focus into the distance and instead looks only at close objects (because the stable is often a visually limited environment with dim light), then it may have a tendency to be shorter sighted (Alison Harman, personal communication 2001).

COLOR VISION

Leblanc & Bouissou[17] showed that mares, when presented with their own and an alien foal, used visual recognition from a distance to identify their offspring. However, when the mare was presented with foals of similar coat color, other sensory responses were required for identification. Notwithstanding this interesting exception, horses have relatively little need for color vision. The equine retina does, however, provide both morphological and electrophysiological evidence for color vision. Although rods dominate, both cones and rods are present in the retina, and there is clear functional duality of responses indicative of cones and rods.[18]

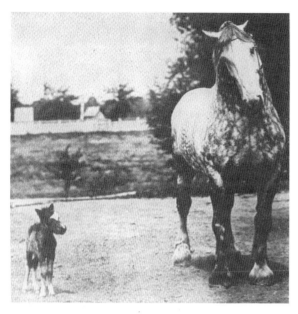

Figure 2.8   Horse raising and tilting its head to look at a pony foal. (Reproduced with permission of Animal Science Dept, Iowa State University.)

Ganglion cell density per 250 × 250 micron square

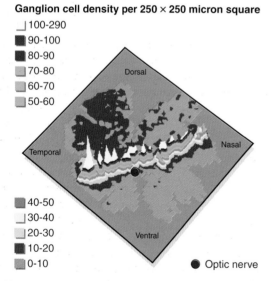

Figure 2.9   The distribution of ganglion cells on a flat-mount of a horse retina. High concentrations are represented by the peaks. (Reproduced with permission of Alison Harman.)

ranging between 150 and 200 cells/mm^2.[11] This arrangement of a visual streak gives the horse a very narrow, but panoramic view. The reason the horse cocks its head sideways is to 'look' at an

It has been suggested that, like all mammals (with the exception of primates, some of which are trichromats), horses are dichromats[19] and that they struggle to discriminate between green and grays of similar brightness. Smith & Goldman[18] suggested that the color discrimination of the horse has no neutral point at which color can be distinguished from gray. Their horses responded to blue, green, red or yellow versus gray at any brightness.

Different colors, from the short-wavelength purples and blues, through the spectrum to the long wavelengths can be tested using color boards arranged in pairs. If the horse distinguishes between colors correctly it finds that it can push the board to reveal a food reward (see the case study at the end of this chapter). However, the problem is ensuring that one adequately controls for brightness or luminance.[20] Early studies on color vision in horses trained horses to choose between a colored stimulus and a gray one.[18,19] In an attempt to eliminate brightness cues, several gray stimuli were used for comparison with each color. Conflicting results from these studies suggest problems with methodology and raised the possibility that horses may be better than humans at discriminating between gray panels of different luminance.

A more recent study[20] first established the range of horses' ability to discriminate brightness of achromatic stimuli and then measured the color discrimination of several animals within this range. Brightness cues may well have played a part at the top end of the range of luminance differences but cannot do so at the bottom end. Using this method, the authors demonstrated that two horses were able to distinguish red and blue across the range of luminance differences but were unable to distinguish green and yellow from gray at the lower end of the scale, indicating that the horses were not seeing these colors well, if at all. [20]

So there could be two reasons why findings from studies of equine color vision seem to contradict one another. The first is methodological: horses in the earlier studies may have been able to discriminate on the basis of 'brightness'. The second is that there may be wide variation between horses so that, for example, some can see yellow and not red and some can see red and not yellow (Alison Harman, personal communication 2002).

Investigations of equine responses to color discrimination tests can be further thwarted by lack of motivation in the horses. Horses have been trained to use the color of a central panel to signal a correct (left or right) lever-pressing response.[21] However, discrimination performance was better when the combinations were differentially reinforced by two types of food than when by a single reinforcer. Interestingly, the stimulus color of the preceding trial interfered with discrimination performance on a given trial.

It seems that future exploration of equine vision, and perhaps even the painting of obstacles for horses in competitions, including show-jumping, should take account of these findings. Retrospective studies of the competition performance of 72 show-jumpers attempting to jump a total of 343 obstacles showed that the number of faults at a particular obstacle depended on obstacle-type, height and arrangement but also color. For example, obstacles of two contrasting colors were jumped without fault more often than those of one (light or dark) color.[22]

Given that cones are maximally sensitive to particular wavelengths of light as determined by their opsin content, analysis of pigment provides the clearest evidence for dichromatic vision in horses. Microscopic studies of the retina support evidence from recent behavior studies,[23] by showing that there are two peaks in the spectral sensitivity of equine cones at 428 nm and 539 nm.[24] This translates into two basic hues: pastel blue and yellow. It is important to remember that, for dichromats, there are no intermediate hues as there are in the visual world of trichromats, such as humans. Instead, when colors from the two ends of the dichromatic spectrum are mixed, the result is a desaturated version of one of the basic hues or an achromatic region (white or gray). These differences are represented most clearly by the color wheels in Figure 2.10.

FOAL VISION

Consistent visual stimulation during neonatal life is required for proper development of the

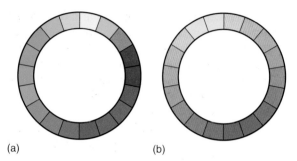

(a) (b)

Figure 2.10 The differences between (a) the dichromatic color vision of the horse and (b) that of trichromats, such as humans, are most notable in the number of different colors seen.[24] (Reproduced with permission of Joseph Carroll.)

visual pathways.[4] When a foal is born the eyes are open and it is assumed that there is some degree of visual function. Important functions of the visual system develop after eye opening. In humans or cats, for example, limited or no input to one eye renders it amblyopic or functionally blind, since no allocation is made for its input in the visual cortex. Similarly the development of a binocular field, i.e. both eyes are in register, takes place some time after birth (up to several weeks in cats, 5 years in humans). This is the 'critical period' during which the input to the visual cortex becomes fixed. We do not know what this period is in equids, but by extrapolation from cats and humans, it probably occupies the first few months (Alison Harman, personal communication 2002).

It has been suggested that neonatal foals are short-sighted because the muscles used in accommodation are relatively weak.[6] This may account for their apparent reliance upon tactile and gustatory exploration, and their occasional collisions with objects, including fences. Exploring ways in which the eye of the neonatal foal is functionally different to that of the mature horse, Enzerink[25] found that foals developed a menace response (avoidance of a hand raised up suddenly to the level of the horse's eye – a crude indication of ophthalmic health) several days post-partum. It is suggested that with open eyelids and the lack of a menace response, foals could be predisposed to eye trauma. However, the absence of a menace response does not provide sufficient reason to stable foals in the first weeks post-partum for fear of globe trauma. Newborn foals are generally well protected by the mare, and globe trauma is not a common finding in healthy foals. The pupillary light response is evident from birth; however, a functional visual cortex is not required to initiate the response, and therefore a positive response does not exclude a visual defect.[25]

PROBLEMS WITH VISION

Horses with partial blindness are potentially more dangerous than those that are fully blind, because they may suddenly see objects and react with surprise. Horses with impaired vision often flick their ears rapidly during locomotion and show excessive sensitivity to sounds. Extraorbital causes of impaired vision may include lesions in the brainstem, cerebral cortex, optic nerve or superior colliculi as well as electric shock, serum hepatitis, or poisoning (for example with hypericum, lead and selenium). On the other hand extreme sensitivity to light is noted in recurrent uveitis, equine viral arteritis and riboflavin deficiency.

CHEMORECEPTION

In the horse, smell and taste are linked neurologically as they are in many other species.

SMELL

Horses familiarize themselves with foreign objects by smelling them. Social exchange by sniffing one another's breath with or without an open mouth, represents an important part of greeting rituals between horses. Forced exhalations help to drive air from the nasal cavity in advance of deep inhalations that allow the horse to sample odor molecules. Rarely do humans allow sufficient time for horses to gather this sort of information. At the same time, we should remember that because of the combined effect of bathing, using soaps, changing clothes and manipulating all sorts of materials with our hands, our odors are likely to change over time in a way that thwarts their reliability for horses. Horses use odors to recognize familiar foods and those for which they have a particular need.[26] The strategic use of agents, such as peppermint essence, that mask the flavor of food and water can overcome capriciousness when horses are presented with novel resources, for instance as a result of transit, competition or sale.

Olfactory receptors that generate the sense of smell are found in the upper part of the nasal cavity within the mucous membrane. Odorous molecules bind with these receptors and initiate the neural signals that may be processed into strong associations, some social and others sexual. Having a long nose, the horse has a predictably large area of olfactory mucosa (see Ch. 3).

In addition to the conventional olfactory system, the horse contains an accessory olfactory system in the form of the vomeronasal organ (VNO,

also known as the Organ of Jacobson). This paired tubular organ is also present in many other animals. It is found inside the horse's nose within the hard palate and is used to detect pheromones in urine and other moderately volatile odors. The horse uses its VNO during the flehmen response in which it raises its head and rolls back its upper lip (often anthropomorphically labeled a laugh), forcing smell-laden air through slits in the nasal cavity into the VNO (Fig. 2.11). The response is often seen in horses conducting a thorough investigation of other horses' urine and feces but may also occur when they encounter novel flavors and nasal irritants. Although gravity assists in this sampling procedure, it has been shown that the lumen of the tubular portion of the VNO alternatively expands and contracts to pump its content in the direction of the accessory olfactory bulb.[27] In contrast to many other species, the VNO of horses does not open into the oral cavity.[28] Rather than being restricted to exhibition of flehmen only after direct contact of the lips or

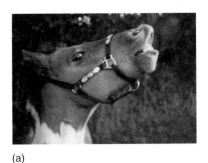
(a)

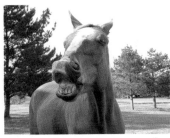
(b)

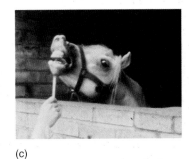
(c)

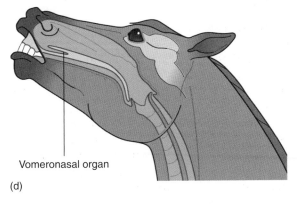
Vomeronasal organ

(d)

Figure 2.11 Flehmen response seen in adult and juvenile horses of both sexes but most commonly observed in mature stallions, especially in response to estrous mares. The typical response includes (a) elevation of the head, rolling back of the eyes, rotation of the ears to the side and (b) eversion of the upper lip. It may also involve (c) some flicking of the tongue and lateral rolling of the head. (d) Section of horse's head showing position of vomeronasal organ during flehmen. (Reproduced with permission of: (b) Jo-Anne Rooker; (c) Francis Burton. (d) Redrawn from Waring 1983[32] with permission.)

tongue with urine, horses are unique in that they can flehmen in response to volatile substances borne in the air.[28]

Colts show more flehmen than fillies but intriguingly foals of both genders show the response more often than do their mothers.[28] This suggests that the response has a role in the development of both sexual surveillance and pheromone processing. Having said that, foals do not appear able to discriminate between estrous and non-estrous urine.[29] As yet, the importance of pheromones in triggering maturational change in adolescent horses can only be inferred from studies in other species. The flehmen response offers a powerful signal to observing horses and seems to have an important role in courtship. Stallions can discriminate between estrous and non-estrous mares, but their ability to do so seems to depend on supportive visual and auditory cues rather than on olfactory stimuli alone.[30,31]

TASTE

Taste, like smell, is a result of interactions of chemical stimuli with receptors on a mucous membrane. These receptors are papillae found on the tongue (Fig. 2.12). The taste sensations perceived by the horse are presumed to be gradations of salt, sour, sweet and bitter.[32]

Just as it is pivotal in the early bonding of a mare with her foal, taste may be used when two horses groom one another.[33] Taste may help horses to determine the caloric content of foods. It also allows animals to discriminate among different foods and exercise their preferences.[34] Studies have shown that horses will learn to avoid a food associated with illness.[35] Gustation may also provide nutritional information about food. For example, if the horse's diet is deficient in salt, it may preferentially select feedstuff higher in salt content over another not so high.[36]

While the sense of taste may also provide information about the toxicity of food, this faculty is far from foolproof.[33] It appears that horses differ individually in their ability to avoid bitter additives and *Senecio* species, including ragwort.[37] This may have practical implications in deciding which horses may safely graze on pastures infested with toxic plants.

Taste also regulates digestive processes that initiate further processes such as enzymatic

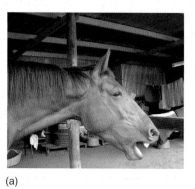
(a)

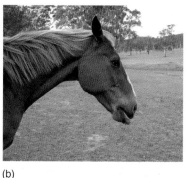
(b)

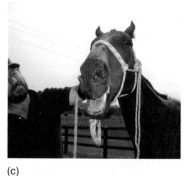
(c)

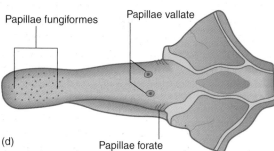
(d)

Papillae fungiformes
Papillae vallate
Papillae forate

Figure 2.12 (a–c) Horses often attempt to get rid of foul-tasting materials (including many oral medications) from their mouths. (d) Distribution on the equine tongue of the papillae that house taste. (Reproduced with permission of: (a & b) Jo-Anne Rooker; (c) Tanya Grassi. (d) Redrawn from Waring 1983[32] with permission.)

secretions. A normal appetite in the horse is determined primarily on the basis of pre-gastric stimuli such as taste, texture and smell.[38] The regulation of feed intake is also highly influenced by taste, and this is of great importance in maintaining the animal's normal body chemical balance. Habituation by gradual exposure to increasingly concentrated solutions of innately aversive chemicals has been reported in horses as an adjunct means of modulating water intake in performance horses.[39]

HEARING

The equine sense of hearing is very well developed. The horse's funnel-shaped ears can move in unison or independently of each other. Using 10 muscles, the ears can be moved around a lateral arc of 180°, enabling accurate location of the source of the sound.[40] Horses with impaired hearing may show more drooping of the ears. The direction in which the ears point helps to indicate in which direction a horse's attention is focused (Fig. 2.13). This seems particularly useful when horses, as group animals, may have their vision obscured

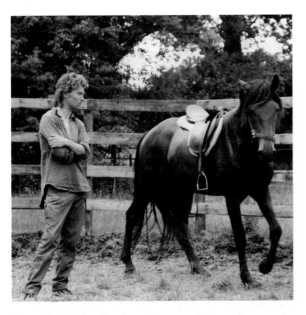

Figure 2.13 The direction of the ears of a horse in a round pen indicates that it has its attention on the handler.

by the bodies of their companions. When outdoors, horses seem to be able to use body positioning in sound detection, e.g. it is suggested that, if they position themselves appropriately, horses can amplify sounds by bouncing them off their shoulders.[6] Horses are able to locate the source of a sound within an arc of approximately 25°. This compares poorly with hunting species such as dogs and humans that are accurate within a degree. However, it seems that horses are well-equipped to hear faint noises. For example, they respond to sounds from up to 4400 meters away.[41]

Horses are better than humans at discriminating between noises of similar loudness. Horses can also protect their ears from very loud noises by laying them flat. The aversive effects of a combatant's squealing during a fight may be tempered by this response. In comparison with the human, the horse is able to hear higher-pitched sounds. A human's range of hearing is between 20 Hz and 20 kHz while a horse's is 55 Hz to 33.5 kHz,[42] being most sensitive to sounds in the range 1–16 kHz, a broader range than most mammals. Horses can therefore hear high-pitched sounds that we cannot, but not some of the lower frequency sounds that we can hear. This is thought to arise from the shorter interaural distance horses have compared with humans.[43] Equine sensitivity to ultrasound helps in determining the source of noises. It may be that we should become more sophisticated in our exploitation of this difference, for example in the development of training aids and secondary reinforcers. There seems to be an interaction between visual and auditory perception, with an especially interesting correlation across a number of mammalian species between sound localization ability and the width of the field of best vision.[44] Species with small foveae or areae centralis have good localization thresholds while those with large fovea have poor localization thresholds. With its characteristic visual streak the horse falls into the latter category, having a long narrow field of good vision that most probably allows it to pinpoint the likely source of a sound without needing accurate identification of the auditory locus.[23]

There is some suggestion that horses can respond (with nervousness and vocalization) to sounds of very low frequencies, such as geographical vibrations preceding earthquakes.[45] It is thought that they do not 'hear' as such, but can detect the vibrations through the hoof.

Studies have shown that there is no difference in hearing ability between adult mares and geldings.[46] However, there is a significant difference between 'adult' horses and 'old' horses, suggesting that the ability to hear sound of a higher frequency decreases with age.[46]

We do well to talk to horses with whom we seek to form a bond. Unlike the visual and olfactory properties we provide, our voice is constant and is therefore a more reliable parameter that can be used in recognition.

TOUCH

The sense of touch is variable over different areas of the horse's body. The withers, mouth, flank and elbow regions are very sensitive areas. Some horses dislike their ears, eyes, groin and bulbs of the heels being touched. As herd animals it is important that they are sensitive to the presence of others at their sides. This may help them to move as a cohesive social group in times of danger and to initiate bouts of mutual grooming (see Fig. 2.14

and Chs 5 and 10). When riders use their legs to move horses beneath them they are capitalizing on this innate sensitivity.

The vibrissae around the eyes and muzzle have a rich afferent nerve supply.[47,48] The apparently disorganized beard of vibrissae in the neonatal foal is thought to facilitate location of the teat.[6] Vibrissae inform the horse of its distance from a given surface and may even be able to detect vibrational energy (sound). Together with the lips, they gather tactile information during grazing and head-rubbing. Horses are said to test electric fences with these whiskers before touching them. It has been suggested that the inability to detect fixed objects is a contributory factor to facial trauma in horses subjected to road transport subsequent to whisker trimming (Amy Coffman, personal communication 2002). Because vibrissae can be identified as anatomically different from normal hair coat, the trimming of whiskers has been outlawed in Germany (Andreas Briese, personal communication 2002). In the mouse, it has been shown that each vibrissa has its own small region of sensory cortex, a so-called whisker barrel, one per whisker, each of which can be clearly seen in brain sections (Alison Harman, personal communication 2002). This dedication of a portion of

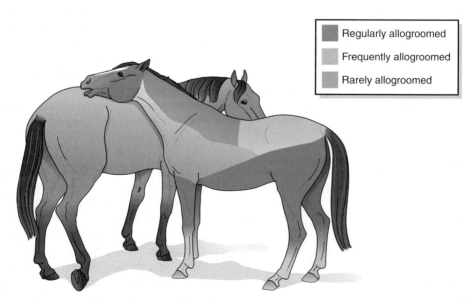

Regularly allogroomed

Frequently allogroomed

Rarely allogroomed

Figure 2.14 Mutual grooming map. (Redrawn after Feh & de Mazieres 1993[49], with permission from Elsevier Science.)

the cortex to each vibrissa indicates that they must be extremely important sensory instruments which should not be removed for cosmetic purposes.

Pain results in the release of pain mediators that act on the specific nociceptors. The nociceptors generate electrical potential in response to traumatic stimulation such as tissue-damaging pressure, intense heat, irritating chemical substances and skin abrasion.[50] As the severity of the stimulus intensifies, there will be an increased frequency of action potential generation. The sensory cortex in the brain (see Ch. 3) creates the perception of pain and makes the horse aware of the strength and position of the pain stimulus. In response to pain there may also be activation of the sympathetic nervous system, causing a range of physiological responses. A painful stimulus also gives rise to a behavioral response and an emotional component that may include fear and anxiety.[6]

Sensitivity of the skin varies according to the thickness of the horse's coat, thickness of its skin and receptor density in different areas. There are distinct receptors in the skin that respond to heat and cold (thermoreceptors), touch, pressure and vibration (mechanoreceptors) and pain (nociceptors). It is worth noting that a common feature of all skin nociceptors is that they become less responsive if the stimulus is repeated at frequent intervals[50] (see Habituation, in Ch. 4).

The distribution of different types of sensory end organs changes in different parts of the body. When practitioners twitch their patients' upper lips (see Ch. 14) they are capitalizing on the fact that this area is rich in three types of nerve endings that detect touch, pressure and pain. The mechanism by which this helps to pacify fractious animals is discussed further in Chapters 3 and 15. It is worth remembering that the buccal mucosa is as sensitive as the skin to tactile stimuli. The discriminative ability horses show when they empty their mouths of fine inedible material taken in during grazing, accounts for the rarity of intestinal foreign bodies in horses compared with, say, cattle. We have exploited this sensitivity by using oral discomfort to control horses. We should respect this sensitivity and avoid the heavy-handed rein-pulling that ultimately destroys it. Given the importance of tactile stimulation for

communication both within human-horse dyads and between horses, it is surprising that this topic has not been more thoroughly explored by equine scientists.

SUMMARY OF KEY POINTS

The horse has:
- almost 350° vision
- a caudal blind spot that accounts for a proportion of startle responses
- dichromatic color vision (i.e. like a color-blind person)
- a sense of taste that discriminates between safe and toxic plants with variable accuracy
- highly developed accessory olfaction
- the ability to hear within and beyond the range of human hearing
- predictable zones of very sensitive cutaneous sensation.

CASE STUDY

Rascal, a 9-year-old cob, is one of a group of horses at Brackenhurst College, UK, being taught to select certain colors in chromatic pairs as part of an investigation of perceptual ability. He can differentiate between white and yellow.

The animals in this study chose between two boxes that were identical, except for the color of a card displayed on the front of each. In Rascal's case a yellow card was on the 'correct' box, which opened to allow the horse to gain the reward, and a white card was on the 'incorrect' box, which was locked. Once successful, a horse can quickly learn *some* other pairs of colors, unless it cannot distinguish between them, or if a color choice has been used in a previous pairing during training. Horses have excellent memories, so they do not easily learn discrimination reversals, even after long breaks.

The horse was first led into the testing arena and helped by the trainer to open the boxes so that the boxes were associated with hidden food rewards (Fig. 2.15). Next day, the horse was allowed to investigate the boxes itself with the trainer walking alongside. Next, the horse learned to approach the devices without being led by a human. It was released from a start line about

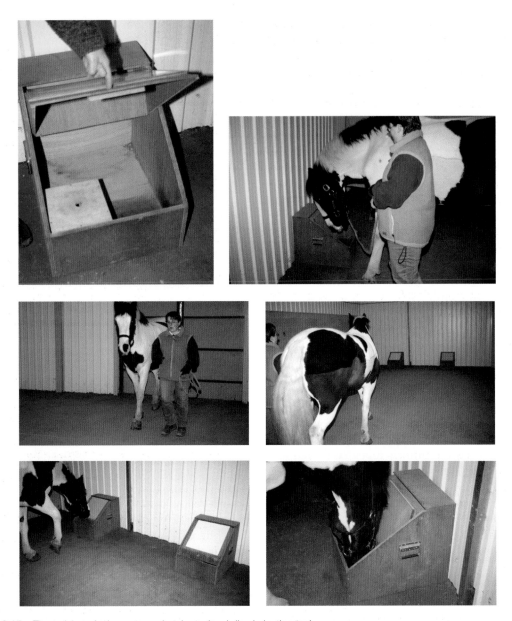

Figure 2.15 The training of a horse to undertake a visual discrimination task.

6 meters from the boxes and allowed to explore alone. Five training sessions, each lasting for about 15 minutes, were given over a period of 3 weeks. Eventually, using only the visual cues, 70% of trained horses confidently selected the 'correct' box every time.

In shaping the final behavior, the trainer randomly assigned the 'correct' choice to a left or right position (with a maximum of three consecutive trials in the same position). This was to make sure that the horse was using the colored card to make a choice and not the position of the box, since spatial cues seem stronger than visual ones for equids.

At first, the horse was encouraged to investigate both boxes to discover that only one of the pair of boxes would open and contained the reward. Later, after obtaining the reward, the horse was not allowed to investigate the other (locked) box, because this negatively punished incorrect selection. If the horse made the 'wrong' choice, it was then allowed to change its choice and go to the other 'correct' box. After four consecutive 'wrong' choices, the horse was guided to the 'correct' box.

As training progressed, the horse was no longer allowed to swap, but was led back to the starting line to try again after an incorrect choice. This increased the 'cost' of failure, making it more important for the horse to get it right first time, and so improved learning.

As opposed to those occasional (often nervous) animals that appear to have no primary motivation to investigate the devices, relaxed horses are most suitable for this type of training. Interestingly, some horses primarily trained as riding animals seem to have preconceptions about being led by humans and do not readily take the opportunity to make choices in the presence of humans. These individuals were reluctant to take the lead and had to be removed from the experimental group.

Clearly, we need more of this type of research because, among other things, it helps us to understand that horses are more than simply draft or riding animals. Many novice observers and even some with equestrian experience are surprised to see horses doing something other than being ridden.

REFERENCES

1. Blake H. Thinking with horses. London: Souvenir Press; 1977.
2. Soemmerring DW. A comment on the horizontal sections of eyes in man and animals. Anderson SR, Munk O, eds. Schepelern HD, transl. Copenhagen: Bogtrykkeriet Forum; 1971.
3. Knill LM, Eagleton RD, Harver E. Physical optics of the equine eye. Am J Vet Res 1977; 38(6):735–737.
4. Roberts SM. Equine vision and optics. Vet Clin North Am Equine Pract 1992; 8(3):451–457.
5. Beaver BV. Equine vision. Vet Med Small Animal Clinician 1982; 175–178.
6. Fraser AF. The behaviour of the horse. Wallingford, UK: CAB International; 1992.
7. Budiansky S. The nature of horses — exploring equine evolution, intelligence and behavior. New York: Free Press; 1997.
8. Saslow CA. Understanding the perceptual world of horses. Appl Anim Behav Sci 2002; 78(2–4):209–224.
9. Crispin SM. Vision in domestic animals. In: Phillipson AT, Hall LW, Pritchard WR, eds. Scientific foundations of veterinary medicine. London: Heinemann Medical; 1980.
10. Timney B, Keil K. Local and global stereopsis in the horse. Vision Res 1999; 39:1861–1867.
11. Harman AM, Moore S, Hoskins R, Keller P. Horse vision and the explanation of visual behaviour originally explained by the 'ramp retina'. Equine Vet J 1999; 31(5):384–390.
12. Saslow CA. Factors affecting stimulus visibility for horses. Appl Anim Behav Sci 1999; 61:273–284.
13. Wouters L, De Moor A. Ultrastructure of the pigment epithelium and the photoreceptors in the retina of the horse. Am J Vet Res 1979; 40:1066–1071.
14. Prince JH, Diesem CD, Eglitis I, Ruskell GL. Anatomy and histology of the eye and orbit in domestic animals. Springfield, IL: CC Thomas; 1960.
15. Farrall H, Handscombe M. Equine vision. Equine Vet J 1999; 31(5):354–355.
16. Sivak JG, Allen DB. An evaluation of the ramp retina on the horse eye. Vision Res 1975; 15:1353–1356.
17. Leblanc MA, Bouissou MF. Development of a test to study maternal recognition of young in horses. Biol Behav 1981; 6(4):283–290.
18. Smith S, Goldman L. Colour discrimination in horses. Appl Anim Behav Sci 1999; 62:13–25.
19. Pick DF, Lovell G, Brown S, Dail D. Equine colour perception revisited. Appl Anim Behav Sci 1994; 42:61–65.
20. Macuda T, Timney B. Luminance and chromatic discrimination in the horse (Equus caballus). Behav Process 1999; 44(3):301–307.
21. Miyashita Y, Nakajima S, Imada H. Differential outcome effect in the horse. J Exp Anal Behav 2000; 74(2):245–254.
22. Stachurska A, Pieta M, Nesteruk E. Which obstacles are most problematic for jumping horses? Appl Anim Behav Sci 2002; 77(3):197–207.
23. Timney B, Macuda T. Vision and hearing in horses. J Am Vet Med Assoc 2001; 218(10):1567–1574.
24. Carroll J, Murphy CJ, Neitz M, et al. Photopigment basis for dichromatic color vision in the horse. J Vision 2001; 1:80–87.
25. Enzerink E. The menace response and the pupillary light reflex in neonatal foals. Equine Vet J 1998; 30(6):546–548.
26. McGreevy PD, Hawson LA, Habermann TC, Cattle SR. Geophagia in horses: a short note on 13 cases. Appl Anim Behav Sci 2001; 71:119–215.
27. Whitten WK. Vomeronasal organ and the accessory olfactory system. Appl Anim Behav Sci 1985; 14:105–109.
28. Crowell-Davis SL. Developmental behavior. Vet Clin North Am Equine Pract: Behav 1986; 573–590.
29. Weeks JW, Crowell-Davis SL, Heusner G. Development of a differential flehmen response in Equus caballus. Appl Anim Behav Sci 2002; 78(2–4):329–335.
30. Anderson TM, Pickett BW, Heird JC, Squires EL. Effect of blocking vision and olfaction on sexual responses of haltered or loose stallions. J Equine Vet Sci 1996; 16:254–261.

31. Houpt KA , Guida L. Flehmen. Equine Pract 1984; 6(3):32–35.

32. Waring GH. Horse behavior: behavioral traits and adaptations of domestic and wild horses, including ponies. Park Ridge, NJ: Noyes; 1983.

33. Kiley-Worthington M. The behaviour of horses in relation to management and training. London: JA Allen; 1987.

34. Houpt KA, Wolski T. Domestic animal behavior for veterinarians and animal scientists. Ames: Iowa State University Press; 1982.

35. Houpt KA, Zahorik DM, Swartzman-Andert JA. Taste aversion learning in horses. J Anim Sci 1990; 68:2340–2344.

36. Salter RE, Pluth DJ. Determinants of mineral lick utilization by feral horses. Northwest Sci 1980; 54: 109–118.

37. Marinier SL, Alexander AJ. Selective grazing behaviour in horses: development of methodology and preliminary use of tests to measure individual grazing ability. Appl Anim Behav Sci 1991; 30(3–4):203–221.

38. Ralston SL. Controls of feeding in horses. J Anim Sci 1984; 59(5):1354–1359.

39. Murphy K, Wishart S, Mills D. The acceptability of various flavoured solutions by Thoroughbred horses. The role of the horse in Europe. Equine Vet J Suppl 1999; 28:67.

40. Vallencien B. Comparative anatomy and physiology of the auditory organ in vertebrates. In: Busnel RG, ed. Acoustic behavior of animals. Amsterdam: Elsevier; 1963:522–556.

41. Busnel RG. On certain aspects of animal acoustic signals. In: Busnel RG, ed. Acoustic behaviour of animals. Amsterdam: Elsevier; 1963:69–111.

42. Heffner RS, Heffner HE. Hearing in large mammals: horses (Equus caballus) and cattle (Bos taurus). Behav Neurosci 1983; 97:299–309.

43. Heffner HE, Heffner RS. Sound localization in large mammals: localization of complex sounds by horses. Behav Neurosci 1984; 98:541–555.

44. Heffner RS, Heffner HE. Visual factors in sound localization in mammals. J Comp Neurol 1992; 317: 219–232.

45. Penick J Jr. The New Madrid earthquakes of 1811–1812. Columbia: University of Missouri Press; 1976.

46. Ödberg FO. A study of the hearing ability of horses. Equine Vet J 1978; 10(2):82–83.

47. Talukdar AH, Calhoun ML, Stinson AW. Microscopic anatomy of the skin of the horse. Am J Vet Res 1972; 31:1751–1754.

48. Van Niekerk HP. Ethological studies within the man–horse relationship. J S Afr Vet Assoc 1980; 51(4):237–238.

49. Feh C, de Mazieres J. Grooming at a preferred site reduces heart rates in horses. Anim Behav 1993; 46:1191–1194.

50. Swenson MJ, Reece WO, eds. Dukes' physiology of domestic animals, 11th edn. Ithaca, NY: Cornell University Press; 1993.

3

Behavior and the brain

Caroline Hahn

INTRODUCTION

'From the brain, and from the brain only, arise our pleasures, joys, laughter and jests, as well as our sorrows, pains, griefs and tears ….' (Hippocrates ~500 BC)

Only relatively recently has it been accepted that the 'mental state' of humans and animals, the emotional, instinctive and cognitive foundations of behavior, are inseparable from their somatic aspects. This artificial schism between psychology and neurology began more than four centuries ago when the philosopher René Descartes was trying to study the human body. The catholic church expressed its dissatisfaction with this study of God's handiwork, and in response Descartes struck a deal with the church – human existence was divided into two realms: the physical body, which he would study, and the mental– spiritual realm, which would remain the exclusive domain of the church. This artificial construct dividing the mental and physical has guided much of scientific and medical thought ever since, to the detriment of human and animal patients.[1] Increasingly powerful molecular tools are being used by neuroscientists to elucidate the relationship between anatomy, physiology and specific functions in perception, thought and movement. Classical psychiatric diseases are not (yet) clearly defined in horses, but an appreciation of basic neuroanatomy and neurophysiology is fundamental to understanding the influence of neuropathology and psychopharmacology on equine behavior.

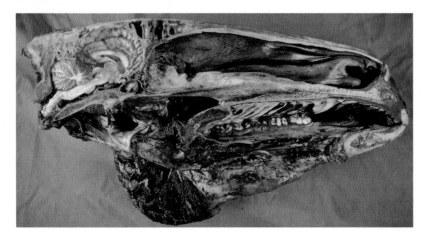

Figure 3.1 Photograph of a sagittal section of the equine head. The equine brain weighs about a third of the human brain (or about 0.1% of the horse's body weight). (Photograph courtesy of Keith Ellis.)

FUNDAMENTALS OF FUNCTIONAL AND BEHAVIORAL NEUROANATOMY

The nervous system processes external stimuli into neuronal impulses resulting in neurotransmitter release, and integrates these with internal drives and emotional stimuli to direct the actions of motor units. These enable the animal to react to its environment and influence the behavior of others. The function of the nervous system fundamentally depends on a group of specialized cells called neurons – polarized, elongated cells that are uniquely capable of extremely rapid, intercellular communication. Neurons have a receptor region (the dendritic zone), a cell body (soma) containing the nucleus, and an axon conducting impulses from the dendritic zone to synapse with other neurons (Fig. 3.2). The cell bodies collectively make up the 'gray' matter of the central nervous system (CNS), whereas the axons are found in 'white' matter. The shape, size and position of the soma as well as the length and branching of the proximal and distal processes differ greatly between neuronal populations. Brainstem axons may have a length of only a few micrometers, whereas the recurrent laryngeal nerve (the nerve that supplies the larynx) is over 3 meters long! Axons often project in groups or bundles that collectively form tracts in the CNS and nerves in the peripheral nervous system. Neurons only make up a small proportion of the total number of cells in the nervous system; the majority are neuroglial cells [Gr. *glia,* glue] such as astrocytes, cells with important supportive and metabolic functions.

MAJOR COMPONENTS OF THE CENTRAL NERVOUS SYSTEM

This section serves to introduce the fundamentals of neuroanatomy, a subject that has been comprehensively addressed by de Lahunta[2] and reviewed by Kaplan & Sadock[3] and Behan.[4] The CNS consists of the brain and spinal cord (Fig. 3.3). The brain includes the two cerebral hemispheres, which are roughly mirror images of one another, and the brainstem, a narrow structure through which all the pathways entering and leaving the two hemispheres must pass and which comprises the centers that control breathing, heart rate, eye movement and many other critical functions. Caudal to the cerebral hemispheres is the cerebellum, a structure that helps to control movement and balance. The caudal part of the brainstem flows into the spinal cord, the point of exit for nerves on their way out to innervate muscles and the point of entry for sensory fibers returning from the body's sensory organs. All the nerves outside the central nervous system are collectively called the peripheral nervous system. The two cerebral hemispheres

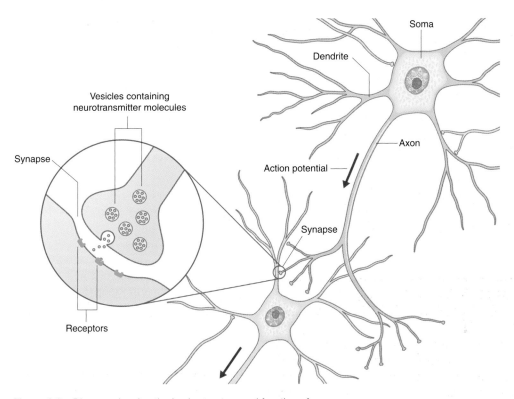

Figure 3.2 Diagram showing the basic structure and function of neurons.

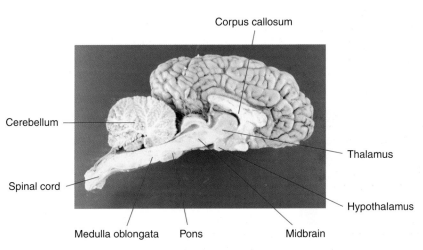

Figure 3.3 Sagittal section of equine brain outlining the major components of the brainstem. (Photograph courtesy of Keith Ellis.)

are built around a connecting system of hollow spaces called the ventricular system. The ventricles are filled with cerebrospinal fluid (CSF). This clear fluid also bathes the surface of the CNS, providing mechanical support to the CNS, and playing an important role in maintaining a constant chemical environment. CSF is produced by modified blood vessels known as the choroid plexus located inside the ventricles.

There are four major divisions of the CNS:

- forebrain, composed of the cerebral hemispheres, basal nuclei, hypothalamus and thalamus

- brainstem, composed of the midbrain, pons and medulla oblongata
- cerebellum
- spinal cord.

Neurons of similar function are grouped together in 'laminae' in the cortex, 'nuclei' in the brainstem and 'columns' in the spinal cord. Axons from sensory and motor nerves enter and leave the CNS as spinal nerves from the spinal cord and cranial nerves from the brain.

FOREBRAIN

Cerebrum

The cerebrum is the most rostral (forward) division of the brain and is divided into two cerebral hemispheres (Fig. 3.4). Cell bodies of the neurons in the cerebrum are located in two general areas: on the outside surface of the cortex (folded into gyri and sulci) and deep to the surface in the basal nuclei (Figs 3.5 and 3.6). Evidence from human studies suggests that the cerebrum is the region of the brain responsible for perception, emotion, voluntary movement and most learning. These functions will be considered in more detail later.

The tremendous number of neurons in the cerebrum have axons arranged in large fiber bundles. Notably the internal capsule serves as the major projection pathway to connect the cerebrum with the brainstem, and the corpus callosum consists of axons connecting the left and

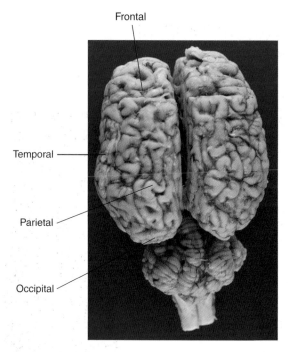

Frontal

Temporal

Parietal

Occipital

Figure 3.4 Cerebral lobes.

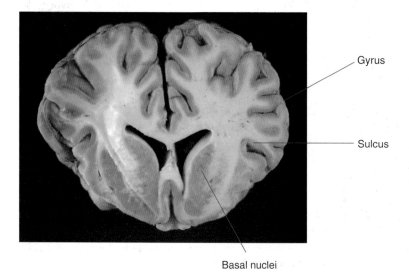

Gyrus

Sulcus

Basal nuclei

Figure 3.5 Transverse section of cerebrum at the level of the basal nuclei. Neurons in the forebrain are aggregated on the surface of the cortex and in the basal nuclei.

right cerebral hemispheres across the midline. Only one cranial nerve (see Table 3.1) – the olfactory nerve, which transmits sensations of smell – is associated with the forebrain (this really is not a 'nerve' at all; in the horse it is a relatively large structure, and it probably received its name on account of its diminutive nerve-like appearance in the human brain).

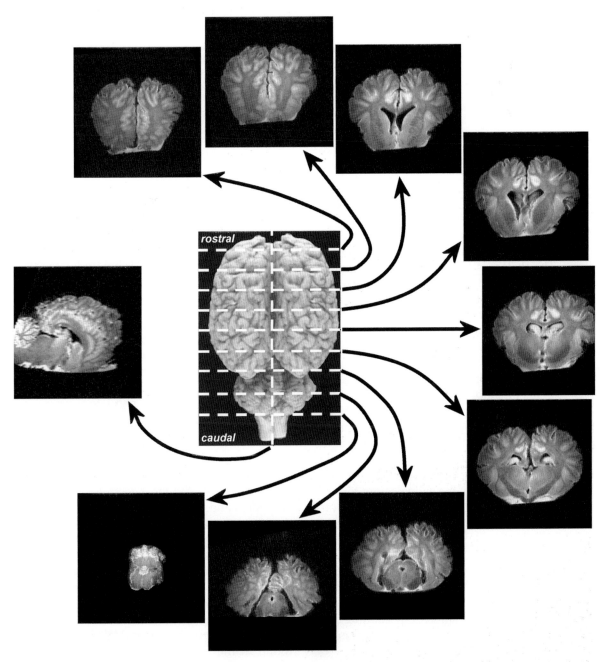

Figure 3.6 One sagittal and nine transverse sections of a T2-weighted proton density magnetic resonance imaging (MRI) scan of an equine brain. (With permission of Luke Henderson, Kevin Keay and Paul McGreevy.)

Table 3.1   Cranial nerves

Number	Name	Brain division	Major function
I	Olfactory	Cerebrum	Smell
II	Optic	Diencephalon	Vision
III	Oculomotor	Midbrain	Eye movement, pupillary constriction
IV	Trochlear		Eye movement
V	Trigeminal	Pons	Sensory from head, muscles of mastication and temporal muscles
VI	Abducens	Medulla oblongata	Eye movement
VII	Facial		Facial movement
VIII	Vestibulocochlear		Balance, hearing
IX	Glossopharyngeal		Taste and pharyngeal movement
X	Vagus		Muscles of larynx and control of viscera
XI	Spinal Accessory		Muscles of neck
XII	Hypoglossal		Tongue movement

Thalamus and hypothalamus (diencephalon)

The most prominent components of the diencephalon are the thalamus and the hypothalamus. The thalamus functions as an integrating system to relay pathways to and from the brainstem and higher centers in the cerebrum. With the exception of impulses from the olfactory nerve, all impulses heading to the cerebrum must synapse in the thalamus; reciprocal fibers there play a critical role in the filtering of sensory input, and in abnormal states they may generate false signals or inappropriately suppress sensation. The thalamus may also serve directly as the site of conscious perception of some sensations[5] and plays a pivotal role in the maintenance of consciousness, the focusing of attention, and the initiation of sleep.[6]

The hypothalamus is the higher center for regulation of autonomic motor activity. It functions without direct voluntary control, but is influenced by the cerebral cortex. There is evidence that stimuli associated with emotionally relevant events may have a significant effect on hypothalamic hormonal regulation. These hormonal consequences seem to influence further behavior and responses in relevant situations, especially aggression and sexual behavior.[7] Seasonal polyestrus behavior of mares is initiated by stimulation of the pineal gland by light, either natural or artificial, causing a reduction of melatonin secretion.

This in turn allows gonadotropin-releasing hormone (GnRH) to be secreted by the hypothalamus, ultimately resulting in the secretion of estrogen and estrus behavior (the exact connection between decreased melatonin production and increased GnRH levels is not understood).

BRAINSTEM

Despite its small size, the brainstem is arguably the most important part of the nervous system. It is the link between the cerebral cortex and the spinal cord and it contains the nuclei of most of the cranial nerves and the regulatory centers for cardiac and lung function.

Midbrain

The midbrain is the most rostral portion of the brainstem and contains the pathways connecting the brainstem and cerebrum. It contains the red nucleus, an important nucleus containing 'upper motor neurons' that initiate the gait of horses (these are neurons in the brain that innervate and control the lower motor neurons in the brainstem or spinal cord). Two of the three nuclei controlling eye movement – cranial nerves (CNs; see Table 3.1) III (oculomotor) and IV (trochlear) – are found in the midbrain. The dorsal components of the midbrain (rostral and caudal colliculi) are linked with reflex functions such as blinking and,

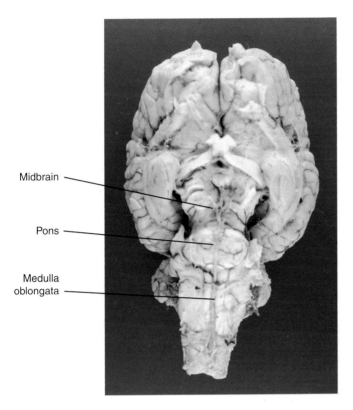

Figure 3.7 Ventral surface of equine brain outlining prominent cranial nerves. (Photograph courtesy of Keith Ellis.)

Midbrain

Pons

Medulla oblongata

in concert with other structures, reacting (shying) to visual or auditory stimuli.

Pons

The pons lies caudal to the midbrain. The pons is the portion of the brainstem that contains the motor neurons of the trigeminal nerve (CN V), responsible for the muscles of mastication (CN V is also the afferent system for facial sensation, but those neurons are distributed throughout the brainstem).

Medulla oblongata

All of the ascending and descending pathways (directional terms that strictly speaking are only correct for upright primates) between the spinal cord and the brain pass through the medulla oblongata, and the nuclei of the last seven cranial nerves (CNs VI–XII) as well as the sensory nuclei involved in proprioception are located there (Fig. 3.7).

CEREBELLUM

The cerebellum lies dorsal to the pons. It modulates the tone and relative degrees of contraction of opposing muscles needed for smooth motion, by integrating complex inputs from the brainstem, cerebrum and spinal cord. The reason for the 'jerky' movement of foals is because the cerebellum is still developing (but is far, far more developed than the neonatal human brain!). Functional imaging studies in humans have shown the cerebellum to be active during mere imagination of motor acts.[8] Foals suffering from a degeneration of the cerebellum, 'cerebellar abiotrophy', are strikingly incoordinated, with strong, jerky movements and prominent tremors, particularly of the head, just before initiating a movement (intention tremors).

SPINAL CORD

The spinal cord is the most caudal part of the central nervous system. It receives and processes sensory information from the viscera, skin, joints, limbs and trunk, and controls movement of the body, parasympathetic outflow to urogenital structures and sympathetic outflow to the entire body. Neural networks in the spinal cord, referred to as 'central pattern generators', produce the rhythmic movements of specific gaits such as trotting, pacing or galloping, even when isolated from the brain and sensory inputs. Supraspinal sensory, and neuromodulatory influences, modulated by training, interact with the central pattern generators to shape the final motor output.[9] The gray matter containing the neurons has a roughly H-shaped outline in the center of the spinal cord. Motor neurons are found in the ventral horn, while sensory neurons are present in the dorsal horn. Ascending sensory information passes along fiber tracts (funiculi) to sensory nuclei in the brainstem and cerebellum. Upper motor neurons in the brainstem control movement by innervating lower motor neurons in the ventral horn of the gray matter of the spinal cord, resulting in muscle contraction.

BEHAVIORAL NEUROANATOMY

One organizational principle of the nervous system is the use of parallel processing, in which sensory, motor and cognitive functions can be served by more than one pathway.[10] Simplistically, the brainstem and thalamic reticular activating system provide arousal and initiate attention; the caudal part of the forebrain integrates perceptions, and, at a conscious level, the frontal cortex initiates voluntary movement and executes plans.

THE CEREBRUM

The cerebral cortex has achieved maximal prominence in humans where, were it spread out flat, it would measure about $45\,cm^2$. In order to fit within the confines of the skull, the cortex of phylogenetically advanced animals such as primates and horses is folded into grooves (sulci) alternating with prominences (gyri). The brains of more 'primitive' mammals, such as rodents, have a smooth surface. The neuronal layers of the cortex form the gray matter, while the underlying white matter is composed of axons traveling to and from the gray matter.

The cerebral cortex is divided into two hemispheres, which have a contralateral relationship with the body – for example impulses originating in the left hemisphere affect the right half of the body. Within the cortex, human studies have suggested a hemispheric dichotomy of emotional representation, with the left hemisphere housing the analytical mind and the right hemisphere appearing to be dominant in functions involving emotion.[11] This may well apply to horses to some extent.

The hemispheres are somewhat arbitrarily divided into four lobes (see Fig. 3.4) named for the overlying bones: frontal, occipital, parietal and temporal. There is a rough correspondence between these loosely defined anatomical regions and their function, a relationship that is most obvious in humans but appears to hold reasonably well for horses. The parietal lobe contains primary somatosensory and motor areas, while the occipital lobe is almost exclusively committed to visual processing. The temporal lobe includes the primary auditory cortex in addition to structures involved in memory, including the hippocampus and the amygdala. The temporal and frontal lobes influence emotions, and epilepsy of the temporal lobes can manifest solely as behavior alterations, such as unprovoked aggression and extreme irrational fear, hyposexuality and tail chasing in small animals.[12,13] Temporal lobe epilepsy has not been shown to occur in the horse, but one could reasonably expect that it does.

The frontal lobe, and particularly the prefrontal cortex, plays a very significant role in the coordination of goal-directed behavior and evaluates the effect of such behavior via reinforcement/punishment outcomes. The frontal lobe also allows the conscious initiation of movement (although once a gait is 'initiated' it is controlled largely by the brainstem and spinal cord of the horse). In most behaviors, sensory systems project to association areas where sensory information is interpreted in terms of memories and motivations. Training horses would not be possible without this system.

EVOLUTIONARY BRAIN DIVISIONS

A further, and rather more functional, classification recognizes three divisions of cerebral cortex: the archicortex, paleocortex and neocortex. These are distinguished on a developmental evolutionary basis and by the number of layers of neurons.

The archicortex and paleocortex are phylogenetically old regions and consist of three layers of cells (laminae) as opposed to the six laminae that characterize the neocortex. The archicortex is composed of medial structures included in the limbic system, such as the hippocampus and amygdala, and is involved mostly with emotion or behavior. The paleocortex is represented by one lobe on both sides of the brain, the piriform lobes, concerned with smell. The neocortex comprises the rest of the cerebral cortex and includes somatosensory and motor areas, visual and auditory cortical areas, and the association cortex. The association cortex is devoted to the collection of information, prioritization of its relative importance and decisions about suitable responses. Horses have representatives of each type of cortex.

In humans, the association cortex appears to be responsible for the ability to think, create, conceptualize and problem solve, and in comparative neuroanatomical studies, the massive size of the frontal lobes is the main feature that distinguishes the human brain from that of other primates. It has been proposed that cognitive abilities of particular species are directly correlated with the challenges of securing food, and that grazing ungulates are to some degree removed from the evolution of higher mental abilities in terms of food procurement. This is reflected in the relatively small size of the equine forebrain compared with that of social carnivores and primates. In terms of solving problems, horses are considerably slower to solve novel problems through rule-learning abilities than species such as primates and higher carnivores.

THE LIMBIC SYSTEM

The components of the limbic system are hard to define, as various authors include different structures and areas in their definitions. It is usually agreed that it consists of those structures forming the border ('limbic') of the rostral end of the brainstem. This includes subcortical nuclei such as the hypothalamus and amygdaloid complex as well as the hippocampus, [Gr. *hippocampos*, sea-horse] an ancient, horseshoe shaped, rolled-up gyrus located within the temporal lobes. In amphibians and reptiles the limbic structures are devoted in large measure to processing olfactory input, a role superseded in mammals by important functions in memory, learning and social and emotional behavior.[14]

Olfaction remains an important sensory system, and olfaction receptor genes are the largest family of genes currently known to exist. Each receptor protein in the nasal mucosa is highly selective and will bind only a select group of odorants. Horses have a large and well-developed olfactory system which plays a role in appetite and food intake, sexual desire, mating, recognition of friends and foes and the accompanying emotional changes associated with these experiences. An associated sensory apparatus is the vomeronasal organ (VNO), an elongated pouch-like structure ventral to the rostral nasal meatus and lined with olfactory receptors. Scent information, particularly from pheromone molecules, is detected in the VNO (assisted by the 'flehmen' response; see Ch. 2). Olfactory signals do not synapse directly in the thalamus but project directly to the frontal lobe and the limbic system. The strong association between odors and memory is rooted in this ancient function of the limbic system.

One nucleus in the limbic system, the amygdala, receives fibers from all sensory areas and appears to assign emotional significance to memories as well as mediating the expression of emotions associated with self-preservation such as fear.[14] Surgical removal of the amygdala results in a loss of fear, changes in social behavior and aggressiveness.

The reciprocal connections between the amygdala and the neocortex could provide the means by which conscious thought and learning can suppress reflex emotional responses such as fears. Certain sensory inputs may trigger a very strong reaction, the flight response, which has evolved as a protection from predation. Horses' ability to hear a wider range of high-frequency tones, such as the sound of twigs broken by the paws of a stalking predator, are naturally linked to an evasive (bolting) response. This is highly relevant to the training of horses, in which natural fearful responses have to be overcome.

MEMORY

Learning mechanisms and memory are fundamental to how the brain processes information (see Ch. 4). There is no universally agreed model of how memory works, but it is agreed that a memory is a set of encoded neural connections. Encoding can take place in several parts of the brain, and neural connections are likely to be widespread. Genetically determined positional cues probably steer growing fibers towards the general target with which to synapse, but fine-tuning of the pattern of projections is accomplished by activity-dependent mechanisms. Synaptic relationships are constantly being remodeled through increases or decreases in the size and strength of individual synapses, as well as the formation of new synapses and the elimination of unnecessary ones. This plasticity of cortical representation may not only underlie learning but may allow for recovery from brain lesions.

A widely held hypothesis is that learning occurs through long-term potentiation, and this has recently been confirmed in rat models.[15] 'Long-term potentiation' produces changes in synapses that are necessary to acquire and store new information. Synapses become increasingly sensitive so that a constant level of presynaptic stimulation becomes converted into a larger postsynaptic output. Certain forms of long-term potentiation have been shown to depend on the activation of NMDA receptors (see following sections). Long-term potentiation can be demonstrated in vitro by recording electrical potentials of single hippocampal neurons, and can be prevented by applying NMDA receptors antagonists to the preparations.

The three brain regions that appear to be critical to the formation of memories are the medial temporal lobe and certain thalamic and basal forebrain nuclei. Aside from sensory projection areas, specific areas of cerebral cortex can be damaged with little specific change in learned behavior. Thus these neural substrates are not necessarily the locations in which memory representations are stored but are areas thought to be critical to the normal functioning of the system. It is by modifying the synaptic connections between neurons that processors for most brain functions, including emotion, motivation and motor function, are built.[16]

Two basic time-scales of learning have been identified: short-term memory and long-term memory (some classifications also include an additional two time scales: immediate and intermediate memory). Neural activity related to short-term memory has been observed in many brain areas, but the mechanism by which this activity can outlast a transient sensory stimulus is still unknown. The transfer of short-term memory (which is easily disrupted) to long-term memory (a more stable anatomical or neurochemical change in the nervous system) depends on the hippocampus and related structures in the medial temporal lobe. Damage to the hippocampus results in an animal's inability to store recent memories but does not interfere with memories already consolidated before damage occurred.

Cognitive psychological studies have suggested that there are two further distinctions within the domain of long-term memory: the conscious recall of information (explicit memory), and the unconscious use of information about motor skills and procedure (implicit memory). Explicit memory relies on a set of structures in the medial temporal lobe, particularly the hippocampus, diencephalon and gyri in the temporal lobe. The learning of motor skills, allowing movements to be made more quickly and accurately with practice, requires constant feedback from the sensory and association areas for completion, but with practice these become encoded within a number of cortical areas as well as the basal nuclei and the cerebellum.[17] The learning of basic strides by foals as well as the complex responses we expect from horses following sensory cues from the rider, require the formation of long-term implicit memory traces.

NEUROPHYSIOLOGY AND NEUROCHEMISTRY

Neuroanatomy does not in itself explain how the brain controls behavior. Insight into the effect of neuropathology on behavior, as well as the action of neuropharmacologic drugs, requires an appreciation of the function and underlying physiology of the nervous system.

ELECTROPHYSIOLOGY

Emotions and behavior are ultimately determined by the release of specific neurotransmitters (reviewed in the following sections), which influence the activity of other neurons. Their release is made possible by the electrophysiological activity of excitable cells in the nervous system. Regardless of cell size and shape, transmitter biochemistry or behavioral function, almost all neurons receive and convey information using electrical signals, the so-called action potentials. Action potentials are rapid, transient all-or-none impulses caused by sodium ions entering the axon and potassium ions rushing out. This changes the difference in electrical potential between the inside and outside of the axon. In most neurons the essence of neuronal processing occurs in the regulation of whether or not an action potential is generated. Action potentials are generated at a specialized trigger region within the origin of the axon, and from there are conducted down the axon in one direction only at rates of 1–100 m/s (360 km/hour!). Near its end, the tubular axon divides into fine branches that form synapses, with other neurons and with effector organs such as muscle.

The ease with which an action potential can be initiated in an individual neuron depends on the relative difference in concentration of sodium and potassium ions inside and outside the axon. The difference is maintained by the action of ion pumps and ion channels. Variation in the resulting electrical difference results in neurons having various thresholds, excitability properties and firing patterns. In the resting state ion channels are closed, but they open in response to the binding of a number of specific molecules at the synapse, or secondary to changes in the membrane potential. Excitatory neurotransmitters act to open cation channels and increase the likelihood of the generation of an action potential. Inhibitory neurotransmitters on the other hand, open anion (chloride) channels that reduce the electrical difference between the inside and outside of the axon membrane and decrease the likelihood of the generation of an action potential. The modulation of the Na^+/K^+ pump is believed to be one of the fundamental mechanisms for learning,[18] by manipulating long-term potentiation.

At the distal end of the axon, the action potential influences other neurons by affecting the synapse. When an action potential reaches the presynaptic terminals of the appropriate synapses, neurotransmitter-containing synaptic vesicles fuse with the presynaptic membrane and release their content into the synaptic cleft. The neurotransmitters bind with specific molecules in the postsynaptic membrane, the receptors, which cause an alteration in the transmembrane potential to either increase or decrease the likelihood of an action potential being generated by the postsynaptic cell.

A single transmitter can produce several distinct effects by activating different types of receptors, and there is now considerable evidence that synapses can be modified functionally and anatomically during development by experience and learning. Training ('schooling') of laboratory animals has been shown to produce measurable changes in synaptic interactions.[15]

NEUROTRANSMITTERS

Neurotransmitters are classically defined as substances that are synthesized in a neuron, released into the synaptic cleft and then exert a defined action on the postsynaptic neuron by modulating cellular excitability. They are absolutely cardinal to the normal function of the nervous system, and it is worth spending a little bit of time reviewing their function. Their physiology and pharmacology have been well reviewed by

Kaplan & Sadock[3] and Dodman et al.[12] Abnormal levels of neuropeptides have unequivocally been shown to be involved in human psychiatric disorders, and it is also clear that the relative amount and location of neurochemicals can all influence 'abnormal' behavior. Rarely if ever can a solitary and unambiguous shift in one neurochemical cause these conditions. Instead changes in the action of several neurotransmitters or their interaction with receptors are necessary.

Three classes of neurotransmitters classically transmit information in the nervous system: biogenic amines, amino acids and neuropeptides (Table 3.2). Recent data have led to the identification of several novel classes of neurotransmitters, including nucleotides, prostaglandins and gases such as nitric oxide. Some neurotransmitters have in addition been shown to influence gene expression. The field of neurochemistry has breached the bounds of the mere study of chemical mediation of nerve impulses and has developed into a broad discipline that overlaps neuroanatomy, developmental neurobiology and behavioral genetics.

It is appropriate at this stage to review the classification and function of some of the principal neurotransmitters which are known to have a role in modifying behavior.

Biogenic amines

The biogenic amines are bioactive amines, derivatives of ammonia (NH_3) in which one or more hydrogen atoms have been replaced by hydrocarbon groups. This includes dopamine, adrenaline (epinephrine), noradrenaline (norepinephrine), serotonin, acetylcholine and melatonin. A common feature of all biogenic amine neurotransmitters is that they are initially synthesized in the axon terminal by enzymes produced in the cell body and transported down the axon. After release, a significant amount of noradrenaline, serotonin and dopamine in the synaptic cleft is taken up again by a presynaptic transporter protein to be repackaged into vesicles, or degraded by the enzyme monoamine oxidase. A number of psychopharmacologic agents affect amine reuptake, synthesis or degradation.

Table 3.2 Classification[a] of neurotransmitters

Neurotransmitter class	Components	Neurotransmitter
Biogenic amines	Quaternary amines	Acetylcholine, Histamine
	Catecholamines	Adrenaline (epinephrine)
		Noradrenaline (norepinephrine)
		Dopamine
	Indolamines	Serotonin, Melatonin
Amino acids	Excitatory	Glutamate
	Inhibitory	GABA
	Inhibitory and excitatory	Glycine
Neuropeptides	Calcitonin gene related peptide	
	Substance P	
	Vasoactive intestinal peptide	
	Opioids	Endorphins, Enkephalins
	Hypocretin	
	Many others	
Nucleotides	Adenosine	
Prostaglandins	Arachidonic acid	
Gases	Nitric oxide	
	Carbon monoxide	

[a]There is no clear consensus on the classification of neurotransmitters, and the list of examples is not exhaustive. Additional neurotransmitters are constantly being added.

Adrenaline and noradrenaline

Adrenaline and noradrenaline, along with dopamine, are classified as catecholamines and are synthesized from the precursor tyrosine in a common biosynthetic pathway. Although adrenaline is in higher concentration in serum and is the catecholamine that causes the sweating and increased heart rate when horses are stressed or excited, noradrenaline is more abundant in the brain. Noradrenergic neurons in the medulla project to the hypothalamus and control cardiovascular and endocrine functions, while equivalent neurons in the reticular formation of the pons mainly provide projections to the spinal cord that modulate autonomic reflexes and pain sensations. A further group in the locus ceruleus in the dorsal part of the pons has wide projections to the rest of the CNS. Although the exact function of the locus ceruleus is unknown, increased activity in this region is associated with anxiety, and it is particularly active in animals undergoing stress. Noradrenergic activity in humans is correlated with aggressive behavior, and specific adrenergic receptor blockers have beneficial effects in violent patients.[19] Antidepressant drugs such as the tricyclic antidepressants and monoamine oxidase inhibitors increase levels of noradrenaline by blocking its reuptake and catabolism. Their use is indicated in narcoleptic horses (see following sections), but potentially serious adverse effects may be seen with large doses.[20]

Dopamine

Dopamine-secreting neuronal groups in the substantia nigra in the midbrain send major ascending dopaminergic inputs to the forebrain, including the cerebrum, limbic system and basal nuclei. An important role of dopamine in human medicine concerns the control that dopamine receptors in the basal nuclei have on the initiation of motor responses and the regulation of movement (affected in Parkinson's disease and Tourette's syndrome). The significant association between Parkinson's disease and depression suggests that the dopamine nigrostriatal tract is involved in control of mood as well as motor control. The only example of selective basal nuclei pathology in horses is equine nigropallidal encephalomalacia following ingestion of yellow star thistle (*Centaurea solstitialis*). Pan-necrosis of the basal nuclei result in devastating dystonia and rigidity of the muscles of mastication in affected horses.

Pathways to the frontal and temporal cortices have been implicated in emotion, thought and memory storage. A strong association has been found between high levels of detachment and a particular subtype of dopamine receptor, D_2 receptors.[21] Drugs that selectively bind D_2 receptors have anti-aggressive effects in human patients.[22] Lesion studies indicate that dopaminergic systems innervating the basal nuclei contribute to feeding, drinking and other motivated behaviors in a crucial way, and their pharmacologic blockade impairs feeding behavior.[23,24]

The dopaminergic systems may be particularly involved in the brain's reward system, leading to addiction, not only to abused drugs such as nicotine, amphetamines and cocaine which directly increase dopamine levels, but also to the biochemical rewards associated with equine stereotypic behaviors. There is evidence that high levels of dopaminergic activity within the basal ganglia play an important role in many stereotypies.[25] Dopaminergic activity is modulated by many neurotransmitters, including endogenous opioids and glutamate, and exogenous NMDA receptor blockers have been shown to suppress crib-biting in horses.[26]

Serotonin

Serotonin is principally produced by neurons in the rostral pons and midbrain. It is synthesized from the amino acid tryptophan, and oral intake of tryptophan supplements may increase serotonin levels in the brain. It has been used to 'sedate' horses and may have a very mild effect; however, other work indicates that tryptophan may actually stimulate horses rather than having a sedative effect.[27] Serotonin (5-HT) – or its precursor, 5-hydroxytryptophan (5-HTP) – may induce sleep and, importantly, appears to reduce anxiety. The 5-HT system is the mediator of learned and sustained fear responses, and decreased 5-HT levels have been associated with violent psychopathological behavior in humans.[28] Potent hallucinogens such as lysergic acid diethylamide (LSD) are structurally similar to 5-HT. It has been argued that serotonin plays a role in the behavioral facilitation system that initiates responses to the environment, and the behavioral inhibition system that arrests ongoing behavior. A decrease in serotonergic transmission leads to an inability to adopt passive or waiting attitudes, or to accept situations that necessitate or create strong inhibitory tendencies. This is particularly relevant to frustrating situations such as encountered by horses kept in what are essentially unnatural environments. Stereotypic behavior patterns in human medicine, often grouped in a classification known as obsessive–compulsive disorders, appear to be partially attributable to decreased 5-HT and abnormal endorphin metabolism. Parallel examples of ritualistic and stereotypic behaviors, including wind-sucking and crib-biting in horses are recognized in veterinary medicine.[29] Many antidepressants, discussed further in the following section, such as the tricyclic antidepressants and fluoxetine (Prozac®) block serotonin reuptake transporters, thus increasing the amount of serotonin in the synaptic cleft.

Acetylcholine

This is a very prominent neurotransmitter in both the central and peripheral nervous system, as it is the major neurotransmitter of the parasympathetic branch of the autonomic nervous system as well as the preganglionic synapses of sympathetic neurons. Neurons in nuclei of the thalamus and brainstem project to the cortex and limbic system and affect behavior patterns. Acetylcholine, one of the principal neurotransmitters involved in the propagation of aggressive, predatory behavior, is important in regulating wake and sleep cycles and has been shown to increase the strength of synaptic connections in the hippocampus. Cholinergic enhancement has been shown to improve memory performance in humans.[30]

Amino acids

Amino acids are molecules containing both an amine and a carboxylic acid group. Amino acid neurotransmitters are the most abundant in the brain. The major excitatory neurotransmitter is glutamate, opposed by the major inhibitory neurotransmitter γ-aminobutyric acid (GABA). A simplified way to look at brain biochemistry is as a balance between those two neurotransmitters alone, with all other neurotransmitters simply being involved in modulation of that balance.

GABA

GABA is the primary neurotransmitter in intrinsic neurons that function as local mediators for inhibitory feedback loops. Major tranquilizing and anticonvulsant agents, including benzodiazepines (e.g. diazepam) and barbiturates act primarily through GABAergic mechanisms. A further inhibitory neurotransmitter, which is predominantly active in the spinal cord, is the amino acid glycine.

Glutamate

It is now generally agreed that glutamate is the major excitatory neurotransmitter in the brain, and it is believed that 70% of the fast excitatory CNS synapses use glutamate as a transmitter. There are five types of glutamate receptors of which N-methyl-D-aspartate (NMDA) is the best understood because it may play a crucial role in learning and memory as well as in aggressive and defensive behavior.

Glutamate has recently gained unparalleled prominence in the field of excitotoxicity (for review see Hahn & Mayhew[31]). Oxygen metabolism results in the generation of free-radical molecules which can result in considerable subcellular damage. Neurons appear to be at particular risk of free-radical damage, and excitotoxicity is now thought to be a potential contributor to the pathogenesis of a large number of diseases, including equine motor neuron disease.[32]

Peptides

An ever growing list of neuroactive peptides, such as calcitonin gene related peptide (CGRP), substance P, vasoactive intestinal peptide (VIP) and hypocretin (see subsection on narcolepsy) act as neurotransmitters or, more commonly, modulate pre- or postsynaptic transmission. Nevertheless the actual molar concentration of any given peptide in the brain is maximally two to three orders of magnitude lower than that of the biogenic amines, acetylcholine and amino acids. Unlike classical neurotransmitters that are synthesized at the synapse, neuropeptides are synthesized in the cell body, from where they are transported down the axon. Neuropeptides thus take a comparatively long time to replenish, cannot be recycled, and have a longer duration of action than the amino acids or biogenic amines.[33]

Opioids

Opioids are a prominent member of the neuropeptide group. The opium poppy was cultivated in lower Mesopotamia in 3400 BC, where it was referred to as the 'joy plant', but it was not until the 1970s that this large family of neuropeptides, the endogenous opioids (endorphins), were isolated from brain extracts. Four classes of endogenous opioids are now recognized, and they are principally involved in the regulation of stress, pain and mood, in addition to potentiating effects on adrenergic and glutamatergic neurotransmission. They are known to have a major role in social affiliation and caring behavior in humans, and there is good evidence for opioid peptides mediating defensive and defeat responses during conflict. Opioid receptors are found closely associated, both functionally and anatomically, with dopaminergic and serotonergic neurons, and are distributed in regions such as the limbic system, hypothalamus and basal nuclei. Endorphin systems are probably involved in the effectiveness of the twitch (see Ch. 14), since its action is blocked by naloxone and its application increases plasma concentrations of β-endorphin.[34] A tandem role of endorphins and serotonin has been suggested in stereotypies and has received considerable attention in the study of crib-biting, not least because it may contribute to the phenomenon of emancipation (see Ch. 8).

EQUINE PSYCHOPHARMACOLOGIC AGENTS

The availability of chemical restraint has revolutionized the number and type of procedures that can be performed on standing horses. The following is a summary of a few of the commonly used behavior-modifying pharmacologic agents used in horses (see Table 3.3).

Phenothiazines

Phenothiazine tranquilizers were introduced into clinical veterinary medicine in the 1950s. Phenothiazines such as acepromazine (and older compounds, including chlorpromazine and promazine hydrochloride) interfere principally with the central actions of dopamine but also affect noradrenaline and adrenaline, resulting in mild brainstem depression. This class of drugs is no longer used to sedate animals heavily, but their calming effects have been valuable in calming unfriendly and apprehensive animals. Individual responses are extremely variable, and there is generally a markedly reduced effect on excited horses. Acetyl promazine maleate given at 0.03 to 0.1 mg/kg i.v. or i.m. has reduced some stereotypies (by reducing all activity?), and the same drug at higher doses eliminated suspected opioid-induced pacing postoperatively.[35] They interfere with the central actions of the excitement-producing catecholamines, adrenaline, noradrenaline and dopamine.[36] Phenothiazines however have no analgesic properties and they decrease gastrointestinal tone and secretions due to CNS depression and anticholinergic actions. Priapism and paraphimosis (penile protrusions) are a recognized risk of using phenothiazines in geldings and particularly stallions. The mechanism is unknown but is attributed to blockade of adrenergic and dopaminergic receptors centrally and peripherally.

Table 3.3   Doses and schedules of administration of selected equine psychopharmacologic agents

Agent	Psychopharmacologic use	Dose and schedule[a]	Comment
Phenothiazine (acepromazine)	Minor tranquilizer	0.02–0.1 mg/kg i.v.	Care: hypotension, paraphimosis
α₂-agonist (xylazine)	Sedative/analgesic	1.0–2.0 mg/kg i.v.	
Opioid (butorphanol)	Analgesic/sedative	0.05–0.1 mg/kg	Care: excitement, particularly if used alone
Benzodiazepine (diazepam)	Sedative/anticonvulsant	Foal: 5–15 mg i.v., may repeat in 30 min Adult: 0.2 mg/kg i.v.	
Reserpine	Long-term sedative	2–5 mg p.o. once *or* 0.5 mg i.m., repeated 1 week later	Erratic behavior, obtundation and anesthetic deaths
Phenobarbitone	Anticonvulsant	2–4 mg/kg b.i.d. for long-term therapy	
Cyproheptadine	Headshaking	0.3 mg/kg b.i.d. q12 h then, after 7 days, 0.4–0.5 mg/kg q12 h	Responses very variable
Carbamazepine	Headshaking	20–30 mg/kg q6 h	Half-life is around 90–100 min so horses should be test exercised within 2 hours of any particular dose. If not effective, can try in combination with cyproheptadine, but care: sedation

[a]The doses are derived from reference material and should be modified according to veterinary clinical assessment. A number of the drugs have additional applications at different doses not discussed in this text.

α₂-agonists

Agonists of the α₂ subgroup of adrenoreceptors were developed as antihypertensive agents for use in humans, and are now far more commonly used for veterinary procedures in horses than are phenothiazines, because they result in more consistent and profound sedation. The behavioral effects of α₂-agonists such as xylazine (Rompun™), detomidine and romifidine are dose related and vary from subtle calming to profound sedation accompanied by head drooping and ataxia. Exaggerated reflex kicking responses have been associated with their use, even in profoundly sedated horses, an effect that is reduced when α₂-agonists are combined with opiates such as butorphanol. α₂-agonists are commonly used with ketamine, a dissociative anesthetic, to induce anesthesia. Pharmacologically the α₂-agonists are classified as analgesics as well as sedatives[37] and result in sedation by binding to central and peripheral presynaptic inhibitory α₂-receptors. These are inhibitory to the release of noradrenaline and thus act to hyperpolarize the postsynaptic neuron.[38]

Opioids

Opioids are exogenous substances that bind specific subpopulations of central and peripheral opioid receptors, and at standard doses have analgesic properties without loss of proprioception or consciousness. The classification of opioid drugs has changed as the molecular pharmacology of opioid receptors has been clarified, but it has traditionally been based on their action on the three main classes of receptors: μ, κ and δ. Thus morphine, fentanyl, codeine and heroin are classed as 'agonists' while butorphanol (Torbugesic™) is categorized as an agonist-antagonist compound due to its effect on κ and μ receptors, respectively. The agonist-antagonist agents have fewer undesirable side effects such as excitation.

Opioid agonists and agonist-antagonists are used in equine medicine for their sedative and analgesic action, and common practice is to mix them with an α_2-agonist or phenothiazine, particularly to prevent the α_2-associated 'reflex' kicking. An example of a pure opiate antagonist is naloxone, notably used in veterinary medicine in trials designed to establish whether endogenous opioid blockade will result in diminished stereotypic behavior. Naloxone administered i.v. had a dose-related effect on eliminating crib-biting for up to 2 days, but it also resulted in abdominal distress.[35] However, resting behavior was also significantly increased in crib-biting horses, and it may be that the stereotypy reduction was due to a sedative effect of the opiate antagonist.

Benzodiazepines

The most prominent benzodiazepine is diazepam (Valium™), a drug noted for its anxiolytic, sedative, anticonvulsive and muscle-relaxing properties. It is used frequently for sedation in foals and is the drug of choice for the treatment of status epilepticus. Benzodiazepines, along with barbiturates, open axonal chloride channels thus hyperpolarizing membranes and leading to inhibition of CNS function.[39] Along with barbiturates they potentiate GABA receptors and increase mean GABA channel opening times.[40]

Phenobarbitone

Phenobarbitone is a long-acting barbiturate used in the management of seizures and occasionally as a tranquilizer. The primary mechanism of the action of barbiturates is to increase inhibition by acting indirectly as GABA agonists, increasing the neuronal threshold of electrical excitability. It is the initial drug of choice for treating seizure disorders in horses and can initially result in profound sedation.

Reserpine

Reserpine is an alkaloid extracted from the root of *Rauwolfia serpentine*, a climbing shrub indigenous to India. It was introduced into veterinary medicine the 1950s and its calming properties were exploited for management and training purposes.

It has essentially been dropped from clinical use as a tranquilizer. Reserpine causes depletion of biogenic amine levels in the brain, including serotonin, noradrenaline and dopamine. Because noradrenaline is an excitatory neurohormone in the brain, its depletion explains the calming or tranquilizing effect of reserpine in the horse.[41] It is still available in oral and injectable preparations as an antihypertensive and antipsychotic drug in human patients, and is on occasion used to calm nervous horses. There is apparently a large variability in the pharmacokinetics of reserpine in horses, and adverse reactions, including erratic behavior and obtundation, and anesthetic deaths due to hypotension, have been recorded. Reserpine should be avoided in stallions and should not be administered prior to surgery.

Fluoxetine

Folk medicine has long used extracts from the flower and leaves of St John's wort (*Hypericum perforatum*) to treat mild depressive disorders, but it is only recently that the ability of St John's wort to inhibit serotonin and dopamine reuptake has been recognized. The antidepressant and anti-obsessional actions of fluoxetine (Prozac®) are similarly thought to be linked to its ability to block presynaptic uptake channels and act as a selective serotonin reuptake inhibitor (SSRI). Fluoxetine has fewer of the anticholinergic, sedative and cardiovascular side effects than the classic tricyclic antidepressant drugs, probably because of comparatively lower opiate, catecholamine and dopamine membrane receptor binding.[42] It is the most commonly used specific 5-HT reuptake blocker in companion animal medicine, and is used in an oral preparation to treat stereotypies, aggression and fear and anxiety.[43,44] Fluoxetine has not been evaluated in horses, but its use is likely to increase given the prominence of the drug in human and small-animal medicine.

Cyproheptadine

Cyproheptadine is a specific serotonin receptor antagonist with histamine receptor blocking and anticholinergic and sedative effects. It may also stimulate ACTH secretion and has a role in altering pain sensations. It is used in human medicine for treatment of severe anorexia nervosa, and encouraging results have been reported in the use of cyproheptadine for the treatment of horses with hyperadrenocorticism[45] and headshaking,[46] a condition that may involve altered pain perception.

Carbamazepine

Carbamazepine is a tricyclic anticonvulsant that increases serotonin levels by blocking the neuronal serotonin transporter.[47] It can be used in the treatment of most types of human epilepsy, although its anti-seizure mechanism of action is incompletely understood. Carbamazepine in humans is increasingly being used for its anti-aggressive effects and to treat a variety of neuropsychiatric disorders. It has been successfully employed as a treatment of trigeminal neuralgia in humans, an effect that may explain its efficacy in ameliorating the signs of headshaking.[48] There are a great many reports in the literature of paradoxical and severe side effects of this drug in human patients,[49–51] and care is advised in its use in veterinary medicine.

THE NEUROLOGICAL EXAMINATION

The first steps in evaluating behavior cases involve obtaining a detailed history and performing a medical examination to rule out any underlying clinical condition. The behavior changes noted as abnormal by the owner may be associated with pain, metabolic changes, weakness or sleep attacks. A systematic neurological examination is considered fundamental to a psychiatric investigation of human patients presenting with recent-onset psychosis or acute changes in mental status.[52] Similarly it is appropriate to have an appreciation of diseases of the equine nervous system known to alter behavior of the horse. A detailed neurological examination including assessment of mentation, cranial nerves and sensory and motor systems should be included in the investigation of any horse presented with a history of a recent

change in behavior, or suspected of having an altered state of mentation.

The physical examination is designed to disclose signs of general disease or pain that may have an influence on behavior, while the objective of the neurological examination is to determine if the change in behavior could be explained by an underlying neurological deficit, and to define the anatomical portion of the nervous system responsible for the clinical signs. This is an absolute prerequisite to allow reasonable differential diagnoses to be formulated. Readers are referred to Mayhew[53] for a detailed description of how to perform and interpret the neurological examination of the horse.

The neurological examination consists of a careful evaluation of behavior, mental status, cranial nerve function, gait and postural reactions. Because the clinician is unable to ask for voluntary responses, the neurological examination of the horse involves testing simple and complex reflex pathways and interpreting the site of the lesion in light of the anatomy of the reflexes tested. A simple reflex arc consists of a sensory neuron, one or more interneurons and a motor neuron which innervates muscles effecting the response. Reflexes occur without connections from ascending or descending central tracts, although input from higher centers classically inhibits excessive reflex movement. Discrete areas of the nervous system are extremely specialized, and by accurately localizing clinical signs the anatomical location of a lesion can be determined. This requires an assessment of all the principal components of the nervous system, and abbreviating the neurological examination is discouraged. If it is determined that neurological deficits other than a subtle change in behavior are present, then it is appropriate to proceed with further diagnostics before initiating protocols to treat a primary behavioral problem.

BEHAVIOR AND MENTAL STATUS

As explained in the introductory chapter, the owner of the horse should be questioned about the onset of the behavioral change, the nature of the signs, and any previous or associated clinical problems. The signalment of the animal has to be taken into consideration, and the presence of possible external triggers, such as auditory or tactile stimuli, should be explored (see Ch. 1). Importantly, the mental status of the animal must be assessed, since neuropathological lesions inducing a change in behavior can also be expected to affect the general function of the cerebral hemispheres as well as neural activity in the brainstem and diencephalon.

The various terms that describe alterations of mental status in horses include obtundation, stupor, coma, hyperactivity and aggression. Further signs of a subtle change in sensorium comprise continual yawning, asymmetric drifting or circling and, in foals, lack of recognition of the mare. More severe forebrain disease may lead to head pressing (Fig. 3.8), head deviation and propulsive walking or circling, aggression and self-mutilation, adopting bizarre postures and leaving food in the mouth. These signs usually reflect disturbances in the diencephalon and forebrain, and often implicate some portion of the

limbic system.[2] Large, space-occupying lesions in the cerebral hemispheres may result in locomotor or postural disturbances. If the lesion is unilateral the animal may circle toward the side of the lesion (because, for that patient, the spatial field contralateral to the lesion 'ceases to exist'?). Lesions of localized regions of cortex, for example the occipital lobe, can result in a specific sensory loss such as blindness with normal pupillary light responses (central blindness). Lesions of the frontal lobes may result in behavioral changes such as lack of recognition of familiar people or objects, while damage to the temporal lobe can result in changes in eating behaviors, sexual habits, and temperament.

Seizures are a clinical sign strongly indicating the presence of forebrain disease. They result from multiple, synchronous discharges from a population of neurons producing a variety of undirected, uncontrolled, unorganized movements or changes of mentation. The seizure may be preceded by an aura (actually a part of the seizure but one that does not include involuntary movement) in which the horse is distracted from its environment or is restless. The actual seizure is called the ictus, and in horses is expressed by involuntary changes in muscle tone or movement. The wave of abnormal neurophysiological activity can remain in one region causing, for example, rhythmic movement of muscles of the face, or can spread to the other cortical hemisphere. If there is a generalized excitation, lower motor neurons in brainstem and spinal cord can become involved, resulting in a generalized seizure with rigidity, recumbency and tonic and clonic limb movements (Fig. 3.9). The animal loses consciousness during a generalized seizure, but recovers in a few minutes. This may be followed by a post-ictal phase of obtundation and temporary blindness which can last for hours or, in the case of foals, days.[53]

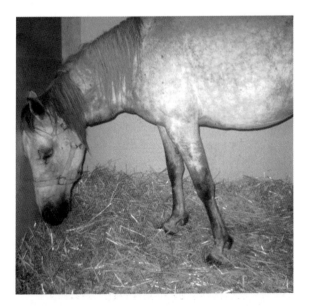

Figure 3.8 Horse showing intermittent somnolence and head pressing as a result of liver failure and hepatoencephalopathy caused by pyrrolizidine alkaloid (ragwort) toxicity. (Photograph courtesy of Joe Mayhew.)

CRANIAL NERVES

Because of the close anatomical relationship between the forebrain and the brainstem, diseases affecting the prosencephalon often also

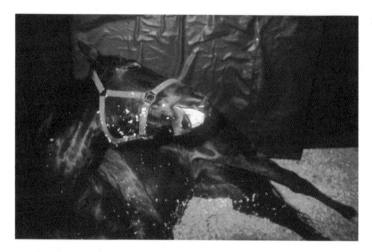

Figure 3.9 Horse with a *Streptococcus equi* cerebral abscess in early tonic phase of generalized seizure. (Photograph courtesy of Joe Mayhew.)

result in dysfunction of one or more cranial nerves. The examination of cranial nerves consists of the evaluation of a series of reflexes and responses involving one or more cranial nerves (see Table 3.1).

The head should be initially examined for asymmetries of posture, facial expression or muscle mass. A head tilt (lateral deviation of the poll), suggests the presence of a vestibular disturbance, and this can be emphasized by applying a blindfold. Ptosis, weak eyelids on palpation, pulling of the muzzle to one side or decreased ear tone are signs of facial nerve (CN VII) paresis. Temporal or masseter muscle atrophy is seen with pathology of the motor branch of the trigeminal nerve (CN V). Atrophy or severe weakness of the tongue is caused by hypoglossal (CN XII) paresis. The function of the sensory branches of CN V is tested by reflex responses to light pricking of the ears, lips or nasal mucosa. Animals with diffuse cerebral dysfunction or focal parietal lobe pathology may show signs of nasal hypalgesia even when CN V is not affected.

The eyes deserve close attention as the ocular muscles are innervated and controlled with great precision. Vision requires intact eyes, optic nerves (CN II) and central visual pathways. Most of the objects viewed with one eye are perceived in the contralateral occipital lobe, but impulses subsequently cross to the opposite hemisphere via the corpus callosum.[54]

Vision is assessed by making a threatening gesture towards each eye, resulting in blinking (the menace response). Care must be taken not to stimulate the cornea or the palpebrae with air current. While the precise central relay of this reflex is not known, it is thought to include several different brain regions including the visual pathways as well as the motor cortex, pons, cerebellum, facial motor nucleus, facial nerve and orbicularis oculi muscle in the eyelid. The menace response is probably mediated by subcortical neural circuits as suggested by work on both rodents[55] and human[56] and non-human primates.[57] Suddenly appearing, 'looming' visual stimuli activate midbrain circuits that produce conjugate eye, head and neck movements away from the source of the stimulus.[55] Foals up to 2 weeks of age, and animals affected by cerebellar disease, may not respond to this test of vision by blinking. They should nevertheless react to a menacing stimulus by retracting the eyeball, resulting in a brief protrusion of the third eyelid, and/or by pulling away the head.

Eye movement is assessed by moving the head from side to side and looking for normal nystagmus, with the fast phase occurring in the direction of movement. Abnormal, horizontal or vertical nystagmus indicates a lesion in the vestibular system, which influences the cranial nerves innervating the external muscles of the eye: CNs III, IV and VI. Strabismus (abnormal eye position) in horses is rarely due to dysfunction of the latter nerves and is more likely to be caused by mechanical interference with eye movements, but ventral strabismus noted after raising the head is common with ipsilateral vestibular disease.

The pupils should be observed for size and symmetry, and the pupillary light response (CN II and III) assessed by observing pupillary constriction after shining light into the eye. Consensual responses are difficult to evaluate in horses, due to the lateral placement of the globes, and instead the light is swung briskly from eye to eye, observing for a further constriction of the pupil when the light is directed into the pupil previously constricted by the consensual response. Normal pupillary light responses in the presence of blindness suggests pathology of the occipital cortex (central blindness).

The obvious presence of the nictitating membrane is notable, and could indicate the presence of enophthalmos, such as can be caused by sympathetic denervation (Horner's syndrome) or, classically, tetanus.

GAIT AND POSTURAL REACTIONS

CNS disease resulting in behavioral changes may also cause gait and postural reaction deficits if the brainstem and associated ascending and descending tracts are affected. Ataxia (lack of coordination due to a deficit in proprioception pathways) and weakness (due to upper motor neuron pathology) can underlie changes in gait that can not be explained by musculoskeletal lesion. Ataxia is assessed by determining the responses to postural reactions, maneuvers designed to accentuate more subtle deficits. The horse should be examined when walking in a straight line, circling tightly, being led up and down a slope with the head extended. Stepping on the opposite foot, pivoting on a limb, increased or decreased joint movement and excessive circumduction of a limb may be signs of neurological disease. Laterally pulling on the tail while walking is a sensitive test for weakness caused by the interruption of the connection between upper motor neurons in the brain and lower motor

neurons in the spinal cord, so called upper motor neuron weakness. Hopping the horse, by flexing one thoracic limb and pushing the animal to the opposite side, can accentuate both ataxia and weakness of subtle thoracic limb signs.

NEUROLOGICAL DISEASES WITH BEHAVIORAL SIGNS

Diseases diffusely affecting the forebrain can be associated with changes in behavior. However, this is highly unlikely to occur in the absence of further clinical signs such as failure to recognize familiar companions, continual yawning, facial twitches (partial seizures) and drifting to one side when blindfolded. More severe disease can in addition be expected to result in circling toward the affected side, obtundation, head-pressing and generalized seizures. Focal lesions in the midline of the brain affecting the ventromedial hypothalamic nucleus or rostral hypothalamus, or bilateral damage of the hypothalamus or limbic systems, may further cause aggression or disturbances in eating, drinking or sexual behavior.[7] It should be remembered that CNS neoplasia is extremely rare in the horse! The following is a brief discussion of diseases of the horse that result in clinical signs which include changes in behavior, but readers are urged to further consult more comprehensive texts.[53,58,59]

HYDROCEPHALUS

Hydrocephalus is a condition marked by an excessive accumulation of CSF resulting in dilation of the cerebral ventricles and raised intracranial pressure. It may result in enlargement of the cranium (Fig. 3.10) and atrophy of brain parenchyma. This can be secondary to some obstruction of CSF normal circulation or its site of absorption into the venous system. On occasion hydrocephalus, even with a severe loss of cortical tissue, is found as an incidental finding in foals with apparently normal behavior. Hydrocephalus is uncommon in adult horses compared with other domestic animals, as neoplasia is exceedingly rare

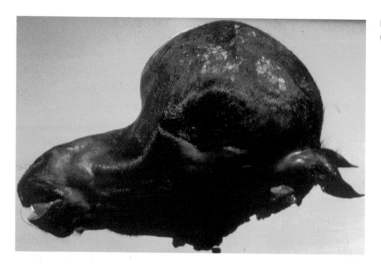

Figure 3.10 Hydrocephalus in a foal. (Photograph courtesy of Joe Mayhew.)

in the brain of this species. It can be associated with massive cholesterol accumulation in the choroid plexus, cholesterinic granulomas, believed to result from choroid plexus congestion and hemorrhage.[60] These can be massive structures and surgical removal has not been reported.

INFECTIOUS DISEASES

Bacterial meningitis

This is rarely seen in adults but is not uncommon in foals, in which it is usually associated with failure of passive transfer of immunoglobulins. Physical and neurological examination findings can include fever, obtundation, ataxia, aimless wandering, abnormal vocalization, collapse and seizures. The prognosis is poor. Attempted therapy consists of long-term antibiotic administration and intensive nursing care.

Diffuse encephalomyelitides

Numerous viruses across the world cause encephalitis or, more commonly, encephalomyelitis (inflammation of the brain and spinal cord), in horses. Most are caused by arboviruses (*arthropod-borne* viruses), which include viruses from a number of families using an insect or tick vector.

Most but not all occur in warm climates, as the vector can survive through the winter. The most prominent of these are the alphaviruses (Eastern, Western and Venezuelan viruses) which are found in the Americas. A variety of other arboviruses such as Semliki Forest, Japanese B, St Louis encephalitis, Equine Infectious Anemia and Equine Encephalosis viruses, however, also result in cerebral disease in horses.[59] Aujeszky's disease (pseudorabies) has occasionally been reported to cause disease in horses,[61] and Borna disease,[62] Hendra virus[63] and West Nile virus have recently received attention.[64] Clinical signs vary in severity depending on the virus, but the majority result in clinical signs attributable to diffuse disease, which may include fever, blindness, ataxia, seizures and hyperexcitability. The prognosis depends on the specific virus involved and is especially poor for Eastern and Venezuelan encephalitis.

A rare virus that deserves additional mention because of its public health significance is rabies, a disease that accounts for thousands of human deaths worldwide each year. The disease can initially cause diverse clinical signs in horses, including lameness, colic, tetanus and peripheral neuropathies.[65] In a group of experimentally infected horses the most frequently observed clinical sign was muscle tremors, with pharyngeal spasm or pharyngeal paresis, ataxia and lethargy or somnolence also being commonly observed.[66] The virus passes from the tissues at the bite wounds via peripheral nerves to the CNS by retrograde axoplasmic flow. Once in the CNS the virus disseminates widely in the brain and spinal cord, resulting in a variety of clinical signs. In the brainstem ('dumb') form, obtundation and dementia with ataxia, drooling and pharyngeal paralysis occur, while the cerebral ('furious') form is characterized by vocalization, photo- and hydrophobia, hyperesthesia and seizures, as well as changes in behavior marked by aggressive and destructive behavior. The behavioral changes are believed to be principally due to pathology of the limbic system, and reflect a strategy by the virus which serves to enhance the likelihood of transfer of the agent.[67] Viral pathology centered on the spinal cord results in ascending paralysis, and this form, more often than the cerebral and brainstem form, seems to result in asymmetric self-mutilation.

Diffuse disease with cerebral signs has also been reported due to bacteria such as the spirochete *Borrelia burgdorferi*, which causes Lyme disease.[68] Protozoal diseases, including equine protozoal myeloencephalitis in the Americas[69] and trypanosomiasis in tropical and subtropical countries,[70] can on occasion present primarily with forebrain disease.

Brain abscess

Primary brain abscesses in horses are rare but do occur following a history of strangles (*Streptococcus equi*, subspecies *equi*) or during an acute septicemic infection in foals (Fig. 3.11). A thorough physical examination may determine whether pyogenic disease or multiple foci are present, and cerebrospinal fluid often has increased inflammatory cells and mildly increased protein levels. Displacement and compression of the neural tissue by the abscess, and the resulting disruption of the vasculature and creation of secondary vasogenic edema, leads to brain swelling and increased intracranial pressure. Compulsive circling, obtundation, symmetric or asymmetric central blindness and gait changes often follow.

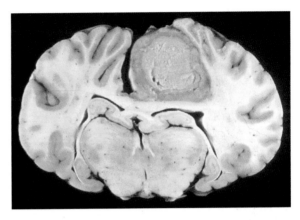

Figure 3.11 Transverse section of equine brain at the level of the thalamus. Cerebral abscesses in the cingulate gyrus are due to *Streptococcus equi* infection (strangles). (Photograph courtesy of Joe Mayhew and Alexander de Lahunta.)

Treatment with antimicrobial therapy is rarely rewarding, and surgical drainage should be considered if the abscess is found to be accessible following a computed tomographic scan.

Parasitic encephalomyelitis

Verminous encephalomyelitis can be due to the aberrant migration of an endoparasite normally found in horses, or due to the presence of a parasite not usually present in horses. Clinical signs usually reflect the random migration of the organism, classically *Strongylus vulgaris*, in the brain or spinal cord. Some nematodes such as the filarioid *Setaria* spp. and the rhabditoid *Halicephalobus gingivalis*, can result in diffuse forebrain disease with behavioral signs such as blindness, circling, obtundation and head pressing. In addition to the direct tissue destruction caused by the migrating parasite, the presence of the organism (usually *Strongylus vulgaris*), in the brachiocephalic arteries can result in a thromboembolic shower to the ipsilateral cerebrum. The resulting acute-onset seizures, obtundation and changes in mentation can be severe. The diagnosis is made on the basis of the history and neurological examination findings and may be supported by serum and CSF neutrophilia or eosinophilia. Treatment is based on anti-inflammatory and anti-parasitic therapy, and the prognosis depends on whether clinical signs were caused by the thromboembolic shower or actual parasite migration (worse prognosis).

METABOLIC DISORDERS

Hepatic encephalopathy

Liver failure is a prominent cause of cerebral dysfunction in the horse and can be due to primary hepatic pathology or, rarely, shunts bypassing the liver; these connect the portal circulation from the intestines to the systemic circulation (portosystemic shunts) in foals.[71] Liver pathology can be acute following Theiler's disease (serum hepatitis), acute toxicosis with mycotoxins or pyrrolizidine alkaloids (found in plants such as ragwort), liver abscessation, suppurative cholangitis or cholelithiasis. Horses with acute liver failure classically present with obtundation, anorexia, and with CNS derangements such as head pressing and aimless wandering (see Fig. 3.8). Icterus and elevation of liver-specific serum biochemistry values are normally a feature of acute liver failure. In chronic liver failure, hepatic insufficiency occurs because hepatocellular compromise is such that the functional reserve of the organ is exceeded.[72] Weight loss is often the most prominent feature of chronic liver failure, and icterus and elevated serum liver enzymes may not be prominent. The most common cause of chronic hepatic failure is exposure to hepatotoxic plants, particularly those containing pyrrolizidine alkaloids, e.g. ragwort). See Savage[73] and Barton & Morris[74] for detailed discussions of the etiologies of liver pathology in horses.

The clinical manifestations range from minimal changes in behavior and motor activity to overt obtundation, anxiety and coma, consistent with a global depression of CNS function. This appears to arise as a consequence of a net increase in inhibitory neurotransmission due to an imbalance between GABA and glutamate receptor agonists.[75] Of the many compounds that accumulate in the circulation principally as a consequence of impaired liver function, ammonia is considered to play an important role in the onset of hepatic encephalopathy.[76] Ammonia is excitotoxic, as it is associated with impaired reuptake of glutamate into nerve endings and astrocytes. This increases the concentration of glutamate in the synapse, ultimately leading to a down-regulation of NMDA receptors and decreased activity of this essential excitatory neurotransmitter (see subsection on aminoacid neurotransmitters, above). At the same time increased inhibitory neurotransmission occurs, due to increased brain levels of benzodiazepines and GABA receptors and the direct interaction of ammonia with one of the GABA receptors. In addition astrocyte metabolism of ammonia to glutamine facilitates plasma-to-brain transport of aromatic amino acids such as tryptophan and tyrosine, direct precursors of the inhibitory neurotransmitters serotonin and dopamine.

Central nervous system energy deprivation

Hypoxia, ischemia and hypoglycemia result in a fall of intracellular energy levels and neuronal necrosis. Neurons in specific anatomical areas in the forebrain and brainstem, including specific populations in the cerebral cortex, hippocampus, amygdala, thalamic nuclei and cerebellum, are especially vulnerable. Excitatory neurotransmitters, principally glutamate, are important final mediators of neuronal death in hypoxia and ischemia.[77]

Hypoglycemia

Significant hypoglycemia produces transient behavioral signs such as confusion and obtundation. In adults it can be associated with hepatic failure, or hyperinsulinism due to inappropriate administration of insulin in treating hyperlipemia or pancreatic neoplasia. Hypoglycemia is more prevalent in foals and can be found secondary to septicemia, potentially due to depletion of glycogen stores, impaired gluconeogenesis and increased peripheral glucose utilization. It is also found in foals with a decreased milk intake, particularly while in intensive care, and is associated with seizures.

Anesthetic hypoxia/anoxia

Respiratory or cardiac failure during anesthesia can lead to hypoxic brain damage. Central blindness and obtundation can be immediate sequelae. If such animals are euthanized, they are found to have an encephalopathy that can be mapped to those areas of the brain sensitive to energy deprivation of neurons[58] such as the superficial cortical laminae.[78] Long-term nursing can be rewarding, and aggressive therapy with the free-radical scavenger dimethyl-sulfoxide is appropriate.

Hypoxic ischemic syndrome

Hypoxic ischemic (neonatal maladjustment) syndrome is a well-recognized but poorly understood disorder of neonatal foals (Fig. 3.12). It affects full-term foals with normal maturity, although a very similar syndrome may be present in full-term, dysmature foals.[79] Affected

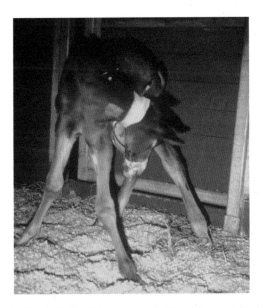

Figure 3.12 Foal with hypoxic ischemic syndrome having a partial seizure. The foal eventually recovered. (Photograph courtesy of Joe Mayhew.)

individuals typically are normal immediately after birth but within a few hours to days postpartum become disinterested in nursing, may wander aimlessly and rarely make peculiar vocalizations, so-called 'barking'. Further deterioration is marked by recumbency, seizures and obtundation leading to coma and death. The neuropathological findings vary with the duration of clinical signs but typically include ischemic neuronal necrosis and patchy, focal and diffuse hemorrhages, sometimes accompanied by edema in specific sites of the brain and occasionally spinal cord. The pathogenesis is unknown but the lesions suggest an hypoxic and/or ischemic insult around the time of birth,[80] such as premature breakage of the umbilicus when mares rise from the ground in response to human interference. Therapy involves controlling any seizures with diazepam and extended, intensive nursing care.[53] Diagnosis is complicated by concurrent septicemia and hypoglycemia.

LEUKOENCEPHALOMALACIA

Long-term ingestion of corn affected by the fungus *Fusarium moniliforme* can result in single cases or outbreaks of leukoencephalomalacia. Liquefactive necrosis of cerebral white matter classically leads to acute onset of signs of dementia, obtundation, central blindness, incoordination, facial paralysis and death in a few hours to a day. Mildly affected horses that recover may have permanent cognitive deficits. The toxins responsible are secondary metabolites of the fungi, principally fumonisin B1,[81,82] causing vascular lesions in the white matter of subcortical regions as well as in the cerebellum, brainstem and spinal cord. Hepatic disease frequently coexists.[58] Confirming the source of an outbreak is complicated by the fact that corn samples commonly contain fungal spores.

EPILEPSY

Seizures, transient and involuntary changes in behavior or neurological status due to abnormal electrical discharges in forebrain neurons, may be related to the syndromes discussed above. In small animals, seizures can manifest as anything from a subtle alteration in alertness to a generalized tonic-clonic event. Subtle behavioral changes may be manifested during auras, while profound behavioral alterations including hysteria, rage and 'fly biting' can be the primary clinical sign during some forms of seizures (partial complex seizures) depending on the seizure focus.[13,83] In humans and dogs partial complex seizures are based in the limbic system, and the amygdala is known to be particularly sensitive to seizure activity. Horses have a relatively high seizure threshold and, unlike in humans and dogs, idiopathic juvenile-onset epilepsy in which no brain lesion can be identified has not been shown to occur. Recurring seizures have been reported in adults, associated with organic lesions, and particularly in foals that may have benign epilepsy that they grow out of.

Seizures have a tendency to occur when the horse is undisturbed, and the first indication of epilepsy in a horse may be unexplained injuries which occur overnight. Any episode which compromises the awareness of an animal as large as a horse must be considered extremely dangerous, and it is strongly recommended that a horse not be ridden unless it has been seizure free without medication for at least 6 months.

NARCOLEPSY

Narcolepsy is an incurable, non-progressive sleep disorder characterized by striking transitions from wakefulness into rapid eye movement (REM) sleep without passing through slow wave sleep (see Ch. 10). In humans the clinical features include overwhelming episodes of sleep, excessive daytime somnolence, hypnagogic hallucinations, disturbed nocturnal sleep, cataplexy (sudden loss of muscle tone) and sleep paralysis. A syndrome that has the clinical appearance of narcolepsy has been noted in older horses (usually when undisturbed, e.g. in the back of a paddock) and Shetland and miniature horse foals.[84] The clinical signs can range from buckling at the knees, usually when the horse is quiet, to total

collapse and areflexia with maintenance of some eye and facial responses and normal cardiovascular function.[53] The syndrome resolves in some foals. Demonstrating the existence of narcolepsy in horses by classical electroencephalographic techniques may prove to be very difficult, as ongoing work (Colette Williams, personal communication) indicates that horses, unlike humans and dogs, may normally be able to go into REM sleep directly from a period of arousal. This may make eminent sense for a prey species as it would enable the horse to inspect its surroundings before becoming recumbent and losing muscle tone in REM sleep. In humans, some breeds of dogs and miniature horses, an hereditary background has been demonstrated. Canine[85] and human[86] narcolepsy is associated with dysfunction of a group of neurotransmitters involved in sleep regulation and satiety, the hypocretin system. In narcoleptic foals, narcoleptic episodes are often associated with nursing, and it is intriguing that the hypocretin system is involved in the regulation of sleep as well as appetite. The tricyclic antidepressant imipramine has resolved the signs of narcolepsy in horses for many hours[87] but is rarely indicated for long-term management.

HEADSHAKING

Headshaking is a condition in which the horse shakes its head in the absence of obvious external stimuli, and with such frequency and violence that it becomes difficult to ride, or the horse appears to be distressed. Headshaking is most often noted in middle-aged horses during spring or summer and is anecdotally associated with horses asked to use gaits with sustained neck flexion, such as dressage animals. The syndrome appears to be progressive in many cases, with increases in severity and loss of the characteristic seasonality. A great deal of research has been applied to this frustrating condition, but the etiology is far from clear.

Several causes have been suggested, including middle-ear disorders, ear mites, cranial nerve disorders, guttural pouch mycosis, dental periapical osteitis, allergic rhinitis and vasomotor rhinitis;

however, only very rarely can it be shown that correction of the abnormality leads to elimination of the headshaking.[88] Clinicians in California examined the role of light on headshaking behavior of horses and determined that the condition appeared to be light-stimulated in approximately 60% of the horses. It was suggested that the close association of the optic and trigeminal nerves in the midbrain may allow optic stimulation to cause referred itching, tingling or electric like sensations in areas innervated by branches of CN V, a condition similar to 'photic sneezing' in man.[46] The majority of horses with idiopathic headshaking showed some improvement or resolution of signs after oral administration of cyproheptadine.[89] This contrasts with studies performed in Great Britain,[48] in which a photic etiology could not be established and where cyproheptadine alone was ineffective; 65% of those cases however showed a 90–100% improvement following local anesthesia of the root of the maxillary branch of CN V, and combination therapy of cyproheptadine and carbamazepine resulted in very significant improvement in the majority of cases.

It was concluded that a trigeminal neuritis or neuralgia may be the basis of the underlying etiopathology of idiopathic equine headshaking. The etiology, just as in the human equivalent, is not known. The sodium channel-blocking effects of carbamazepine[90] are used to make a diagnosis of trigeminal neuralgia in humans, where similar clinical signs of sporadic or persistent mild to extreme facial pain is associated with the distribution of the trigeminal nerve. In the human condition, 'trigger factors' are a consistent feature; this may correspond with the intermittent seasonal nature of the equine disorder. Human trigeminal neuralgia has a much greater prevalence in multiple sclerosis patients,[91] and the disease may be associated with demyelination, but so far no direct clinical evidence for this has been established.[92] In spite of exhaustive studies on the peripheral portion of the trigeminal nerve, ganglion and sensory trigeminal nucleus, however, no consistent detectable pathology has been identified (Derek Knottenbelt, personal communication 2001).

There are currently no consistently useful therapies, and, although a particular case may respond to single or multiple management or therapeutic measures, the prognosis for cases of idiopathic headshaking is poor. The reported efficacy of the antihistamine hydroxyzine in some headshaking cases[93] may be attributed to the fact that rhinitis due to an allergic response may be the trigger factor rather than the specific pathology underlying this disorder. Furthermore hydroxyzine does possess some sodium channel-blocking effects,[94] so it is difficult to establish whether decreased histamine release or sodium blockade is producing the benefit in these isolated individual cases.

There is much research remaining to be done to understand this distressing disorder that regularly results in euthanasia of otherwise healthy horses.

SUMMARY OF KEY POINTS

- Major components of the central nervous system are the forebrain (cerebral hemispheres and thalamus), the brainstem (midbrain, pons and medulla oblongata), the cerebellum and the spinal cord.
- The brainstem and thalamic reticular activating system provide arousal and set up attention; the caudal part of the forebrain integrates perceptions, and the frontal cortex initiates voluntary movement and executes plans.
- The parietal lobe comprises primary sensory and motor areas; the occipital lobe is concerned with visual processing; the temporal lobe includes areas devoted to memory and hearing; the hippocampus and the amygdaloid nuclei are involved with memory and emotion; the frontal lobe is concerned with planning and control of movement.
- The limbic system is involved with memory, social and emotional behavior.
- Brain regions that appear to be critical to the formation of memories are the medial temporal lobe and certain thalamic and basal forebrain nuclei.
- Behavior is based on neurons receiving and conveying information using action potentials which trigger the release of neurotransmitters.
- The main neurotransmitter classes are the biogenic amines, amino acids, neuropeptides, nucleotides, prostaglandins and gases.
- Psychopharmacologic agents act by modifying neurotransmitters
- The neurological examination is carried out to determine whether the change in behavior could be explained by an underlying neurological deficit, and to define the

anatomical portion of the nervous system responsible for the clinical signs.
* A number of neurological diseases affecting the forebrain produce changes in behavior.

CASE STUDIES

* The author has examined several horses with recent changes in behavior such as becoming 'hot', difficult to ride, unwilling to move forward or being prone to frequent and sudden bucking and bolting. A neurological consult was sought, usually because the owner was concerned that the horse may have a 'brain tumor'. Careful neurological examinations did not reveal changes in mentation or other neurological signs in any of these cases. Several of these horses were euthanized and a postmortem examination further failed to determine morbid neuronal pathology.
* (Courtesy of Professor Joe Mayhew) An adult Thoroughbred mare known to be 'difficult' was brought to a farrier for corrective shoeing. During shoeing she became very belligerent, pushing through handlers, not standing still and acting aggressively. She was dealt with as a 'difficult' and 'badly behaved' horse by the farriers until, after about one hour of this, the experienced groom realized that the behavior was pathological. She was examined by a veterinary surgeon who found severe icterus. STAT liver enzyme analysis confirmed the diagnosis of acute liver failure and she was euthanized.

ACKNOWLEDGMENTS

The author would like to thank Professor Joe Mayhew for many years of instruction, and Mr Keith Ellis for remarkable tolerance and exceptional photography.

REFERENCES

1. McMillan FD, Rollin BE. The presence of mind: on reunifying the animal mind and body. J Am Vet Med Assoc 2001; 218(11):1723–1727.
2. de Lahunta A. Veterinary neuroanatomy and clinical neurology. Philadelphia: WB Saunders; 1983.
3. Kaplan HI, Sadock BJ. The brain and behavior. Kaplan and Sadock's synopsis of psychiatry. Baltimore: Williams & Wilkins; 1998.
4. Behan M. Neuroanatomy. Basic science course in veterinary and comparative neurology and neurosurgery, Madison, WI; 1998.
5. Peele TL. The neuroanatomic basis for clinical neurology. New York: McGraw-Hill; 1977.
6. Newman J. Thalamic contributions to attention and consciousness. Conscious Cogn 1995; 4(2):172–193.
7. Van de Poll NE, Van Goozen SH. Hypothalamic involvement in sexuality and hostility: comparative psychological aspects. Prog Brain Res 1992; 93(93):343–361.
8. Luft AR, Skale JM, Stefanou A, et al. Comparing motion- and imagery-related activation in the human cerebellum: a functional MRI study. Hum Brain Mapp 1998; 6(2):105–113.
9. MacKay-Lyons M. Central pattern generation of locomotion: a review of the evidence. Phys Ther 2002; 82(1): 69–83.
10. Kandel ER, Schwartz JH, Jessel TM. Principles of neural science. New York: McGraw-Hill; 2000.
11. Walker SF. Lateralization of functions in the vertebrate brain: a review. Br J Psychol 1980; 71(3):329–367.
12. Dodman NH, Miczek KA, Knowles K, et al. Phenobarbital-responsive episodic dyscontrol (rage) in dogs. J Am Vet Med Assoc 1992; 201(10):1580–1583.
13. Feeney DM, Gullotta FP, Gilmore W. Hyposexuality produced by temporal lobe epilepsy in the cat. Epilepsia 1998; 39(2):140–149.
14. Aggleton JP. The contribution of the amygdala to normal and abnormal emotional states. Trends Neurosci 1993; 16(8):328–333.
15. Rioult-Pedotti MS, Friedman D, Donoghue JP. Learning-induced LTP in neocortex. Science 2000; 290(5491):533–536.
16. Rolls ET. Memory systems in the brain. Annu Rev Psychol 2000; 51:599–630.
17. Willingham DB. Systems of memory in the human brain. Neuron 1997; 18:5–8.
18. Brunelli M, Garcia-Gil M, Mozzachiodi R, et al. Neurobiological principles of learning and memory. Archives Italiennes de Biologie 1997; 135(1):15–36.
19. Elliott FA. Propanolol for the control of beligerent behavior following acute brain damage. Ann Neurol 1977; 1:489–491.
20. Peck KE, Hines MT, Mealey KL, Mealey RH. Pharmacokinetics of imipramine in narcoleptic horses. Am J Vet Res 2001; 62(5):783–786.
21. Breier A, Kestler L, Adler C, et al. Dopamine D2 receptor density and personal detachment in healthy subjects. Am J Psychiatry 1998; 155(10):1440–1442.
22. Hector RI. The use of clozapine in the treatment of aggressive schizophrenia. Can J Psychiatry 1998; 43(5):466–472.
23. Galey D, Simon H, Le Moa M. Behavioral effects of lesions in the A10 dopaminergic area of the rat. Brain Res 1977; 124(1):83–97.
24. Johansson AK, Bergvall AH, Hansen S. Behavioral disinhibition following basal forebrain excitotoxin lesions: alcohol consumption, defensive aggression, impulsivity and serotonin levels. Behav Brain Res 1999; 102(1–2):17–29.
25. Dodman NH. Veterinary models of obsessive-compulsive disorder. In: Jenicke MA, Baer L, Minichiello WA, eds. Obsessive-compulsive disorders: practical management. St Louis, MO: Mosby; 1998:318–334.
26. Rendon RA, Shuster L, Dodman NH. The effect of the NMDA receptor blocker, dextromethorphan, on cribbing in horses. Pharmacol Biochem Behav 2001; 68(1):49–51.

27. Bagshaw CS, Ralston SL, Fisher H. Behavioral and physiological effect of orally administered tryptophan on horses subjected to acute isolation stress. Appl Anim Behav Sci 1994; 40(1):1–12.
28. Lee R, Coccaro E. The neuropsychopharmacology of criminality and aggression. Can J Psychiatry 2001; 46(1):35–44.
29. Overall KL. Self-injurious behavior and obsessive-compulsive disorder in domestic animals. In: Dodman NH, Shuster L, eds. Psychopharmacology of animal behavior disorders. Malden, MA: Blackwell Science, 1998.
30. Furey ML, Pietrini P, Haxby JV. Cholinergic enhancement and increased selectivity of perceptual processing during working memory. Science 2000; 290(5500):2315–2319.
31. Hahn CN, Mayhew IG. Equine neurodegenerative diseases – stressed neurons and other radical ideas. Vet J 1997; 154(3):173–174.
32. Divers TJ, Mohammed HO, Cummings JF, et al. Equine motor neuron disease: findings in 28 horses and proposal of a pathophysiological mechanism for the disease. Equine Vet J 1994; 26(5):409–415.
33. Cooper JR, Bloom FE, and Rothe RH. Neuroactive Peptides. The Biochemical Basis of Neuropharmacology. Oxford, Oxford University Press 1996: 410–458.
34. Lagerweij E, Nelis PC, Wiegant VM, van Ree JM. The twitch in horses: a variant of acupuncture. Science 1984; 225(4667):1172–1174.
35. Marsden MD. Behavioural problems. In: Collahan PT, Mayhew IG, Merritt AM, Moore JN, eds. Equine medicine and surgery, vol 1. St Louis, MO: Mosby; 1999:914–931.
36. Muir WW. Standing chemical restraint in horses. In: Muir WW, Hubbell JAE, eds. Equine anaesthesia: monitoring and emergency therapy. London: Mosby Year Book; 1991:247–266.
37. Booth NH, McDonald LE. Veterinary pharmacology and therapeutics. Ames: The Iowa State University Press; 1982.
38. Hedrick MS, Ryan ML, Bisgard GE. Recurrent laryngeal nerve activation by alpha 2 adrenergic agonists in goats. Respir Physiol 1995; 101:129–137.
39. Hubbell JAE, Muir WW. Standing chemical restraint. In: Reed SM, Bayly WW, eds. Equine internal medicine. Baltimore: WB Saunders; 1998:188–189.
40. Birnir B, Eghbali M, Cox GB, Gage PW. GABA concentration sets the conductance of delayed $GABA_A$ channels in outside-out patches from rat hippocampal neurons. J Membr Biol 2001; 181(3):171–183.
41. Tobin T. A review of the pharmacology of reserpine in the horse. J Eq Med Surg 1978; 2:10,433–438.
42. CPS. Compendium of pharmaceuticals and specialties, Canadian Pharmaceutical Association; 1997.
43. Dodman NHD, Shuster R, Mertens L, et al. Use of fluoxetine to treat dominance aggression in dogs. J Am Vet Med Assoc 1996; 209(9):1585–1587.
44. Romatowski J. Two cases of fluoxetine-responsive behavior disorders in cats. Feline Pract 1998; 26(1):14–15.
45. Fey K, Jonigkeit E, Moritz A. Zum equinen Cushing-Syndrom (ECS). Fallbericht, Literaturauswertung zu Diagnostik und Therapie sowie wesentliche Unterschiede zum Cushing-Syndrome des Hundes. Tierarztliche Praxis. Ausgabe G, GrossTiere Nutztiere 1998; 26(1):41–47.
46. Madigan JE, Kortz G, Murphy C, Rodger L. Photic headshaking in the horse: 7 cases. Equine Vet J Suppl 1995; 27(4):306–311.
47. Dailey JW, Reith ME, Steidley KR, et al. Carbamazepine-induced release of serotonin from rat hippocampus in vitro. Epilepsia 1998; 39(10):1054–1063.
48. Newton SA, Knottenbelt DC, Eldridge PR. Headshaking in horses: possible aetiopathogenesis suggested by the results of diagnostic tests and several treatment regimes used in 20 cases. Equine Vet J Suppl 2000; 32(3):208–216.
49. Pellock JM. Carbamazepine side effects in children and adults. Epilepsia 1987; 28(suppl 3): S64–70.
50. Herranz JL, Armijo JA, Arteaga R. Clinical side effects of phenobarbital, primidone, phenytoin, carbamazepine, and valproate during monotherapy in children. Epilepsia 1988; 29(6):794–804.
51. Langbehn DR, Alexander B. Increased risk of side-effects in psychiatric patients treated with clozapine and carbamazepine: a reanalysis. Pharmacopsychiatry 2000; 33(5):196.
52. Sanders RD, Keshavan MS. The neurologic examination in adult psychiatry: from soft signs to hard science. J Neuropsychiatry Clin Neurosci 1998; 10(4):395–404.
53. Mayhew IG. Large animal neurology: a handbook for veterinary clinicians. Philadelphia: Lea & Febiger; 1989.
54. Hanggi EB. Interocular transfer of learning in horses (Equus caballus). J Equine Vet Sci 1999; 19(8):518–524.
55. Westby GW, Keay KA, Redgrave P, et al. Output pathways from the rat superior colliculus mediating approach and avoidance have different sensory properties. Exp Brain Res 1990; 81(3):626–638.
56. King SM, Dykeman C, Redgrave P, Dean P. Use of a distracting task to obtain defensive head movements to looming visual stimuli by human adults in a laboratory setting. Perception 1992; 21(2):245–259.
57. King SM. Cowey A. Defensive responses to looming visual stimuli in monkeys with unilateral striate cortex ablation. Neuropsychologia 1992; 30(11):1017–1024.
58. Summers BA, Cummings JF, de Lahunta A. Veterinary neuropathology. St Louis, MO: Mosby; 1995.
59. Hahn CN, Mayhew IG, MacKay RJ. The nervous system. In: Colahan PT, Mayhew IG, Merritt AM, Moore JN, eds. Equine medicine and surgery. St Louis, MO: Mosby; 1999:863–995.
60. Jackson CA, deLahunta A, Dykes NL, Divers TJ. Neurological manifestation of cholesterinic granulomas in three horses. Vet Rec 1994; 135(10):228–230.
61. Kimman TG, Binkhorst GJ, van den Ingh TS, et al. Aujeszky's disease in horses fulfils Koch's postulates. Vet Rec 1991; 128(5):103–106.
62. Richt JA, Grabner A, Herzog S. Borna disease in horses. Vet Clin North Am Equine Pract 2000; 16(3):579–595.
63. Selvey LA, Wells RM, McCormack JG, et al. Infection of humans and horses by a newly described morbillivirus. Med J Aust 1995; 162(12):642–645.
64. Cantile C, Di Guardo G, Eleni C, Arispici M. Clinical and neuropathological features of West Nile virus equine encephalomyelitis in Italy. Equine Vet J 2000; 32(1):31–35.

65. Joyce JR, Russel LH. Clinical signs of rabies in horses. Compend Contin Ed 1981; 3:56–61.
66. Hudson LC, Weinstock D, Jordan T, Bold-Fletcher NO. Clinical presentation of experimentally induced rabies in horses. Zentralbl Veterinarmed 1996; 43(5):277–285.
67. Johnson RT. Selective vulnerability of neural cells to viral infections. Brain 1980; 103(3):447–472.
68. Hahn CN, Mayhew IG, Whitwell KE, et al. A possible case of Lyme borreliosis in a horse in the UK. Equine Vet J 1996; 28(1):84–88.
69. MacKay RJ. Equine protozoal myeloencephalitis. Vet Clin North Am Equine Pract 1997; 13(1):79–96.
70. Sewell MMH, Brocklesby DW. Animal diseases in the tropics. London: Baillière Tindall; 1990.
71. Hillyer MH, Holt PE, Barr FJ, et al. Clinical signs and radiographic diagnosis of a portosystemic shunt in a foal. Vet Rec 1993; 132(18):457–460.
72. Rose RJ, Hodgson DR. Manual of equine practice. Sydney: WB Saunders; 1993.
73. Savage JC. Diseases of the liver. In: Colahan PT, Mayhew IG, Merritt AM, Moore JN, eds. Equine medicine and surgery. St Louis, MO: Mosby; 1999:816–833.
74. Barton MH, Morris DD. Diseases of the liver. In: Reed SM, Bayly WW, eds. Equine internal medicine. Baltimore: WB Saunders; 1998:707–738.
75. Jones EA. Pathogenesis of hepatic encephalopathy. Clin Liver Dis 2000; 4(2):467–485.
76. Albrecht J, Jones EA. Hepatic encephalopathy: molecular mechanisms underlying the clinical syndrome. J Neurol Sci 1999; 170(2):138–146.
77. Matsumoto K, Graf R, Rosner G, et al. Elevation of neuroactive substances in the cortex of cats during prolonged focal ischemia. J Cereb Blood Flow Metab 1993; 13(4): 586–594.
78. Auer RN, Siesjo BK. Biological differences between ischemia, hypoglycemia, and epilepsy. Ann Neurol 1988; 24(6):699–707.
79. Rossdale PD. Clinical view of disturbances in equine foetal maturation. Equine Vet J Suppl 1993; 14:3–7.
80. Palmer AC, Rossdale PD. Neuropathological changes associated with the neonatal maladjustment syndrome in the thoroughbred foal. Res Vet Sci 1976; 20(3):267–275.
81. Thiel PG. Levels of fumonisins B1 and B2 in feeds associated with confirmed cases of equine leukoencephalomalacia. J Agric Food Chem 1991; 39:109–111.
82. Wilkins PA. A herd outbreak of equine leukoencephalomalacia. Cornell Veterinarian 1994; 84:53–59.
83. Dodman NH, Knowles KE, Shuster L, et al. Behavioral changes associated with suspected complex partial seizures in bull terriers. J Am Vet Med Assoc 1996; 208(5):688–691.
84. Lunn DP, Cuddon PA, Shaftoe S, Archer RM. Familial occurrence of narcolepsy in miniature horses. Equine Vet J 1993; 25(6):483–487.
85. Lin L, Faraco J, Li R, et al. The sleep disorder canine narcolepsy is caused by a mutation in the hypocretin (orexin) receptor 2 gene. Cell 1999; 98(3):365–376.
86. Thannickal TC, Moore RY, Nienhuis R, et al. Reduced number of hypocretin neurons in human narcolepsy. Neuron 2000; 27(3):469–474.
87. Sweeney CR, Hendricks JC, Beech J, Morrison AR. Narcolepsy in a horse. J Am Vet Med Assoc 1983; 183(1):126–128.
88. Lane JG, Mair TS. Observations on headshaking in the horse. Equine Vet J Suppl 1987; 19(4):331–336.
89. Madigan JE. Evaluation and treatment of headshaking syndrome. International Congress on Equine Clinical Behaviour 1996, Basel, Switzerland.
90. Rizzo MA. Successful treatment of painful traumatic mononeuropathy with carbamazepine: insights into a possible molecular pain mechanism. J Neurol Sci 1997; 152(1):103–106.
91. Katusic S, Beard CM, Bergstralh E, Kurland LT. Incidence and clinical features of trigeminal neuralgia, Rochester, Minnesota, 1945–1984. Ann Neurol 1990; 27(1):89–95.
92. Newton SA. The functional anatomy of the trigeminal nerve of the horse. PhD Thesis, Liverpool University, 2001.
93. McGorum BC, Dixon PM. Vasomotor rhinitis with headshaking in a pony. Equine Vet J 1990; 22(3):220–222.
94. Martindale: the extra pharmacopoeia. London: Pharmaceutical Press; 1972–1996.

4

Learning

LEARNING THEORY

Equids can learn remarkable behaviors (Fig. 4.1), but if we are to consider principles in horse training from a rigorous scientific perspective, there is an abiding need to demystify traditional horse training jargon and couch the following discussion in the language of learning theory. With these prerequisites in place veterinarians can be agents of change by counseling owners and trainers on effective and humane approaches to training and retraining. A glossary of equestrian terms appears at the end of this book, so this chapter avoids any such esoteric labels. The original rules of what we call learning theory were first set down by psychologists and behaviorists who used clinically controlled, some would say sterile, stimuli. These days the study of animal learning is increasingly the pursuit of cognitive ethologists. These are the behavioral scientists who, when considering the way in which a member of a species processes information, emphasize the importance of the environment for which that species evolved and determine how the biology of a species can influence its behavior.

THE DEFINITION OF LEARNING

Broadly speaking, a stimulus is any detectable change in an animal's environment. A response is any behavior or physiological event. The usual technical definition of learning or conditioning, as it is often called, is any relatively permanent change in the probability of a response occurring as a result of experience. Importantly, this refers to a response and not a cognitive outcome, such as knowledge.

85

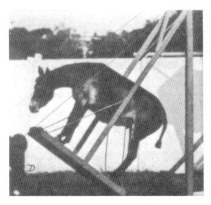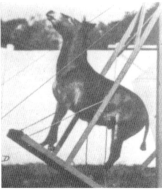

Figure 4.1 Denver, the swinging mule, changing his head and neck position to shift his center of gravity and swing a platform.

Not all changes in behavior are consequences of learning. The reference to a 'relatively permanent change' is added to exclude modifications of behavior by motivational factors, physiological variables or fatigue. A thirsty horse that drinks despite having refused water some hours earlier has changed its behavior but is not considered to have learnt anything in the interim. Instead, its motivation to drink has changed as a result of shifts in variables such as blood volume and the concentration of sodium in body fluids. Similarly, fatigue can change behavior, transforming a rearing colt into a weary slug, but its effects could not be described as relatively permanent.

Sufficient reflexive responses cannot possibly be built into each foal to meet every challenge throughout life, so learning enables young horses to use their experience to update their behaviors according to their developing circumstances. It is likely that horses are particularly attentive when learning to do what they fill most of their days with – grazing. Foals sample their mothers' feces when learning to select safe vegetation types, while adult horses retain the ability to review preferences in diet according to the proximate consequences of consumption.[1]

INTELLIGENCE

The intelligence of animals is difficult to assess. Intelligence may be shown when the animal learns to ignore irrelevant stimuli, just as it also learns to react to significant stimuli. This permits the behavioral developments that make discrimination possible. The horse's integration with its domestic environment is facilitated by this ability to compare and contrast. Most horses can accurately discriminate between stimuli and evaluate them, e.g. they can differentiate sounds, visual features of special significance, the identities of people, and so on.[2]

Veterinarians are often asked to comment on the intelligence of horses. For example, some owners are intrigued to know whether they should credit their horses with the cognitive talents of dogs. Attempts to compare brain to bodyweight to arrive at a quantitative comparison between species are rarely well received by horse lovers since, using this measure, the horse approximately equates with the turtle (see Ch. 3). Furthermore the same ratio credits the shrew with more brain power than the human. One of the core problems here seems to lie in the definition of intelligence, because it is a nebulous construct. It may be preferable to speak of the ability to learn, but even that approach may be flawed when experimental designs fail to select naïve subjects. We should bear in mind that conclusions about equine reasoning abilities (or lack thereof) may be biased because they have been based on observations that appear to have been made almost exclusively with horses that have been trained by negative reinforcement (Amy Coffman, personal communication 2002). It is possible that this may have affected their performance, e.g. by reducing their willingness to risk making mistakes.

Several attempts have been made to compare learning abilities in horses with those of other species and to compare the ability of different breeds of horses.[3,4] All of the tests between species are confounded by the differences in physical ability and sensory acuity between species, as these may account for the differences in perceived 'intelligence'. As soon as one makes such changes, comparisons become flawed. One can see how difficult it is to devise a test that two species can undertake with equity. Experimenters have yet to make the necessary adjustments to stimuli so that members of two species can detect and respond to them with equal ease, speed and motivation. The same criticism can be leveled at experiments that compare the problem-solving ability of breeds within a species or, for that matter, bloodlines within a breed.[5] Selection of breed traits can impair or enhance performance in various ways, including emotionality.

IMPRINTING AND SOCIALIZATION

First described by Konrad Lorenz, imprinting is said to occur when innate behaviors are released in response to a learnt stimulus. Imprinting is more important in precocial species, in which the offspring are less dependent on their mothers for food and warmth, than in altricial species, which often confine their more vulnerable, and often hairless, young to nests. Most imprinting promotes survival of newborn animals and shapes their future breeding activities. Imprinting has a number of characteristics, including a sensitive period. This refers to a window of opportunity during early postnatal life when this unique form of learning is most easily achieved. Although the empirical evidence is sparse, it is suggested by Miller[6] that the time for intensive foal handling is the first 48 hours of life when the 'following response' is learnt. At this time a foal learns to follow its mother, who is normally the nearest large moving creature in its world.

We do well to explore ways in which we can exploit this limited learning opportunity in our companion animals. Many horse breeders recognize the lifelong benefits of socialization programs for newborn foals. Stimuli to which youngsters are exposed during this window period may be more readily accepted as being 'normal' in later life. Waring[7] found that, compared with control foals, neonatal foals that have been extensively handled readily-overcome fear responses to novel stimuli and show more exploratory behavior with less dependence on their dams.

In experimental studies of anserine birds, imprinting seems the least likely of all forms of learning to be forgotten or unlearned. Whether the rules established for birds can be readily applied to horses is the source of some controversy, not least because the process of 'imprint training'[6] does not meet the criteria of true neural imprinting.[8,9] Because studies of imprinting in precocial birds show that the imprinted associations are irreversible and retained for life, there is need for more research in any equine equivalent of this phenomenon.

Just as learning to struggle can start from the earliest experiences, learning to tolerate and be passive in the face of restraint can also be acquired by a foal. Ideally, neonatal training programs should be designed to reduce the prevalence of defensive aggression and are therefore noteworthy for equine practitioners.[6] Whereas less precocious neonates, such as puppies and kittens, have to wait until they are mobile to enter their socialization period, foals can learn from the first moments of life. Because lessons learnt at this stage in an animal's life may be indelible, time spent working with foals may be considerably more efficient than time spent schooling larger, stronger and more dangerous animals in later life. However, in the absence of any evidence that there are significant disadvantages in waiting until the mare and foal have bonded and the foal has gained its strength, there seems to be no need to rush into a program aimed at socializing the youngster.

While conceding that it is not, strictly speaking, a new idea, Miller[6] advocates ritualized habituation of the foal to common stimuli and then sensitization to selected prompts (so-called performance-related stimuli). In this way he fosters passivity while preserving a degree of responsiveness. He advocates multiple manipulation of the foal's body. These he calls stimulations. Between 30 and 50 stimulations of each area are prescribed. Under-stimulation is more likely to be a problem than over-stimulation. Here is a précis of Miller's training recipe:[6]

1. Bring the mare indoors to foal.
2. When she has delivered the foal and the umbilical cord is severed, begin drying the newborn with the mare. This allows the foal to expect humans in its life as much as it does its dam. On day one, pay attention to all of the following areas:

   (a) Rub the foal all over its body, starting at the poll. Concentrate on one region until the foal physically relaxes to the extent that it appears sleepy.

   (b) Repeat this procedure in an established order, such as ears, including ear canals, face, upper lip, mouth, tongue and nostrils.

   (c) This is followed by the eyes, neck, thorax, saddle area, legs, feet, rump, tail, perineum and external genitalia.

3. The next step involves introduction of artificial devices, including clippers and a rectal thermometer. This, along with mock rectal examinations, attracts some controversy. It is perhaps surprising that when the recipe calls for 50–100 wiggles of the lubricated gloved finger, it seems to make no allowance for individual differences; this suggests that there needs to be more empirical work on these thresholds.

4. Next comes the introduction of what one might generally consider 'unusual stimuli'. Crucially one should take a step back at this point and remind oneself that, although we have selected horses for the tolerance of restraint (among many other traits), there is nothing in the development of the horse that predicates it to accept any of the stimuli consequent to domestication. Head-collars are no more normal to a naïve foal than are motor vehicles.

   The handler goes on to rub the foal's entire body with a piece of crackling plastic until it evokes no panic response. Desensitization of the newborn foal to gunfire, hissing sprayers, whistles, loud music, flapping flags and swinging ropes is also recommended. As one can imagine, the list of stimuli to which a foal can be desensitized is virtually endless.

5. The next day, with the help of an assistant (who ensures the foal does not learn to escape), further desensitization, in spells of no more than 15 minutes, takes place. The foal is positioned head to head with its dam as all areas are subjected to a repeat test and revisited if any evasive response is detected.

6. The girth area is next on the list as the chest is encircled by the handler's arms and squeezed rhythmically until habituation is evident.

7. Sensitization comes after habituation in Miller's schema. The paradigm of pressure being sustained until the horse responds is applied in regular equitation. Its use in neonates seems perfectly valid. With an assistant, he teaches the foal that resistance to pressure applied to the flanks or to the head, via a head-collar, is useless. Reward in this part of the program is given by relieving the pressure (see the subsection on negative reinforcement, p. 96).

Foals learn faster than adults because they have so little to 'unlearn', so the concept of early lessons is wholly sensible. However, even though Waring[10] isolated foals at 5 to 70 minutes of age with no apparent ill-effects, it may be that instead of attempting to muscle in on the bonding that occurs between a mare and her foal, we should focus solely on offering opportunities for appropriate socialization (Fig. 4.2).

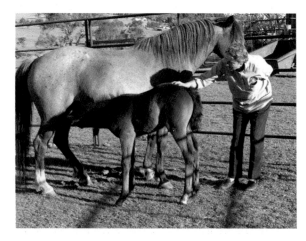

Figure 4.2 Early exposure to humans can be achieved without compromising the mare–foal bond.

While Waring[10] warns that the boldness and 'zealous curiosity' of early handled foals may make them more likely to expose themselves to danger, some ethologists are concerned that the Miller program trains learned helplessness (see p. 340). Others question the ease with which the model can be followed and the efficacy of the intervention.

A study involving 25 treated and 22 control foals examined the effects of a training procedure at 2, 12, 24 and 48 hours after birth on 25 foals and their reaction to stimuli used in the early training procedure, and to a novel stimulus 1, 2 and 3 months later.[11] During the introduction of each stimulus, the behavior of each foal, the time required to complete exposure to each stimulus (foals that were more reactive took longer) and heart rates were recorded. At 1 and 2 months of age, treated foals required less time than control foals to complete exposure to the stimulus and had lower heart rates during exposure. However, by 3 months of age, there were no significant differences between the two groups for any measures.[11] A subsequent study of 9 horse and 6 pony foals cast further doubt on some of the claims made for the Miller program by showing that early handling seems to increase friendliness to handlers and general ease of handling but not acceptance of key interventions.[12] Specifically, this questions the justification for handling techniques intended to teach acceptance of farriery and veterinary procedures, such as nasogastric tubing and the introduction of rectal thermometers (see steps 2 and 3 above).[12]

The perceived need for persistence in application of restraint as part of the Miller regime remains a contentious issue. While fears that the restraint may delay ingestion of colostrum are fuelled by data showing that it increases latency to stand, these should be allayed by the absence of any comparable increase in the latency to nurse.[13] Because restraint of struggling foals may increase their risk of injury, veterinarians should consider this outcome carefully before advocating the Miller system. Similarly they should be mindful that there is insufficient work to demonstrate that handling at later ages could not have similar results.[14]

The suggestion that foals be stimulated until they appear sleepy rather than reactive is central here. We cannot assume that sleepiness is indicative of emotional acquiescence. There is a need for surveillance of foals' physiological response to this intervention. This may allow us to assess any deleterious effects of elements of the training program and refine the entire approach.

Although it may please some readers to note that foals reared without peers are bolder with humans,[15] it is possible for foals to learn to become too familiar with handlers. Grzimek[16] separated a neonatal foal from its own species for 64 days and found that it developed a fear of conspecifics and a social preference for humans over equids. Similarly, Williams[17] noted that artificially reared foals failed to respond to the social signals of conspecifics and sought human company rather than that of other horses. The socialization benefit is an important reason why fostering orphan foals on to nurse mares is preferable to hand-rearing (see Ch. 12).[18] It is not clear how labile the unwelcome consequences of mal-imprinting are in later life. Some owners speak of foals that have mal-imprinted as having a lack of 'respect', e.g. 'because they have no fear, they climb on top of you'. As with any training, the key to finding the best course is to be consistent. If you do not want a horse that takes dangerous liberties in later life, then never reward it for doing so as a foal. Familiarity does not necessarily breed contempt. However, just as a mare disciplines her foal before and during weaning by punishing behavior she finds unacceptable, so the human handler should do the same to avoid the youngster growing up with a litany of inappropriate responses and no 'respect' for humans. This is why sensitization in early handling programs is so important. Sensitization (acting as a precursor to negative reinforcement) trains the foal to move away from tactile stimuli as it must to become a safe and responsive working animal in later life.

The sensitive period during which foals can be influenced by socialisation strategies is not clearly defined. Indeed Mal & McCall[19] concluded that handling throughout the first 42 days of life increased foal performance in the halter-training task compared with handling from 43 to 84 days of age. Interestingly, they suggested that as well as the possible existence of a critical period within the first 42 days of life, the importance of timing in handling may be due to some degree of learned helplessness. Because in free-ranging contexts, foals take their flight cue from their dams and conspecifics, it would be interesting to see how much the process of desensitization described above trains the foal to tolerate all novel stimuli as long as a human is present as a protective cue. There is no evidence that pre-weaning handling has any effect on the post-weaning learning ability of foals[20] but it may well make them calmer.

When Dutch Warmblood youngsters that received additional training from the age of 5 months onwards were tested at 9, 10, 21 and 22 months of age in a novel object test and a handling test, they showed a significant increase in mean heart rate and decrease in heart rate variability measures at all ages, when compared with youngsters that had had regular training.[21] Furthermore, statistical analysis showed that the increase in mean heart rate could not be entirely explained by the physical activity. This suggests a marked shift of the balance of the autonomic nervous system towards sympathetic dominance. This shift was particularly pronounced in control horses during the novel object test. Because these horses showed individual consistency of these heart rate variables at all ages, it is further suggested that, with these tests, non-motor cardiac responses might be useful in quantifying certain aspects of a horse's temperament.[21]

Heird et al[22] found that horses that had been extensively handled learned which way to turn in a maze more slowly than minimally handled horses, but faster than unhandled horses, suggesting that only moderate handling is best from the horse's perspective when in a problem-solving situation without human help. The same authors reported that horses that were continuously handled as weanlings and yearlings were less emotional and more trainable for riding than were horses receiving less early handling.

In conclusion, while noting the helpful efforts of researchers in this domain, we should accept that a great deal of confusion prevails about best practice in the formative years of a horse's life.

This highlights the need for experimental designs that provide data that is more readily applicable to the needs of horse producers and equestrians.

NON-ASSOCIATIVE LEARNING

Imprinting aside, there are two major categories of learning: non-associative and associative. In non-associative learning the animal is exposed to a single stimulus to which it can become habituated or sensitized, while in associative learning, a relationship is established between at least two stimuli. There are two subdivisions under the umbrella of associative learning. These are classical conditioning and operant conditioning. The latter, as we will see, is important for animals to be able to solve novel problems in their environment. The central tenets of learning theory merit detailed consideration by those embarking on behavior modification in practice because the ontogeny and resolution of inappropriate behavior patterns can be explained with reference to learning theory. If we can appreciate how a horse finds benefits from aggressive responses to humans, we can understand why meeting such responses with violence rarely, if ever, helps. If we can understand how to train a horse to bow, we can apply similar techniques to modify the behavior of a horse that has learned to avoid being loaded onto trailers.

The most basic form of learning involves cumulative experience of stimuli by themselves. This gives the horse data about the relevance of stimuli in its environment.

HABITUATION

Habituation is said to have occurred when repeated presentations of a stimulus by itself cause a decrease in the response. It is really the simplest form of learning. Consider the training of a police horse (see case study below) that must be gradually exposed to more and more of the potentially frightening stimuli that it will later encounter when out on patrol. The people delivering these stimuli in training are familiar to it and started their disturbances at a considerable distance from

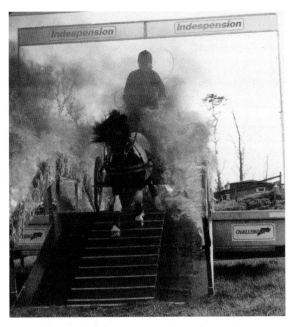

Figure 4.3 Stunt pony, Mr Pie, galloping through fire. (Photograph courtesy of Amanda Saville-Weeks)

it. Only when it ignores the rumpus at a certain noise level and a certain distance are these variables made more threatening and proximate. Similar approaches are used in the training of stunt horses for film and exhibition work (see Fig. 4.3).

The likelihood of habituation and its rate are dependent on the nature of the stimulus, the rate of stimulus presentation and the regularity with which it is presented. When habituating a horse to a stimulus, it is essential that the stimulus be repeated well past the point of habituation. To stop prematurely can teach the animal exactly the opposite of what is desired. Habituated responses show spontaneous recovery when stimulation is withheld. This means that exposure to the relevant stimuli must continue at intervals to prevent the original response (e.g. a flight response) from recurring.

Habituation is central to horse taming and pivotal in early handling regimens. Recent work by Jezierski et al[23] using Konik horses, confirms that habituation to handling can reduce reactivity. Konik horses are a primitive breed unlikely to have been selected to be easily managed by humans.[24]

Horses exposed to daily handling (10 minutes per day over 5 days per week) from 2 weeks of age displayed a reduced heart rate and enhanced manageability compared with horses born and reared up to weaning age in a forest environment free from human contact.[23] The early handling intervention made horses much easier to manage than non-handled foals in a variety of tests given at 6, 12, 18 and 25 months.

Desensitization and counter-conditioning

In behavior modification, the step-by-step process of weakening an unwelcome fear response to a given stimulus or set of stimuli to the point of extinction is often labeled systematic desensitization. If the horse is relaxed when exposed to barely perceptible measures of the causative factors one at a time, it can learn to behave passively rather than fearfully. The emphasis in this approach has to be on the gradual introduction of increasing aliquots of the problematic stimuli. Too fast an advance is marked by a return to the fearful response or an alternative evasion. If this arises, exposure to the stimuli must be returned to the level to which the horse had successfully habituated.

If, rather than simply habituating horses to aversive stimuli, we expose them to pleasant coincidental consequences, counter-conditioning occurs. This helps to facilitate the emergence of an alternative, more appropriate response to the aversive stimulus. Despite encouraging data to support the use of this approach,[25] this is a sadly underexploited strategy in the management of horse behavior. Any veterinarian who appreciates the motivation most equids have to feed should be able to harness this drive to train appropriate behaviors. For example, if one is required to administer eye drops to a horse one can either struggle with it as it wrestles its head away or condition an appropriate head posture using food. The principles of learning theory that apply when horses learn to tilt their heads to nuzzle in the pockets of owners and find titbits can be used for veterinary purposes. For sustained performance, the rewards must outweigh the costs and, because horses learn to avoid aversive stimuli more than some other domestic species such as the dog,[26] this means that the daily value of the reinforcements must eclipse the aversiveness of the total daily dose of eye drops. Unfortunately, for some veterinarians and owners, simple habituation to periorbital palpation is too time consuming and therefore counter-conditioning holds even less appeal. Because they are reliable sources of ocular discomfort, these are the people whom equine ophthalmic patients learn to avoid.

It is important to recognize that simply offering food in the presence of a fear-eliciting stimulus is an inadequate approach since the horse may be chewing a mouthful of food and therefore gaining gratification from it while demonstrating a flight response. Rather than allowing the fearful horse to stuff his head into a bucket of grain during exposure, a simple gratifying distraction, effective trainers use valuable rewards that are small enough to be consumed quickly. These rewards are used when the horse that tends to run away with an elevated head posture offers approximations of a more appropriate response such as turning towards the stimulus and lowering its head.[27] By waiting for the horse to offer the appropriate response rather than forcing it to 'behave' with aversive stimuli, such as buccal discomfort where rein pressure is used, the trainer allows the horse to learn the consequences of its own actions in bringing about a reward. This elegant approach, which allows the horse to have some control over the situation, requires all the features of good training practice, including sensitive shaping technique (see p. 99) and, above all, consistency.[28]

A less sophisticated approach to fearfulness in horses that may, at first glance, seem expeditious, is flooding, which involves the over-exposure to the causative stimuli until the response disappears. A familiar example of flooding is seen in traditional horse 'breaking' when a saddle is strapped to a naïve horse that is then allowed to buck in an attempt to rid itself of the saddle until it stops. Driven by the belief that the horse is not responding because it is no longer fearful, many misguided handlers reach for this approach. Unfortunately the horse has no control over the situation and can learn that it is simply helpless to respond. Where this learning is context specific (see below), the lessons are only partially learned and the horse may emerge with extreme fear responses in slightly different circumstances. Trainers of police horses generally do not use flooding because the horses must offer learned responses in a very wide variety of contexts (see case study at the end of the chapter). Flooding in combination with physical restraint and muscle relaxants such as succinylcholine chloride has been described, with warnings about the dangers of the subjects damaging themselves as they struggle or collapse to the ground.[29] Flooding that leads to apathy may be justified in certain aggressive horses, as an alternative to euthanasia, but for some it remains questionable on welfare grounds.

SENSITIZATION

Sensitization is the opposite of habituation in that there is an increase in a response after repeated presentations of the stimulus by itself. The stimulus has to be intrinsically unpleasant or aversive. Sensitization usually happens when an individual cannot escape or make an avoidance response to prevent repeated exposure to a stimulus that is intrinsically unpleasant or aversive. This is particularly likely if the subject is highly aroused. If one recalls the magnified unpleasantness of a dripping tap when searching for sleep, the effect of sensitization becomes clear. Sensitization can override habituation. For example, if while completing his training, the police horse described above is involved in a road traffic accident every day for a month, he would reliably become sensitized to motor vehicles and perhaps even become phobic so that just the sound or sight of them might be sufficient to send him into a flight response.

ASSOCIATIVE LEARNING

When horses make links between stimuli and responses or, to use training terms, cues and outcomes they are undergoing associative learning.

CLASSICAL CONDITIONING

Classical conditioning is the acquisition of a response to a new stimulus by association with an old stimulus. It involves coupling a stimulus with an innate behavior or physiological response. It is also labeled Pavlovian conditioning because it has its origins in primarily unrelated saliva collection experiments conducted by Ivan Pavlov.

Pavlov had spotted his experimental dogs salivating when they heard his technician tinkling a bell as he approached the kennels to feed them. To determine how accurately a dog could develop such associations, Pavlov decided to replace the sound of the bell with more easily varied sounds made by a buzzer and then a metronome. He surgically implanted a tube to collect saliva and measure its rate of production (Fig. 4.4).

Pavlov coupled a novel external stimulus to a physiological stimulus and response. The dog learned to respond to the buzzer, a new stimulus that had previously been irrelevant or neutral. Because its effect was the product of learning, Pavlov called the buzzer a *conditioned stimulus*. The salivation response to the conditioned stimulus is called the *conditioned response*. Before the learning experience, only meat powder, the *unconditioned stimulus*, produced salivation as an *unconditioned response* (Fig. 4.5). Crucially, in classical conditioning, the sound of a buzzer was followed by the delivery of food to the mouth, regardless of what the dog might have done when it heard the buzzer. Classical conditioning enables the animal to associate events over which it has no control. This increases the *predictability* of an environment. The more frequently and consistently the neutral stimulus is paired with the unconditioned stimulus, the more rapidly the association will be made. In some cases, usually involving the most fundamental pain or pleasure, the association is formed with a single experience.[30]

A good example comes from horse-breeding units. Learning about sex seems especially likely as a consequence of classical conditioning. Some stallions get aroused when they hear the sound of the bridle used to control them in the service pen. Their excitement increases when they are led to the

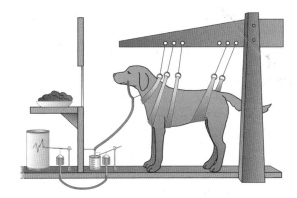

Figure 4.4 Illustration of one of Pavlov's dogs in its experimental apparatus used for measuring the rate of salivation as an indicator of the strength of associations between conditioned stimuli and food.

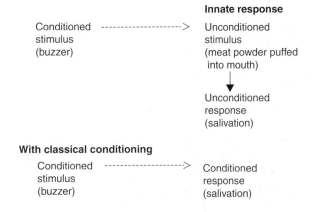

Figure 4.5 Classical conditioning.

service barn – hence, through classical conditioning another reliable environmental cue becomes associated with copulation. Racetrack grooms use classical conditioning when they whistle each time they see their charges urinating. Once the association between the whistling and urination is made, the horses urinate on cue for post-race urine tests (see Ch. 9). Riders use classical conditioning when they replace pressure cues with previously neutral signals such as changes in their position (seat).

Pavlov recorded an interesting footnote to his studies: he noted that his dogs would race ahead of their handlers to get to the experimental area. They would not wait for a stimulus that made their mouths water, they would actively try to put them-selves into situations and perform activities that led to rewards. This was a result of trial-and-error learning and brings us neatly to the other impor-tant category: operant conditioning.

OPERANT CONDITIONING

An operant response is a voluntary activity that brings about a reward. In operant conditioning, the buzzer might still be presented but the dog must make a particular response before food is con-sumed. In other words, there is a special link (what learning theorists call a contingency) between a particular behavioral response and a food reward.

While Pavlov was concentrating on the physio-logical responses of dogs in harnesses, Thorndike[31] was studying the behavioral responses of cats in puzzle boxes. Instead of delivering food inde-pendently of behavior whenever a signal had been presented, Thorndike delivered it once his ani-mals had responded. In a body of work intended to discredit the notion that animals are capable of reason, Thorndike[31] described the behavior of a naïve cat in a specially designed box (Fig. 4.6).

Without any food or other home comforts, life was rather dull and unsustainable in the puzzle box. The cat could get out – but only by pulling a trigger. Motivated to access food outside the box, Thorndike's cats would eventually learn to escape by operating the trigger that released the door latch. Once out of the box, they would get their food. Thorndike called this trial-and-error learning, but this label has largely been replaced by the terms instrumental learning and operant conditioning. The animal sees a cue (the trigger), performs a response (pulling) and gets a reward (liberty and food). The effect of the reward is to strengthen the correct response. This is known as reinforcement. The term reinforcement refers to the process in which a reinforcer follows a particular behavior so that the frequency (or probability) of that behavior increases.

On successive occasions in his free-operant studies (see below), Thorndike noted that the cat's latency to escape fell but only very gradually. The absence of a sudden drop in the latency to learn was sufficient evidence for Thorndike to assert that

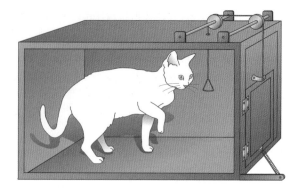

Figure 4.6 Illustration of one of Thorndike's cats in a puzzle box.

his cats were not using thought or reason to solve the problem. Thorndike's work was followed by that of Skinner,[32] who maintained that almost any response could be learned by an animal that is given opportunities to operate within its envi-ronment to obtain a desired outcome.

Rocky, the 8-year-old Irish Draft horse in Chapter 1 (see Fig. 1.10), learned within 4 weeks of being at a new home that unlocking the bolt on his stable door allowed him to enrich his environ-ment. He learned that the behavior had a pleasant result. However, he does not attempt to escape if a chain is slung across the threshold of his door-way and loosely tied with a single strand of twine. It appears that the open door affords him a better view and, for the time being at least, satisfies his motivation to observe the activity on the yard.

Operant or instrumental conditioning consists of presenting or omitting some reward or punish-ment when the animal makes a specific response.[33] The likelihood of an association arising depends on the relationship between the first event and the second via stimulus–response–reinforcement chains. Operant conditioning enables an animal to associate events over which it has control. This increases the *controllability* of the environment, which represents the crucial difference between classical (Pavlovian) and operant conditioning. Operant conditioning can have potential benefits for horse welfare by improving choice. In classical conditioning, rewards become associated with stimuli while in operant conditioning they become associated with responses.

Operant conditioning has been studied experimentally in two types of situations: 'discrete trial' situations and 'free operant' situations. In a 'discrete trial' situation, a subject is exposed to the learning task, required to make a response, and then withdrawn from the situation. For example, a horse may have to choose one of two directions, left or right, in a simple T-maze. In a 'free operant' situation, on the other hand, the subject is allowed to operate freely on its environment. For example, a horse placed in a paddock and free to do whatever it likes, can be conditioned by reinforcement under a given set of contingencies. Horses such as those that open their stable doors or dunk their own hay are good examples of free-operant conditioning. Like Thorndike's cats and the rats that pressed levers in Skinner's laboratory, they work within their environment to effect a reward. Several studies suggest that lack of control over aversive events can bring about major behavioral and physiological changes. For example, after being exposed to uncontrollable electric shocks, rats have increased gastric ulceration, increased defecation rates and are more susceptible to certain cancers when compared with individuals that retain control over comparable shocks.

Operant devices can be used to determine the preference animals have for certain environmental parameters. Horses have been trained to break photoelectric beams to turn on lighting in their accommodation and, using this device, have demonstrated a preference for an illuminated environment.[34] Others have been trained to nuzzle buttons to access resources (Fig. 4.7).

Conditioned horses have been used to study the effects of psychotropic pharmaceuticals. For example, horses were trained to interrupt a light beam for a reward of oats.[35] Horses developed their own individual response rates, which remained stable at between 5 and 35 responses per minute for each horse over a period of months. Reserpine (5 mg/ horse, i.v.) depressed the response rate in all horses tested. This depression was maximal between 3 and 5 days after treatment and lasted for up to 10 days. In part, the lasting nature of the drug accounts for its appeal to those seeking to modulate equine flight responses, especially during

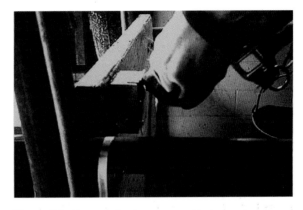

Figure 4.7 Horse performing an operant task: pressing a button with its muzzle. (Photograph courtesy of Katherine Houpt.)

traditional breaking (2.5–10 mg s.i.d. or b.i.d. orally for up to 30 days[36]) (see also Ch. 3).

TRAINING AND BEHAVIOR MODIFICATION

Learning allows animals to use information about the world to tailor their responses to environmental change. By avoiding pain and discomfort, animals can make their life more pleasant. Even invertebrates such as flies, slugs and ants show impressive forms of learning when avoiding unpleasant stimuli. When animals cannot evade pain or aversive stimuli, they become distressed; but if this is chronic in nature, they develop learned helplessness and fail to make responses that were once appropriate.

We manipulate animals' experience to train them. Training generally means drawing out desirable behaviors and suppressing undesirable innate behaviors to institute novel responses.

In training horses we have exploited their need as prey animals to avoid discomfort and, for that matter, threats of discomfort.[26] Crudely speaking, we apply pressure to attain the desired response and remove it when we get the desired responses. The aim of training is to install signals (cues) that result in predictable behavior patterns. When the association between pressure, response and timely release becomes highly predictable, a habit emerges. If a habit does not develop, it could be that the animal has learned that there is no response that can reliably cause the pressure to be released. Unfortunately, it is possible to identify many horses in all spheres of ridden and draft work that have developed such learned helplessness and are often labeled 'stubborn' (see Ch. 13).

The ability of horses to learn is one reason they are useful to humans and directly influences their monetary value to humans.[33] The changing role of the horse demands a greater emphasis on humane treatment and the development of more sophisticated research into horse education. In this context, veterinarians and equine scientists can play an important role as innovators countering traditional horse-lore that resists technological advances.

Training naïve animals is generally preferable to training animals with inappropriate experience.[22] If an animal is pre-exposed to a conditioned stimulus for a number of trials before structured conditioning commences, i.e. before reinforcement, the acquisition of a conditioned response to that stimulus will be retarded. The animal has simply learned to ignore the stimulus because it has no important consequences.

With a sound grip on learning theory, all practitioners can apply therapeutic behavior modification programs that identify the motivation, remove the rewarding aspects of the unwelcome behavior and reinforce a more appropriate alternative. If the strategy does not work, one can be sure that training has been insufficient to establish the new associations or that the reinforcement for the new response is insufficient to overcome gratification from the existing behavior.

Training horses, whether under-saddle or in-hand, stabled or in the paddock, basic, advanced or remedial, usually involves operant principles. Before giving a reward, the trainer must wait until the animal produces the desired activity. Rewarding the desired behavior relates to the Law of Effect, which states that whatever behavior immediately precedes reinforcement will be strengthened.

REINFORCERS AND PUNISHMENTS

Be it positive or negative, reinforcement will always make a response more likely in future.

Table 4.1 Punishment versus reinforcement – effect of the treatment

Response becomes more likely in future	Response becomes less likely in future
Positive reinforcement – titbit reinforces begging	Positive punishment – applying tension on the rein increases discomfort in the mouth
Negative reinforcement – easing tension on the rein reduces discomfort in the mouth	Negative punishment – complete removal of food extinguishes begging

Conversely, positive or negative punishment will generally make a response less likely in future (Table 4.1).

Both punishment and negative reinforcement can be applied as consequences of behavior and so are central to operant conditioning. Many trainers claim not to use negative reinforcement but are instead simply confused by a term that may have unpleasant connotations. In this context, negative refers to the removal of something from the animal's world, while positive refers to an addition. So, when trainers reinforce a behavior with the removal of something unpleasant, they make the behavior more likely in the future. For example, if a trainer stops tapping a horse with a whip (see case study in Ch. 13) when it moves in the correct direction, he makes the horse more likely to move away from the whip when the tapping resumes. The 'move away' response has been negatively reinforced. To an extent, punishment and negative reinforcement are interrelated (Fig. 4.8) since, by definition, an animal must know that a stimulus is aversive in order for its removal to be reinforcing.

Negative punishment or omission forms an important part of our attempts to improve or modify responses. Most readers will agree that a horse being encouraged to perform a new behavior in the *manège* will first attempt to use an established response. The absence of reinforcement at that point makes repetition of an unwanted established response less likely. If reinforcement has been omitted, the horse been negatively punished. This forces any horse labeled as having either any

Operant conditioning

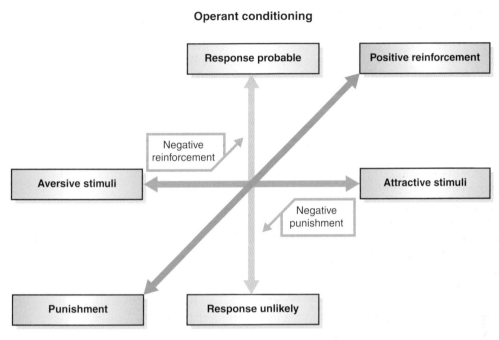

Figure 4.8 Reinforcement and punishment can be considered on the same continuum.

talent or even a temper to try new solutions to its problem. An educated horse has learned that it can use a variety of responses to solve the problems presented by hand and leg signals. It is consistency in both the presentation of such problems and the provision of consequences that distinguishes good trainers.

In the interests of clarity, I encourage all trainers and animal educators to consider carefully their use of these terms. Punishment is not in itself a dirty word. Nor is negative. Both negative punishment and positive punishment can be extremely mild. The degree to which one relies on either reinforcers or punishers and the consistency with which one applies them are what matter to the animal.

USING REINFORCERS

A reinforcer is anything that increases the frequency of the particular behavior that it follows. A response will increase in strength when followed by a reward. The merit of a reinforcer can be measured only in terms of the degree to which it makes the behavior more likely in future. If a trainer's

saying 'good boy' in response to a horse's leg-yielding has no effect on the horse's future behavior then, according to this definition, reinforcement has not occurred. The trainer's words have had a neutral or even confusing effect. The definition does not describe how or why some events act as reinforcers. Whether some event is called a reinforcer is purely a matter of the effect it had.

Consideration of the type of reinforcer is important. Discrimination performance in horses improves if there is a differential outcome in reward.[37] In a discrimination task where the color of the center panel signaled that either a left or a right lever response was correct, horses performed best when different reinforcers (food pellets for one lever; chopped carrot for the other) were linked with each lever, than when reinforcers were randomly assigned or identical.[37] Therefore *many* different contextual features associated with both stimuli and reinforcers can be integrated to maximize differentiation and thus enhance performance.[24]

Palatable foods are generally more reinforcing if they are not normally part of the horse's diet.

Horses that have been exposed to these foods may perform with a higher level of consistency for this type of reinforcer. Because they can recognize these types of food as highly palatable and receive them infrequently, they seem more motivated to work for them. However, this is less effective in naïve horses because of neophobia (literally, fear of the new).

Significantly, horses work to avoid negative reinforcement, even when this interferes with their access to positive reinforcement.[24] In practical terms, this has meant that although such rewards appear frequently in experimental protocols, little attention has been paid to the merits of reinforcing desirable behavior with positive reinforcers. The problem is that it is difficult to deliver food immediately after the horse offers a desirable response. Therefore devices that instantly deliver rewards to the mouth allow the time between performance of the desired behavior and its reinforcement to be minimized, effectively enhancing the speed of learning.

Food is not the only reward that can be used. The other obvious one is water, when given to subjects that have been kept thirsty. For example, although questionable on humane grounds, this approach is acknowledged as one of many effective means of motivating a horse to enter a trailer.

Reinforcers can be either primary or secondary. Primary reinforcers are any resources that animals have evolved to seek. If the animal's motivation is correctly predicted, food, water, sex, play, liberty, sanctuary and companionship can all be used as primary reinforcers. Secondary reinforcers are stimuli that are not intrinsically rewarding but that have become associated with the kind of primary resources listed above. These associations make great sense in evolutionary terms since an auditory, olfactory or visual cue that has become reliably linked with a primary reinforcer will hold an animal's interest much longer than a neutral stimulus.

Consider the way horses are often praised with tactile stimuli: they can either be scratched at the withers or patted on the neck. Horses have evolved to find grooming one another rewarding. Indeed, when horses indulge in the familiar 'I'll scratch your back if you scratch mine' occupation, reduced heart rates suggest that they may be getting pleasure or stress reduction from the stimulation. So, a scratch on the correct part of the withers can represent a primary reinforcer. By comparison, the far more common practice of patting horses on the neck is reinforcing only if the owner has coupled the pat with something pleasant.[2] Because horses have not evolved to be motivated to behave in certain ways for pats on their necks, the intervention has to be conditioned as a secondary reinforcer.

REINFORCEMENT SCHEDULES

Until a behavior is firmly fixed as a conditioned behavioral response, the trainer must be consistent in applying signals and in granting rewards. If consistent reinforcement is not provided for correct responses, the horse's behavior becomes unpredictable. As we see in Chapter 13, this is especially important when using pressure/release pairings. Horses cannot be expected to learn well if exposed to delayed reinforcement, as they do not relate the reinforcement to the behavior. Immediate comfort or immediate relief from discomfort is what works for horses.

Once a behavior is consistently elicited as a conditioned response, it can be enhanced by means of a variable reward schedule. The desired behavior can then be rewarded unpredictably. It is also necessary to obtain the same results in multiple locations in order for the behavior to become generalized and for context specificity (see later) to be overcome.

Myers & Mesker[38] showed that a horse could respond to different fixed-ratio positive reinforcement schedules (in which partial reinforcement is delivered on the basis of the number of correct responses made) and fixed-interval positive reinforcement schedules (in which reinforcement only becomes available again after some specified time has elapsed). They reported that few reinforcements were required under each new presentation schedule to get predictable response rates from the horse. Their results ranked horses' responses to the different reinforcement schedules as similar to the responses of tropical aquarium fish, guinea pigs and octopi.

SHAPING BEHAVIOR

Although Skinner's findings with his lever-pressing rats may seem to represent common sense, his school of thought has produced some intriguing principles. Perhaps one of the simplest yet most powerful of these is shaping. This is the concept of reinforcing successive approximations to the final response. The technique allows a trainer to move from a situation where it is impossible to reinforce a desired response (because that response never occurs) to one where the response is occurring, being reinforced, and increasing in reliability. If trainers wish to reinforce particular responses, they can either wait for the behavior to occur spontaneously, which can be readily reinforced if the behavior occurs frequently, or they can shape the behavior pattern. In seeking to train complex behaviors or those that occur uncommonly in an animal, the trainer will usually opt to reinforce successive approximations of the final behavior (Fig. 4.9).

Crucially, shaping relies on sparing and grading the reinforcement so that the animal does not stagnate. So, for example, when training a horse to approach a target (in so-called target training) a reward is given only when the horse travels closer to the paddle or stick (or whatever is being used as a target) or does so with more speed than on previous occasions. A common characteristic among good trainers is their ability to recognize an opportunity to reinforce improved 'approximations'. While poorer trainers complain that their animals fail to understand what is being asked of them and feel that the animals have peaked in their training, superior trainers have the sense and patience to capitalize on each tiny improvement as the only way of moving toward the final response.

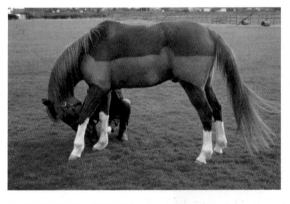
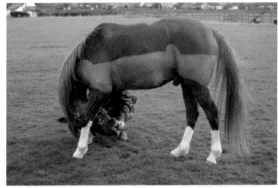
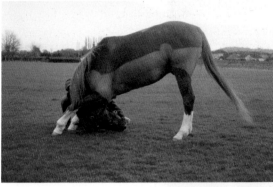
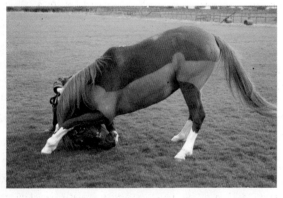

Figure 4.9 Arabian gelding being shaped to bow. Generally, at each successive iteration of the behavior, the reward is withheld until the horse shows an improvement on its previous best. (Reproduced by permission of the University of Bristol, Department of Clinical Veterinary Science.)

While shaping a new behavior or, for that matter, modifying an existing one, it is important to reward target behaviors as soon as they happen. Any delay in rewarding the improvement will lessen the effect of that reward. This may be because it allows the subject to perform another response during the delay interval and it is then potentially this response that is reinforced. An example might be rewarding a horse for jumping a fence very cleanly by giving him a sugar cube. To administer the sugar while riding, you would have to bend forward and place it in front of the horse's mouth. Since this could not be achieved safely you would probably slow down or even halt. Instead of learning to jump ever more cleanly, the horse would predictably learn to slow down and halt, these being the behaviors closest to the reward.

CLICKER TRAINING

Perhaps the most popular example of a secondary reinforcer is the sound made by a so-called 'clicker', the handy device used by thousands of trainers worldwide.[39] Clickers develop an association for the animal that allows the trainer to *bridge* the gap between the time at which an animal performs a response correctly and the arrival of a primary reinforcer (most commonly a food reward). Essentially the clicker comes to mean 'Yes, that's good – expect a reward any second now'. When a clicker is first used, the correct association is established by making the sound just before giving a delicious reward. Repetition assures the animal of the signal's reliability.

As discussed in subsequent chapters, clicker training can be extremely helpful in remedial behavior modification. Moreover, after traditional operant conditioning has established desirable responses, clicker training is suitable for refining them (Fig. 4.10). The benefits of positive reinforcement as applied in clicker training should not be underestimated. There are many impressive accounts of successful clicker training, including the use of the device to train a sour dressage horse to work with its ears pricked forward. It would be interesting to examine the effect of such a cosmetically palliative approach on the physiological stress responses in such animals. If nothing else, clicker training may be more humane than traditional negative reinforcement training. With clicker training, 'what you click is what you get', therefore if your observations and timing are not perfect you will inadvertently shape some behaviors you do not want. So poor timing can make clicker training ineffective. In contrast, poor timing in traditional negative reinforcement training can amount to abuse (see Ch. 13).

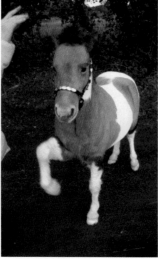

Figure 4.10 Pony being clicker trained to perform Spanish Walk.

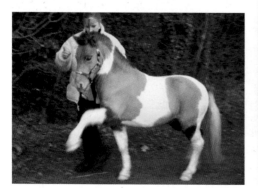

Any secondary reinforcer can be instituted in this way. The only significant feature of a commercial clicker device is that the sound it makes is sharp and distinctive. The brevity and clarity of a clicker facilitates precise reinforcement of brief behaviors, such as the bringing forward of the ears. Being pocket-sized or attachable to keyrings, clickers are convenient, but by no means unique. Indeed, as long as they cannot be confused with words that appear in common parlance, human vocalizations (so-called clicker words) are even more readily available. Some horses are fearful of the click per se and are therefore candidates for such alternative secondary reinforcers. The use of clicker training principles for shaping and modifying unwanted behaviors, such as reluctance to load, merits serious consideration. By deconstructing a response we can demonstrate to the horse that its fears may have been unjustified.

Secondary reinforcers are most effectively established when presented before or up until the presentation of a primary reinforcer. Simultaneous presentation of a reward and a novel secondary stimulus is less likely to work because the primary reinforcer will block or overshadow the new stimulus. Similarly, presentation of the secondary stimulus after the primary reinforcer is unproductive, because although an association will exist between the two, it does not help the animal to predict the arrival of a reward.

The speed or strength of learning increases with the size and attractiveness of the reinforcer. This is why horses will learn to run faster to the sound of a rattling bucket than they will to the rustling of a haynet. Many horses respond well to carrots as the primary reinforcer in a clicker training protocol but only if carrots are not routinely offered in regular meals. The relationship between motivation and the reinforcing value of any food should be considered here. However, as we have seen, a degree of familiarity is altogether desirable since some horses will not work for novel foods regardless of their apparent suitability. So when selecting primary reinforcers experienced trainers observe the horse's responses to determine the reinforcing value of a novel reward.

Horses show a rapid decline in interest in responding for the secondary reinforcer only, and

the temporal link between primary and secondary reinforcers is also critical.[39] Thus the fundamental rules of learning theory apply, and trainers who build the firmest association between the primary and secondary reinforcers by ensuring that the 'clicker never lies' (i.e. it always predicts the arrival of a primary reinforcer) can most effectively shape desirable behaviors. The use of secondary reinforcement seems to increase a horse's interest in performing novel tasks,[39] and this creativity in the horse's approach to problem solving accounts for the growing appeal of clicker training in behavior modification programs, especially where traditional remedial approaches have failed (see Chs 13 and 15).

When shaping alternative responses, practitioners find that continuous reinforcement schedules rapidly increase the response rate of new behaviors.[39] However, once the behavior has been shaped and is under stimulus control (see below), intermittent reinforcement can be used (with a resultant increase in the resistance to extinction).

CONTIGUITY

The principle of contiguity states that events that are temporally close will become associated. Giving a sugar lump to a horse two minutes after a pat on the neck will not develop a useful association. The lump has to arrive within seconds of the pat if the latter is to become reinforcing.

The time interval between stimuli is not necessarily the most important criterion for the establishment of an association. Events far apart in time can still be associated as long as there is a high predictive link between them. The best example of this is food aversion learning that helps animals to avoid food items that have previously made them ill. Novel flavors are more likely to be associated with later sickness and therefore the horses may be alert to this possibility when they consume novel foods.

Operant conditioning has been used to indicate the behavioral effects of drugs. Since the reward is usually food, a decrease in the rate of responding suggests that the drug administered is either a depressant or an anorexic agent. Food aversion learning has also been used by scientists interested in the consequences of proprietary drugs on horse welfare. The aversive effect of drugs can be calibrated by the degree to which food associated with it is subsequently avoided.

PUNISHMENT

Horses can learn from both unpleasant and pleasant experiences. Haag et al[40] found that there was significant correlation between a pony's rank in learning ability to navigate through a maze for a food reward and its rank in learning ability to avoid mild electric shocks. When shocks are used to teach a horse how to navigate through a maze, subjects take significantly longer to make their choices than horses who were not punished and simply found their way through by trial-and-error. So punishment can stifle creativity and impede a horse's innate problem-solving skills. One should bear this phenomenon in mind when horses that are familiar with human handlers are asked to solve problems in the presence of humans. It is possible that horses have learned that it is best not to offer creative solutions to problems since this can lead to punishment.

Punishment decreases the likelihood that a behavior will be repeated. Positive punishments are those that are instinctively recognized by the horse as detrimental. For example, a horse who bites at a human's arm and in doing so impacts on a spiky object concealed in the sleeve, experiences a positive punishment that is clearly linked to the unacceptable action. Negative punishments involve the removal of desired things in response to particular behaviors. In free-ranging adult horses, resources are rarely withdrawn as a result of an individual's behavior. This may be why negative punishment is not an important feature of equestrianism. The chain of association between events is weaker if the events involve removal of consequences.

Negative reinforcement involves the conditioning of preceding signals that predict the potentially aversive stimulus. Punishment, on the other hand, is more complex in that it represents a form of backward chaining because any signaling of

the aversive stimulus is either absent or follows the undesirable behavior. Trainers who use punishment to eliminate undesirable behavior must ensure that the wrong association is not created. The unthinking rider who thrashes a horse for knocking down a fence runs the risk of associating fence jumping, be it clean or sloppy, with being hit. Rather than correctly associating a painful consequence with the undesirable behavior, many animals learn to fear the trainer or the training area (Fig. 4.11).

Despite some of the problems that are associated with the use of punishers, they remain popular. Free-ranging equids communicate with their companions using aggression and reliable threats of aggression. This may make horses innately tolerant of such negative stimuli but is no excuse for physical abuse by humans.

The punishment procedure makes the onset of an aversive stimulus contingent on a particular

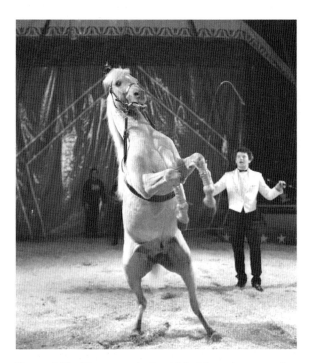

Figure 4.11　Horses can be taught that the only means of escaping aversive stimuli (the whip) is to rear. Discomfort is apparent on the face of this animal as the tight side reins thwart his attempts to balance on his hindlegs. (Reproduced with permission of the Captive Animals Protection Society.)

response. The punishment procedure may or may not lead to a reduction in the response. The situation is complicated because the punishing stimulus also elicits other responses that may actually increase the performance of the 'punished response'. Whipping a horse for bolting will usually serve to rocket it forth once more. Bit pressure is usually increased prior to such whippings and with discomfort in both the mouth and on the flank, the horse enters a conflict situation (see Ch. 13).

Presentation of aversive stimuli will usually produce an overall suppression of behavior in general. Therefore, a reduction in performance of a response may have nothing to do with the specific link between the response and the 'punishing' stimulus. So, in beaten horses, confusion and flight responses are more common than useful, learned associations.

The effectiveness of punishments is limited by a number of other factors, including punishment intensity. The more motivated an animal is to perform an action, the greater the intensity of the punishment required to stop it.

Warnings of punishment could be useful, just as clickers are predictors of reinforcement. Therefore it seems likely that both horses and riders could benefit from a device that warns them of the imminent rein pressure. There is evidence that horses can learn to take evasive action when they hear noises that warn of aversive stimuli. Early data suggest that reins that stretch and make a noise before reaching the limit of their elasticity and causing discomfort in the mouth are good for horse welfare and indeed rider education.

CONTINGENCY

Contingency is a measure of the extent to which two events are related, ranging from complete consistency – so that if one event occurs then the other will follow, even if after a considerable time – through completely independent, to a consistent negative relationship where the occurrence of one event indicates the non-occurrence of the other. Most forms of conditioning, except perhaps taste aversion learning (see later), require both contingency and contiguity (closeness in time) between two events (in the case of classical conditioning) or between a response and a reinforcer (in the case of operant conditioning). Contiguity and contingency should not be confused with one another. As indicated above, it is possible for there to be a very strong contingency between two events that do not occur close together in time. Conversely two events can sometimes occur close together in time but overall there can be a weak or zero contingency between them (independence). In many ways one can think of contingencies as consistent links between events that transcend time. Effective training requires the application of both contiguity and contingency.

The contingency between the response of the horse and its subsequent reinforcement relies on an attentive trainer. To use clicker training as an example: effective linkage of the primary and the secondary reinforcers relies on the arrival of a primary reinforcer being contingent on the sound of a click but, as we have seen, contingency varies with the consistency of the training method. Contingency reaches 100% when the 'clicker never lies'. If a food reward arrives without a click or the clicker is sounded without the subsequent arrival of food then the contingency is weakened.

GENERALIZATION AND DISCRIMINATION

Pavlov found that almost any stimulus could act as a conditioned stimulus provided it did not produce too strong a response of its own. In very hungry dogs, even painful stimuli such as electric shocks delivered to the paws, which initially caused flinching and distress, quite soon evoked salivation if paired with food.

A colored board in front of Pavlov's dogs could be used to present visual images with an infinite variety of colors and shapes. Pavlov carried out exhaustive tests using this apparatus and a variety of tactile, visual or auditory stimuli. He found that if a dog was conditioned to salivate when a pure tone of perhaps 800 Hz was sounded, it would also salivate but to a lesser extent when other tones were given. This is now known as generalization.

The dog generalized its responses to include stimuli similar to the conditioned one, and the more similar they were the more the dog salivated.

Generalization

Stimulus generalization occurs when a response reinforced in the presence of one stimulus is also elicited by similar stimuli. For example, a horse might be trained to nudge an orange panel for a reward. If the color of the panel is changed to yellow the horse will still nudge, though possibly at a lower rate. We capitalize on stimulus generalization when we use mature educated horses (so-called schoolmasters) to educate novice riders. The horse generalizes the rider's cues to others it remembers from previous, preferably better, riders and obligingly executes the required maneuver. Generalization is at play when horses learn to offer the same responses that they have developed in the home schooling *manège* to, say, a dressage arena at a competition. This demonstrates that the trained maneuvers are not context specific to the stimuli that surrounded the animal during its early learning at home. Barrier trials in racing are useful in a similar fashion since they give young race-horses the opportunity to transfer appropriate responses from starting stalls at the training center to starting stalls in general.

Stimulus generalization works against us when we encounter horses that 'hate vets'. Such animals have learned to generalize the stimuli from one human wearing veterinary smells and bearing needles to all humans that meet the same criteria. But by recognizing and mimicking the stimuli horses use to identify vets and making appropriate associations with them, owners can train horses to tolerate and even enjoy vets.

Discrimination

The opposite process to generalization is discrimination. Horses naturally discriminate to some extent, otherwise they would respond equally to all stimuli. Discrimination can be accelerated if, as well as rewarding the right stimuli, the horse is slightly punished when it responds to others. This

is called conditioned discrimination and has been of enormous benefit in working out the sensory capabilities of animals (see the case study of Rascal performing a visual discrimination task in Ch. 2).

Commands used to cue a behavior can be the product of discrimination. When a horse learns that certain cues set the stage for a specific response, the cues (i.e. the commands, signals or aids) are labeled discriminative stimuli and the horse is said to be under stimulus control. By rewarding horses for responding appropriately to stimuli that are less and less obvious, we can foster the power to discriminate between the stimuli that are rewarded and all other background information that would otherwise prevail. Discrimination is what allows us to train dogs to detect drugs, pigs to locate truffles and chickens to identify images of familiar feathered friends. A similar process is at play when we train horses to respond to smaller and smaller cues in training. To obey a trainer's leg signal to pirouette, a horse must first be persuaded to rotate on a much larger surface with the use of much less subtle stimuli. All horses can learn to discriminate. Unfortunately, however, only the good trainers learn to deliver cues with sufficient subtlety to capitalize on this ability.

Whether positive or negative, reinforcers are effective only if the recipient is motivated appropriately. Relative to normal or fat horses, poor body condition may make horses less likely to err in discrimination tasks for food rewards.[41] Rather than true learning ability differences, this seems to reflect the lack of motivation in replete horses.

Although the only data available are from experiments using stimuli such as cards and panels that are arguably less salient to horses than, say, grazing-related stimuli, the ability of horses to discriminate is impressive (for example, see Sappington & Goldman[42]). It appears that, although horses can learn complex discrimination problems based on sameness,[43] we have yet to show that they can generalize this learning to situations involving novel stimulus presentation.[44]

While stimuli that have become generalized may be ignored, those that are enhanced are more likely to elicit a response. Stimulus enhancement describes the process by which an animal's attention can be drawn toward a given stimulus and increase the animal's motivation to approach the stimulus.[45] For example, the sound of a rattling bucket will prompt experienced horses to approach the bucket and eat.

EXTINCTION

Extinction occurs if the learned response occurs but is no longer followed by reinforcement or if a conditioned stimulus is always presented without the unconditioned stimulus. The effect of these procedures is an eventual reduction in response strength, as measured, for example, in rate of response. If horses do not get their expected rewards, they are less likely to behave in ways that have previously paid off. The behaviors drop out and extinction is said to have taken place. This is what happens when horses that nip and nuzzle humans for food stop doing so because they are never rewarded. Often extinction is accompanied by not simply an absence of the learned responses but a reversion to innate behaviors. Occasionally animals may experiment at this point by adopting sequences of other learned behaviors in an attempt to acquire rewards. Practitioners should plan ahead to determine which of these should be reinforced.

Because extinction does not occur in a vacuum, context-specific stimuli that were present during learning of the unwelcome response can retard extinction. This explains why behavior-modification programs that advocate removal of perceived rewards work best if imposed at the same time as a fundamental environmental shift such as a change of stable.

Frustration effect

There are some intriguing outcomes associated with extinction. Early in extinction it is usual for a so-called 'frustration effect' to occur. This describes the way responses usually get transiently more frequent before they disappear. For example, rather like a human repeatedly pressing the 'on' switch of a faulty television set, a horse that has superstitiously learned to kick the stable door to get food will kick it harder if the feeding delivery is delayed.

One theory proposes that the subject responds faster because it is 'frustrated'. To avoid misinterpreting an extinction-based behavior-modification program as a failure, it is important for therapists to be aware that the frustration effect occurs.

Spontaneous recovery

Presentation of the conditioned stimulus alone causes extinction. Extinction can apply to any behavior that occurs and is no longer reinforced. Both welcome and unwelcome behavioral responses will weaken in the absence of reinforcement. If, after extinction has been completed, the animal is given a break from training and then presented with the conditioned stimulus again, the previously extinguished response may suddenly reappear.[30] This rebound in response strength after a 'rest', following extinction, is called spontaneous recovery. This possibility is sometimes overlooked in behavior therapy designed to eliminate unwelcome behaviors by extinction. If an undesirable behavior makes a return, personnel may forget the strength of the original response when they compare current behavior with previous behavior. So, when the response recurs after a long absence, the owner's conclusion may be slightly damning with remarks like 'the removal of rewards hasn't helped' or 'the animal has regressed'. In fact, this is the typical pattern found in extinction. This is particularly important with originally fearful responses that have been modified by counterconditioning because these responses can show spontaneous recovery if reinforcement is withheld. To prevent the original fearful response recurring, the trainer must continue to expose the animal to the relevant stimuli from time to time.

MEMORY

Memory is the retention or storage of information and therefore the basis for all higher forms of learning. The laying down of memory traces is considered to occur in stages, but can be thought of as a continuum. Fraser[46] rather boldly suggests that the length of time an animal can remember a specific signal of training or command can be taken as some measure of intelligence. However, horses that learn a task most readily are not necessarily those that have the best memories.[5]

Sensory memory refers to memory traces formed within the sensory areas of the CNS (see Ch. 3) whenever any sensory receptor is activated. It has been estimated that only about 2% of sensory input is ever committed to permanent memory. For input to pass from sensory memory to short-term memory there must be some kind of response to the experience. The trace is more likely to be stored if the experience was bad (the speed with which horses learn to avoid electric fences is pertinent here). Animals under the influence of sedatives, tranquilizers, etc. have their sensory experiences dulled and therefore have great problems remembering new experiences. Veterinarians do well to remember this before they prescribe psychoactive drugs for behavior modification. This explains the poor results obtained when horses that are fearful of, say, clippers are treated with acepromazine or detomidine; they show no attenuation of the fear response when presented with clippers after the effects of the sedative have worn off. Similarly, studies on the effect of reserpine on unhandled yearlings[47] suggest that the attenuating effect it has on heart rate response to the presence of handlers is transient. This is state-dependent memory. There is also place-dependent memory which is considerable in horses. When teaching a young horse a new response it is useful to go back to the same spot in the arena to rehearse it. Because confusion often prevails when an animal is in a highly emotional state, an upset and anxious horse does not learn desired responses as well as a calm subject. Hence classical riders advocate the practice of the systematic elimination of resistance. This approach requires that the horse must be calm before being cued to perform. After stress, conflict or confusion during training, the good trainer waits for the calm to return before resuming work. Even though classical riders often apply very subtle stimuli, one can see how the return of calm would be less elusive if one were using positive reinforcement.

We know that primary memory involves continuous neural activity because if anything interrupts the activity (for example, a blow to the head,

drugs, unexpected interruption) then the short-term memory trace is lost. Short-term memory appears to have a temporal sequence, so what goes in first will be replaced by later inputs if the memory is not repeated (learned). This repetition is essential for pushing the memory into the long-term stage.

The mechanism for the long-term storage of memory traces is thought to be biochemical. Being physical, they do not depend on sustained neural activity. Specifically, long-term memory depends on alteration in gene expression, which influences the formation of either persistent proteins or nerve growth factor.

There are many impressive accounts, anecdotal and scientific, of the resilience of equine memory traces.[1,27,48,49] An established means of testing memory in equids is to offer 20 pairs of patterns (Fig. 4.12). The horse is taught that regardless of its position, one of each pair will always yield a food reward when pressed. Deterioration depends on the extent to which horses are taught new associations and perhaps new apparatus in the interim,

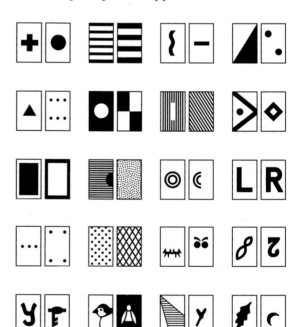

Figure 4.12 Twenty pairs of patterns used for equine memory tests, including those by Dixon[48] and Voith.[49] To obtain food the horse had to select the patterns that appear on the left of each pair in this illustration.

but the reported frequency of correct choices when the same apparatus is presented after 6 months is approximately 85%. Horses and ponies compare well with donkeys and elephants using this experimental paradigm.[10]

An interesting phenomenon is the effect of a period without conditioning, because the temporal distribution of training trials influences equine learning abilities.[50] While this is challenged by data showing that horses learn more quickly and make fewer errors if they are trained daily,[51] it accounts for the effectiveness and popularity of turn-out or spelling periods during the early education of horses, even though plausible mechanisms have yet to be investigated.

The robust nature of equine memory helps to explain the poor performance of horses in discrimination reversal tests[3,33] in which, for example, a turn to the left is reinforced for a given number of trials and then the reverse, a turn to the right, is required.

ADDITIONAL TOPICS IN EQUINE LEARNING

As we begin to appreciate the complexities of studying equine learning scientifically, the role of cognition in adaptive behavior is becoming clearer.

LEARNING SETS

Horses learning to use experimental apparatus such as in the pairs discrimination tests in Figure 4.12 often take time to grasp the concept of discriminating between operant panels. Once they have established the learning set, their responses become more rapid and accurate. Such horses are described as having learned to learn. When they build on a basic groundwork and then begin training more high school maneuvers, dressage trainers report a similar phenomenon. That is, having reached a certain understanding about what is being asked of them, educated horses learn to pay attention to yet finer stimuli and climb a steep learning curve that takes them to Grand Prix level.

INSIGHT VERSUS SIMPLE LEARNING

Using insight, an animal can arrive at a solution without trial and error. The possibility of such complex learning has to be approached with caution since apparently complex patterns of learning can often be explained in terms of simple associative learning. Take, for example, the story of Clever Hans, a horse that lived in Austria in the 1900s.[52] Hailed as an equine arithmetic genius, Hans appeared to be able to count and do basic algebra. When set any puzzle with a number as its answer, Hans would begin to count out the solution with his hoof. He would never tap too many times; always stopping at the right number. This looked like complex learning and was the subject of detailed scientific scrutiny. His owner, Baron von Osten, was justifiably proud of him and their fame spread. They were fêted far and wide until a panel of scientists assembled to determine the status of the horse's IQ. By placing a screen between the horse and any observers, they found his accuracy was entirely dependent on being able to see his audience. A question was posed and the counting commenced. The answer was reached and the counting continued. On and on it went because the horse had received no cue to stop. Hans had learned that he would be rewarded if his foot movements stopped when he detected subtle behavioral changes in human observers. These cues reliably emerged whenever he was set a problem and, of course, they always coincided with the human's anticipation of the arrival of the right answer. It is believed that von Osten leaned forward as Hans approached the correct number and adopted a more upright posture when it had been reached. Furthermore it is thought that his brimmed hat (Fig. 4.13b,c) helped to accentuate this visual cue. Maybe the observers smiled, grimaced, braced themselves or changed their breathing patterns. Whatever they did constituted a sufficient cue for the horse to stop counting.

So, rather than complex learning, simple associative learning could explain the illusion. Hans was responding to tiny physical changes in the behavior of his trainer and observers as they became more tense and anxious that he was about

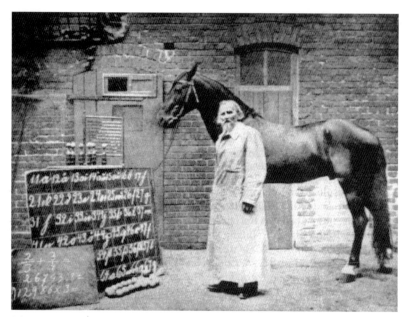

(a)

Figure 4.13 (a) Clever Hans and Baron von Osten. (b–e) Clever Hans undertaking a series of tests intended to demonstrate problem solving without trial-and-error.[52] (Reproduced with permission.)

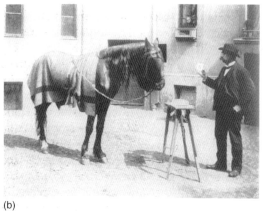

(b)

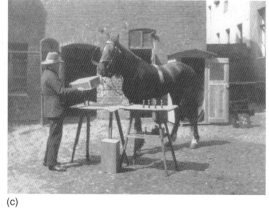

(c)

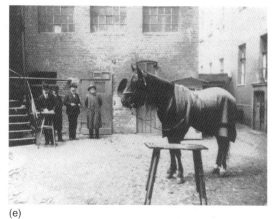

(d)

(e)

to count too many times and disappoint them. He was declared a fraud even though he was in fact a brilliant judge of minute detail who had trained himself to spot these cues and earn rewards. This should serve as testament to visual acuity in the horse. The same principle has subsequently been used many times in entertainment to give the illusion of such unlikely academic brilliance.

MAZE TESTS

Maze tests have been used extensively to measure the learning ability of animals. These typically involve a T-maze, in which an animal is presented with a choice to go left or right; the wrong choice runs into a dead end, the correct choice to an exit out to food, water or an area with other animals (Fig. 4.14).[53] Mazes have merit because they allow the animal to demonstrate its ability without human presence and thus avoid the Clever Hans effect. The absence of humans helps to eliminate other operator effects in horses, especially those that have been previously handled. It is

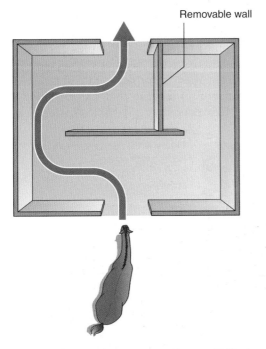

Removable wall

Figure 4.14 A horse about to enter a T-maze. (© Stephen Budiansky. Redrawn, with permission, from Budiansky.[53])

worth noting, however, that the absence of humans is far from absolute in maze studies since they have to lead the horse to the starting point in the maze and retrieve it at the end point. It is important, therefore, to establish baseline results for each individual in an attempt to control for horses that, for example, may prefer not to be left or those that dislike being caught.

Differences between types of horses in maze-learning ability are intriguing. Foals learned which way to turn in a maze in fewer trials than their dams,[54] and the adult horses were particularly slow to learn a reversal, i.e. turning right after learning to turn left. Houpt et al[54] investigated how a foal's early experience with its dam could influence its learning ability. Using a single-choice maze, they compared the learning abilities of foals raised with their dams with those of orphan foals. Although the orphan foals spent more time in the maze during their first exposure to it, the learning abilities of the two groups did not differ.

Previously unhandled and extensively handled horses learned less quickly in a maze than moderately handled horses.[22] This may have been because the previously unhandled horses were still adjusting to being handled, and the extensively handled horses were dependent on human contact to show them the way. In contrast Marinier & Alexander[1] found no correlation between horses' abilities to learn a maze and the extent to which they had been handled earlier. Maze studies suggest that a social rank does not predict problem-solving ability. A study of artificially reared and naturally reared foals[55] that showed the latter group to take longer to solve a maze problem, alluded to the role of dependence on a leader. Perhaps we have yet to recognize the role of bonded pairs in problem-solving situations relevant to free-ranging equids. Other explanations for differences in learning ability in a maze also include the motivation for the reward and inhibition resulting from nervousness.

Many horses begin maze trials with a clear preference for one side or the other. An example comes from Kratzer et al[33] who allowed 37 yearling geldings, fed diets with a range of protein contents, to wander through a T-maze on a daily basis. At the beginning of the experiment when the horses were allowed to freely walk through the maze five times with both exits open, 5 of the 37 horses chose the right side every time, and 5 chose the left side every time. For the next 5 days, the right side was open and the left side was blocked. Therefore horses with a left preference had to return to the bifurcation before completing their trip through the maze. Although on the fifth day of the experiment the mean number of wrong turns per trial fell from 0.65 to 0.27, about 20% of the youngsters still turned left as their initial choice on entering the maze.

SOCIAL LEARNING

The transmission of new information and behavioral strategies among animals is slowly becoming more clearly understood. When we consider the transfer of information between animals it is important to distinguish between social facilitation, stimulus enhancement and true cultural transmission. In social facilitation, innate behaviors are initiated or increased in rate or frequency by the presence of another animal carrying out those behaviors. Horses, for example, are more likely to drink when they see others drinking. Stimulus enhancement is the ethological term that describes the ability of one animal (the so-called demonstrator) to draw the attention of another animal (the observer) to the location of reinforcement opportunity rather than an activity per se. These hard-wired copying responses commonly found in

social animals are distinct from true cultural transmission, which is considered a higher mental ability and describes the observational learning of a novel behavior without trial-and-error experience.

This is taking us into the realms of what is known as observational learning and allelomimetic behavior. In laboratory settings, a variety of species, including chickens, grey parrots, quails, ravens, cats, octopi and chimpanzees, have been shown to pass information about foraging strategies from one individual to another. It makes sense for offspring to learn from their parents and for social animals to learn from one another, for example, what food is safe to consume (see Ch. 8).

As social animals with excellent vision, one would predict that horses would use observations to improve their biological fitness. It makes sense that animals that conform to a form of social order should be able to learn from pre-trained conspecifics; for example, young farm horses were traditionally harnessed alongside a steady mature plough horse to be taught verbal driving commands (Fig. 4.15). But this is associative and not necessarily observational learning. While horses seem good at hard-wired copying, there is no empirical evidence of true cultural transmission. Controlled studies in the horse have provided some evidence that stimulus enhancement may result from the behavior of demonstrator horses as they approach and interact with experimental apparatus that delivers food (Fig. 4.16).[56] However, they have failed to demonstrate

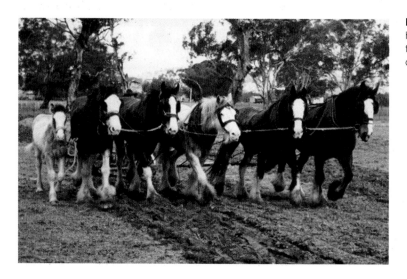

Figure 4.15 Schoolmasters can be hitched with youngsters to assist in the training of draft horses. (Photograph courtesy of Les Holmes.)

that observational learning enhances an individual's ability to perform an operant task[57] or make a choice between two feeding sites.[56] As such they have challenged the notion that stereotypies can be acquired by mimicry.

Studies in other species demonstrate that animals do not observe all conspecifics with the same enthusiasm. It may be that we have failed to ask the right questions of horses that are appropriately related in terms of rank, kinship or affiliation to demonstrators. There are likely to be serious limitations on what can be learned by observation. Feeding behaviors are more likely to be transmitted than those such as maintenance behaviors with less obvious proximate advantages to the performer. Glibly one might add that if horses learned to respond to riders by observing other horses being ridden, dressage arenas would most surely have been constructed with gallery-style stabling all around them.

Obedience trainers report that motivation is enhanced in dogs that are allowed to observe others working with their trainer. This reflects dogs' motivation to play (part of the so-called 'will to please') and the increasing use of rewards, especially toys, in their training. Although the opportunity to observe has little effect on the dogs' ability to complete a task, it certainly seems to enhance their desire to get involved. The equivalent in horses will continue to elude us as long as we persist in using only negative reinforcement. The laudable use of educated horses in training novices to jump is sadly flawed as an example of effective use of observational learning in horse training because it relies on the youngsters' motivation to follow (other horses) rather than to jump per se.

ERROR-FREE LEARNING

In operant-conditioning, the most humane exposure of an animal to correction seems to arise in so-called error-free learning, in which circumstances are modified to reduce the chances of errors being offered. For example, in training horses to jump obstacles, a jumping lane can be used to instill the behavior pattern of negotiating the obstacle without testing the opportunities for evasion and acquiring inappropriate responses. Unfortunately arranging schooling sessions so that opportunities for errors do not arise is far easier said than done. Given this reality and the likelihood that horses are learning all the time, it pays to bear in mind the following maxim:

> Just because you don't intend to teach a horse something doesn't mean that you won't; and just because you are not aware of having taught a horse something doesn't mean that you didn't.[58]

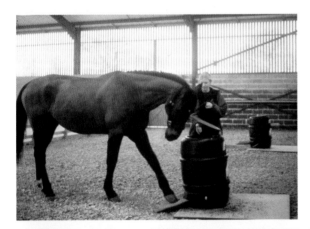

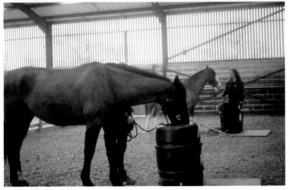

Figure 4.16 Results of tests of observational learning in horses have proved disappointing when compared with those for other domestic species. (Reproduced by permission of the University of Bristol, Department of Clinical Veterinary Science.)

INFLUENCES ON LEARNING

BREED DIFFERENCES IN NORMAL BEHAVIOR

When the learning ability of different breeds is compared we do well to consider breed differences in normal behavior that may create a bias.

While many of the behavioral differences among breeds reflect the uses for which they have been bred[59] (see Table 1.2 on p. 8), the origins of others are rather more obscure. For example, Icelandic ponies are said to have a particularly good homing instinct, though it is not clear whether they have advanced skills or a heightened motivation to return to their home range.

Bagshaw et al[60] reported a breed effect of an oral dose of L-tryptophan on horses' reactions to 15 minutes of acute isolation stress. Arabians were more active and vocalized more in isolation compared with Standardbreds. This study also showed that the Arabian had lower resting serotonin concentrations than the Standardbreds and that Arabians on a separate farm had lower serotonin than 10 Swedish Warmbloods fed the same feed and housed under the same conditions.[60]

If we assume that all horses are equally able to deliver signals from within the equine ethogram, some interesting differences seem to emerge in the extent to which they signal. Standardbreds have been noted to be more likely to demonstrate snapping behavior in estrus than Arabians.[61] This intriguing finding merits further exploration. It is possible that this is a form of displacement behavior that masks behavioral conflict. When 224 adult riding horses' responses to humans were observed and scored on the basis of their posture, French Saddlebreds showed friendly behavior more often than Anglo-arabs, whereas Thoroughbreds were more indifferent.[62]

In addition to the intriguing, intrinsic behavioral differences between breeds, breed differences in learning ability of horses have been reported by several authors. Mader & Price[63] found that Quarter Horses learned a visual discrimination task more readily than Thoroughbreds, a finding attributed to the relative distractability of the Thoroughbreds. However, the importance of the experimental apparatus in reducing fearfulness may have been confirmed by Sappington et al,[3] who found no difference in the learning ability of Quarter Horses, Thoroughbreds and Arabians. Hot-blooded and warm-blooded horses learned an operant task less quickly than cold-blooded horses.[56] As with any comparison of problem-solving exercises for a reward, it pays to consider whether the motivation to access the resource is all one ends up testing. Thoroughbreds are often fussy feeders. Being generally less motivated to eat they may be disinclined to solve problems for food rewards. Thoroughbreds are also more reactive (see the discussion of emotionality in the subsection on temperament, below) and therefore may take longer to approach novel pieces of apparatus calmly. Also, because they tend to be stress susceptible, learning may be reduced as a result of generalized anxiety.

Some intriguing individual differences in temperament, in correlation with the height of facial whorls, have been reported. Horses with a single whorl above or between the eyes are said to be of an 'uncomplicated' nature whereas horses with a single whorl below the eyes are said to be 'unusually imaginative and intelligent'.[64,65] Notwithstanding the problems that arise when one attempts to measure intelligence, these reports merit thorough investigation because similar reports in cattle have been ratified by repeated studies.[66–68]

TEMPERAMENT

A number of temperament tests for horses have now been reported,[69–72] and it is possible that in combination they may form a suite of tests that may be useful in identifying the best horses for certain sorts of work.[73]

It is important to note that emotionality (or nervousness) has an influence on behavior. McCann et al[74] scored emotionality in 32 Quarter Horse yearlings based upon their response to a series of procedures, including standing in a chute, being identified and being released from the chute. The nervous yearlings tended to have a higher overall activity index than the normal yearlings. This correlated with heart rates. Escape tendencies, reactivity to people, behavior after release and overall emotionality contributed to the horses' being classified as highly nervous, nervous, normal or quiet. Emotionality of the horses affected their frequency of eating and drinking, defecation, locomotion and contact with the other members of the group.

It seems that the learning ability of an individual horse is profoundly influenced by emotionality.

Fortunately it is becoming clear that measurement of emotionality as an outcome of avoidance learning tests is possible and that early detection of this quality in yearlings gives a reliable prediction for life and is more consistent than responses in reward learning tests.[75] It may be that time spent grading young horses in this way could reap economic benefits for the industry in the long term.[75] Tailoring training schedules and ultimately jobs to meet the individual emotional profiles of horses rather than assuming that all of them can do a single form of work may save time and money. Having said that, care must be taken to avoid oversimplifying equine temperament tests, because they do not show significant interrelationships.[76] It is suggested that several different qualities of a horse's personality must be assessed before predictions of its working performance can be made with any confidence. So, tests used to predict a horse's performance as, say, a show-jumper must include its response to novel objects, handling, avoidance learning, reward learning and technique in free jumping.[76] The limitations of these assessments reflect the additional role of physical development, long-term training and the skill of the horse's future riders.[76]

Stallions and colts are generally less timid than mares and fillies.[77] This, along with the absence of reproductive cycles which have the potential to interrupt training schedules[78] and produce variability in competitive performance, accounts for male horses' being favored for show-jumping and eventing. Meanwhile, the dynamic presence of stallions predisposes them for work in elite dressage. Behavioral tests comparing saddle mares with draft mares showed the former to be more fearful, and indicated that pregnant mares demonstrated fewer fear responses than non-pregnant mares.[79]

There are anecdotal reports that dominant horses can be difficult to train because they are more likely than passive, subordinate animals to deploy evasions.[53] However, social dominance appears unrelated to learning ability in visual discrimination,[4] simple maze,[40,54] and avoidance learning tests,[40] suggesting that there is a need for more work in this domain. The individual differences in emotionality and trainability demand the collection of data from a battery of temperament tests.[23,77,78,80–82] Given the wastage that results from behavior problems and the advent of databases for logging the careers of sport-horses, it may be that the time is right for the FEI to develop an international model of breeding stock selection and agree upon a suite of tests that help select breeding stock on the basis of their being tolerant and trainable.

BREED DIFFERENCES IN ABNORMAL BEHAVIORS

Other differences among breeds include a predisposition to stereotypic behaviors. Horses may inherit both sensitivity to stressors and an ability to express a stereotypy.[83] Certain breeds are more prone to stereotypies than others. Usually these are also the breeds that are managed most intensively. Standardbreds are a possible exception here in that they are regularly stabled but show fewer stereotypies than similarly managed Thoroughbreds.[84] Thoroughbreds are particularly predisposed to cribbing and weaving, while Arabians tended to stall walk more.[85] These trends may be of significance to horse trainers since some retardation in learning (specifically persistence in tasks that are no longer rewarding) has been shown to accompany stereotypies in other species.[86]

SUMMARY OF KEY POINTS

- Learning facilitates adaptation to novel environments.
- Horses learn in the same way as other species.
- Horses are remarkably adaptable and tolerant.
- A good lesson provides a novel environment with stimuli to which the horse must learn appropriate responses.
- Habituation is the pivotal technique for overcoming flight responses.
- Most horse training involves operant conditioning.
- Shaping relies on the reserving of reinforcement until an improved response appears.
- Horses are generally trained with negative rather than positive stimuli, but innovations that accentuate the positive are being successfully developed.
- Clicker training offers a simple method for shaping appropriate responses and therefore provides a basic framework for retraining many unwelcome responses, especially in the unridden horse.
- Consistency and timing are the hallmarks of good training.

CASE STUDY

Star is a 6-year-old Thoroughbred being trained to work in the mounted police force. Mounted police perform a wide variety of duties, ranging from park and street patrols to parades, escorts, demonstrations and crowd control at special functions. Whenever on duty, police horses work in pairs and are required to remain calm and steady regardless of highly unusual circumstances. This requires the horse to be relaxed and unflappable, and to remain stationary unless instructed otherwise.

It is central to this training that the horse learns to ignore stimuli from crowds and respond only to those from its rider. It must stand firm under physical pressure from a noisy, pushy crowd and push a pedestrian when so directed by its rider. In other words, the strongest of equine instincts, the flight response, must be modified. When given signals, the horse must learn to follow them precisely, irrespective of jostling people, noises, lights and other distractions. Owners who have encountered unwelcome flight responses, including shying (see Ch. 15), could learn a great deal from this case study.

Horses newly acquired by the police force spend 6 weeks being evaluated by a general trainer. Selection is based on temperament and responsiveness. After 6 weeks of assessment, each horse is paired with a single rider for both training and operational work over a number of years, so that a bond develops between mount and rider that, over time, increases the horse's capacity to cope with new situations. The benefits of this appear in later schooling, where the horse is asked to perform unfamiliar tasks, facilitated through rider reassurance.

Initially, the horses are given basic education, including responses to leg, seat and rein signals. On command, they will then move sideways, forwards or backwards, and it is essential that they will stand for extended periods. They are handled daily during grooming and saddling so that they become accepting of contact on all areas, especially sensitive regions such as groin or head. The basic training program generally continues for 6 weeks before specific behaviors are trained.

There is considerable attrition in the selection and training of police remounts. Of the horses that commence training, 10% go on to perform all desired behaviors adequately while only 5% do extremely well. Flighty or nervous horses are unsuitable for crowd control. Mares and stallions are also avoided, as they are considered rather less predictable than geldings and are regarded as being easily distracted when working with other horses.

The horse is first cued to stand with a pedestrian in front of it touching its neck and chest. Next, the rider makes the horse stand still while the pedestrian applies pressure. Although horses have a tendency to move away from persistent pressure, the rider ensures that the horse responds only to commands from him. The horse is then prompted with leg and rein signals to advance toward the applied pressure, that is, toward the pedestrian.

The next stage is to simulate contact from multiple directions within a crowd by organizing several people to surround the horse (Fig. 4.17). The horse is again cued to respond only to the rider's signals, and walk forward as directed. Discrimination is required in that the horse must learn to discern between pressure on the flank that comes from the rider and that coming from other humans. The most difficult step is training the horse to continue walking even when pedestrians in front of it do not retreat. This is achieved by continuing to apply leg signals until the horse responds.

Gradually other distractions are added to the horse's repertoire, including pedestrians holding or waving strange objects, or broadcasting loud noises. When multiple novel stimuli are used together, the greatest risk is that they will frighten the horse. In other words, advancing too far too quickly is a real danger. If the horse behaves fearfully, the training reverts to the last step with which the horse was comfortable, before the problem step is attempted again. Verbal and physical reassurance from the rider is considered particularly important during this stage.

Training sessions are given every day, with the length of an average training session being

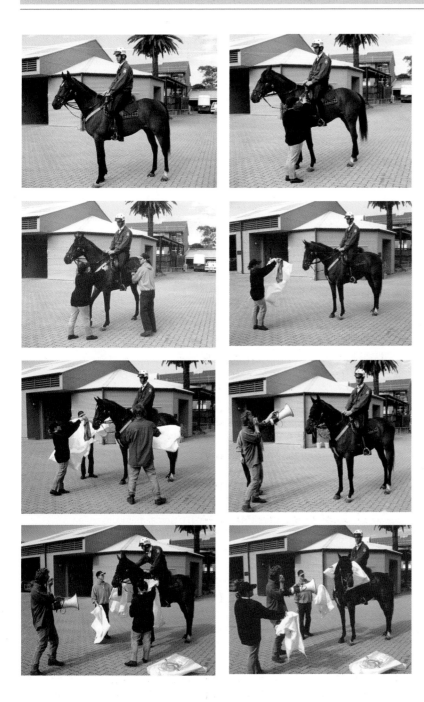

Figure 4.17 Police horse being trained for crowd control.

45 minutes. As horses are worked every day, it becomes an accepted routine, and no specific attempt is made to change motivation prior to a session.

Reinforcement of crowd control responses is not part of a police horse's routine training. Basic training is reinforced whenever horses are ridden, but specific behaviors are only revised in an intensive lead-up to a particular event. Training is then tailored specifically to that event, using appropriate lighting, sound effects and props.

REFERENCES

1. Marinier SL, Alexander AJ. The use of a maze in testing learning and memory in horses. Appl Anim Behav Sci 1994; 39:177–182.
2. Fraser AC. Restraint in the horse. Vet Rec 1967; 80(2):56–64.
3. Sappington BKF, McCall CA, Coleman DA, et al. A preliminary study of the relationship between discrimination reversal learning and performance tasks in yearling and 2-year-old horses. Appl Anim Behav Sci 1997; 53(3):157–166.
4. Mader DR, Price EO. Discrimination learning in horses: effects of breed, age and social dominance. J Anim Sci 1982; 50:962–965.
5. Wolff A, Hausberger M. Learning and memorisation of two different tasks: the effects of age, sex and sire. Appl Anim Behav Sci 1995; 46(3/4):137–143.
6. Miller RM. Imprint training the newborn foal. Colorado Springs: Western Horseman; 1998.
7. Waring GH. Socialisation and behavioral development of newborn American Saddlebred Horses. Paper presented to Deutschen Veterinarmedizinischen Geselschaft, Frieburg/Breisgau, 1972.
8. Hess E. Two conditions limiting control age for imprinting. J Comp Physiol Psychol 1959; 52,516.
9. Budiansky S. The nature of horses: exploring equine evolution, intelligence and behavior. New York: Free Press; 1997:171–174.
10. Waring GH. Horse behavior: the behavioral traits and adaptations of domestic and wild horses including ponies. Park Ridge, NJ: Noyes; 1983.
11. Williams JL, Friend TH, Toscano MJ, et al. The effects of early training sessions on the reactions of foals at 1, 2, and 3 months of age. Appl Anim Behav Sci 2002; 77(2):105–114.
12. Simpson BS. Neonatal foal handling. Appl Anim Behav Sci 2002; 78(2–4):309–323.
13. Diehl NK, Egan B, Tozer P. Intensive, early handling of neonatal foals: mare–foal interactions. Havemeyer Workshop on Horse Behavior and Welfare, Holar, Iceland, 2002:40–46.
14. Macleay JM. Smart horse: training your horse with the science of natural horsemanship. Fort Collins, CO: J and J Press; 2000:101–105.
15. Goodwin D, Hughes CF. Horse play. Havemeyer Workshop on Horse Behavior and Welfare, Holar, Iceland 2002:102–105.
16. Grzimek B. Ein Fohlen, des kein Pferd kannte. Z Tierpsychologie 1949; 6:391–405.
17. Williams M. Effect of artificial rearing on social behavior of foals. Equine Vet J 1974; 6:17–18.
18. Kelly AJ. Practical tips on fostering. In: Harris PA, Gomarsall GM, Davidson HPB, Green RE, eds. Proceedings of the BEVA specialist days on behaviour and nutrition. Newmarket, Suffolk, UK 1999:39–41.
19. Mal ME, McCall CA. The influence of handling during different ages on a halter training test in foals. Appl Anim Behav Sci 1996; 50(2):115–120.
20. Mal ME, McCall CA, Cummins KA, Newland MC. Influence of pre-weaning handling methods on post-weaning learning ability and manageability of foals. Appl Anim Behav Sci 1994; 40(3/4):187–195.
21. Visser EK, van Reenen CG, van der Werf JTN, et al. Heart rate and heart rate variability during a novel object test and a handling test in young horses. Physiol Behav 2002; 76(2):289–296.
22. Heird JC, Lennon AM, Bell RW. Effects of early experience on the learning ability of horses. J Anim Sci 1981; 53:1204–1209.
23. Jezierski T, Jaworski Z, Gorecka A. Effects of handling on behaviour and heart rate in Konik horses: comparison of stable and forest reared youngstock. Appl Anim Behav Sci 1999; 62:1–11.
24. Nicol CJ. Equine learning: progress and suggestions for future research. Appl Anim Behav Sci 2002; 78(2–4):193–208.
25. Gough MR. A note on the use of behavioural modification to aid clipping ponies. Appl Anim Behav Sci 1999; 63(2):171–175.
26. Casey RA. Recognising the importance of pain in the diagnosis of equine behavioural problems. In: Harris PA, Gomarsall GM, Davidson HPB, Green RE, eds. Proceedings of the BEVA specialist days on behaviour and nutrition. Newmarket, Suffolk, UK 1999:25–28.
27. McGreevy PD. Why does my horse …? London: Souvenir Press. 1996.
28. McGreevy PD, Boakes RA. Carrots and sticks: the principles of animal training. Cambridge: Cambridge University Press. In press.
29. Miller RM. Psychological effects of succinylcholine chloride immobilization on the horse. Vet Med/Small Anim Clin 1966; 61:941–944.
30. Lieberman DA. Learning: behavior and cognition. Pacific Grove, CA: Brooks/Cole; 1993.
31. Thorndike EL. Animal Intelligence. New York: Macmillan; 1911.
32. Skinner BF. The behavior of organisms. New York: Appleton-Century-Crofts; 1938.
33. Kratzer DD, Netherland WM, Pulse RE, Baker JP. Maze learning in Quarter horses. J Anim Sci 1977; 45:896–902.
34. Houpt KA, Houpt TR. Social and illumination preferences of mares. Equine Pract 1992; 14(6):11–16.
35. Shults T, Combie J, Dougherty J, Tobin T. Variable-interval responding in the horse: a sensitive method of quantitating effects of centrally acting drugs. Am J Vet Res 1982; 43(7):1143–1146.
36. McDonnell SM. Pharmacological aids to behaviour modification in horses. Equine Vet J Suppl 1998; 27:50–51 (abstr).
37. Miyashita Y, Nakajima S, Imada H. Differential outcome effect in the horse. J Exp Anal Behav 2000; 74(2):245–254.
38. Myers RD, Mesker DC. Operant responding in a horse under several schedules of reinforcement. J Exp Anal Behav 1960; 3:161–164.
39. McCall CA, Burgin SE. Equine utilization of secondary reinforcement during response extinction and acquisition. Appl Anim Behav Sci 2002; 78(2–4):253–262.
40. Haag EL, Rudman R, Houpt KA. Avoidance, maze learning and social dominance in ponies. J Anim Sci 1980; 50:2, 329–335.

41. McCall CA. The effect of body condition of horses on discrimination learning abilities. Appl Anim Behav Sci 1989; 22:3–4, 327–334.

42. Sappington BKF, Goldman L. Discrimination learning and concept formation in the Arabian horse. J Anim Sci 1994; 72(12):3080–3087.

43. Flannery B. Relational discrimination learning in horses. Appl Anim Behav Sci 1997; 54(4): 267–280.

44. Nicol CJ. Equine learning: progress and suggestions for future research. Appl Anim Behav Sci 2002. 78 (2–4) 193–208.

45. McQuoid LM, Galef BG Jr. Social influences on feeding site selection by Burmese fowl (Gallus gallus). J Comp Psychol 1992; 106:136–141.

46. Fraser AF. The behaviour of the horse. London: CAB International; 1992.

47. McCann JS, Heird JC, Bell RW, Lutherer LO. Normal and more highly reactive horses, II: The effect of handling and reserpine on the cardiac response to stimuli. Appl Anim Behav Sci 1988; 19:215–226.

48. Dixon JC. Pattern discrimination, learning set, and memory in a pony. Paper presented at the Midwestern Psychological Association Convention, Chicago, 1966.

49. Voith VL. Pattern discrimination, learning set formation, memory retention, spatial and visual reversal learning by the horse. Thesis, Ohio State University, Columbus, 1975.

50. Rubin L, Oppegard C, Hintz HF. The effect of varying the temporal distribution of conditioning trials on equine learning behaviour. J Anim Sci 1980; 50:1184–1187.

51. Kusunose R, Yamanobe A. The effect of training schedule on learned tasks in yearling horses. Appl Anim Behav Sci 2002; 78(2–4):225–233.

52. Pfungst O. Clever Hans: the horse of Mr von Osten. New York: Holt, Rinehard & Winston; 1965.

53. Budiansky S. The nature of horses: exploring equine evolution, intelligence and behavior. New York: Free Press; 1997.

54. Houpt KA, Parsons MS, Hintz HF. The learning ability of orphan foals, of normal foals and of their mothers. J Anim Sci 1982, 55:1027–1032.

55. Houpt KA, Hintz HF. Some effects of maternal deprivation on maintenance behaviour, spatial relationships and responses to environmental novelty in foals. Appl Anim Ethol 1983; 9(3/4):221–230.

56. Clarke J, Nicol CJ, Jones R, McGreevy PD. Effects of observational learning on food selection in horses. Appl Anim Behav Sci 1996; 50:177–184.

57. Lindberg AC, Kelland A, Nicol CJ. Effects of observational learning on acquisition of an operant response in horses. Appl Anim Behav Sci 1999; 61(3):187–199.

58. Hagerbaumer J. Exploring the equine mind with learning and memory studies. In: The thinking horse. Guelph: Equine Research Centre; 1995.

59. Hausberger M, le Scolan N, Bruderer C, Pierre JS. [Temperament in the horse: factors in play and practical implications] Le temperament du cheval: facteurs en jeu et implications pratiques. 24 journée

de la Récherche Equine, 1998, Institut de Cheval, Paris, France, 1998:159–169.

60. Bagshaw CS, Ralston SL, Fisher H. Behavioural and physiological effects of orally administered tryptophan on horses subjected to acute isolation stress. Appl Anim Behav Sci 1994; 40:1–12.

61. Houpt KA, Kusunose R. Genetics of behaviour. In: Bowling AT, Ruvinsky A, eds. The genetics of the horse. Wallingford, Oxon: CAB International; 2000.

62. Hausberger A, Muller C. A brief note on some possible factors involved in the reactions of horses to humans. Appl Anim Behav Sci 2002; 76(4):339–344.

63. Mader DR, Price EO. Discrimination learning in horses: effect of breed, age and social dominance. J Anim Sci 1980; 50:962–965.

64. Tellington-Jones L, Bruns V. The Tellington-Jones equine awareness method. Buckingham: Kenilworth Press; 1985.

65. Tellington-Jones L. Getting in touch with horses. Buckingham: Kenilworth Press; 1995.

66. Grandin T, Deesing MJ, Struthers JJ, Swinker AM. Cattle with hair whorl patterns above the eyes are more behaviorally agitated during restraint. Appl Anim Behav Sci 1995; 46:117–123.

67. Randle HD. Facial hair whorl position and temperament in cattle. Appl Anim Behav Sci 1998; 56:139–147.

68. Lanier JL, Grandin T, Green R, et al. A note on hair whorl position and cattle temperament in the auction ring. Appl Anim Behav Sci 2001; 73:93–101.

69. Mackenzie SA, Thiboutot E. Stimulus reactivity tests for the domestic horse (Equus caballus). Equine Pract 1997; 19(7):21–22.

70. Anderson MK, Friend TH, Evans JW, Bushong DM. Behavioral assessment of horses in therapeutic riding programs. Appl Anim Behav Sci 1999; 63(1):11–24.

71. Le Scolan N, Hausberger M, Wolff A. Stability over situations in temperamental traits of horses as revealed by experimental and scoring approaches. Behav Process 1997; 41:257–266.

72. Seaman SC, Davidson HPB, Waran NK. How reliable is temperament assessment in the domestic horse (Equus caballus)? Appl Anim Behav Sci 2002; 78(2–4):175–191.

73. Houpt KA, Rudman R. Foreword to special issue on equine behaviour. Appl Anim Behav Sci 2002; 78:83–85.

74. McCann JS, Heird JC, Bell RW, Lutherer LO. Normal and more highly reactive horses, I: Heart rate, respiration rate and behavioural observations. Appl Anim Behav Sci 1988; 19:201–214.

75. Visser EK, van Reenen CG, Schilder MBH, et al. Learning performances in young horses using two different learning tests. Appl Anim Behav Sci 2003; 80(4):311–326.

76. Visser EK, van Reenen CG, Engel B, et al. The association between performance in show-jumping and personality traits early in life. Appl Anim Behav Sci. 2003; 82(4):279–295.

77. Budzynski M, Slomka Z, Soltys L, et al. Characteristics of nervous activity in Arab horses [Polish]. Annales Universitatis Mariae Curie-Sklodowska, EE Zootechnica 1997; 15:165–175.

78. Fiske JC, Potter GD. Discrimination reversal learning in yearling horses. J Anim Sci 1979; 49:583–588.

79. Vierin M, Bouissou MF, Vandeheede M, et al. Development of a method for measuring fear reactions in the horse. 24 Journée de la Récherche Equine, 1998, Institut du Cheval, Paris, France, 1998:171–183.

80. Budzynski M. Repeatability and heritability of the assessment of nervous type in horses [Polish]. Annales Universitatis Mariae Curie-Sklodowska, EE Zootechnica 1983; 1:229–232.

81. Budzynski M. Timidity test to assess the degree of nervousness of horses [Polish]. Medycyna Weterinaryjna 1984; 40(3):156–158.

82. Budzynski M, Soltys L, Slomka Z. The nervous excitability of Hutsul horses [Polish]. Zetzyty Naukowe Akademii Rolniczej im H Kollataja w Krakowie, Sesja, Naukowe 1991; 29:41–45.

83. Luescher UA, McKeown DB, Halip J. Reviewing the causes of obsessive-compulsive disorder in horses. Vet Med 1991; 86:527–530.

84. Luescher UA, McKeown DB, Dean H. A cross-sectional study on compulsive behaviour (stable vices) in horses. Equine Vet J Suppl 1998; 27:14–18.

85. McGreevy PD, French NP, Nicol CJ. The prevalence of abnormal behaviours in dressage, eventing and endurance horses in relation to stabling. Vet Rec 1995; 137:36–37.

86. Garner JP, Mason GJ. Evidence for a relationship between cage stereotypies and behavioural disinhibition in laboratory rodents. Behav Brain Res 2002; 136(1):83–92.

5

Social behavior

SOCIAL ORGANIZATION

Social interactions between horses have been the focus of several recent studies. This is good news for domestic horses because by understanding the relationships between horses, humans can learn to build a better understanding between themselves and their equine companions.

As the nature of social hierarchies in free-ranging horses, the effects of domestication and the significance of behavioral and social needs are better understood, our ability to comment on equine welfare issues is necessarily enhanced. For example, studies of groups of free-ranging horses have provided information on the roles of the stallions, mares and juveniles within their natal groups. This provides the rationale for single-sex grouping of horses in domestic contexts especially where social flux is constant and agonistic interactions must be modulated for the sake of horse safety. Thoughtful planning of social groups can reduce some of the undesirable effects of pair-bonding on ridden work and minimize injuries from conspecifics in the paddock. It is usually better to find the optimal social milieu for horses than take the 'safe' option of isolation in a paddock or, worse still, a stable.[1]

Domestic horses are not the only beneficiaries of studies of free-ranging equids, since the humane control of feral horses is also facilitated with this sort of information. For example, given the importance of a stable social group, the relocation and confinement of feral horses, while sounding reasonably simple, is likely to modify current social structure and range use, ultimately leading to fights and injuries in the short term and the need for more intensive management in the longer term.[2]

GROUPS OF HORSES

Other than occasional solitary individuals (which are more often than not transiently drifting between groups), two main groupings of horses occur within herds: the natal band (or birth band or family group) and the bachelor group (Fig. 5.1).[3] Traditionally, horse herds are thought of as harems, comprising one stallion, his mares and foals and juveniles. This simplistic view fails to embrace the leadership role of mares and the context-specificity of the stallion's rank.

In a group of horses, the lead animal shows the way to resources, such as water, saltlicks and rolling sites, as well as initiating activities, such as grazing or resting. This individual is often an older experienced mare but, depending on the context, the stallion may also direct its herd by herding and snaking, for example when he detects predators or competitors. Increasingly, the importance of mares as the functional core of the group is being recognized, with 25% of them staying permanently in their original natal band[3] and with matrilineal dynasties spanning generations.

Similarly, those mares that disperse into a fresh band often remain within it for life. It is important to note that the stallion may not always be the alpha member of the natal band.[4-6] Similarly, gender has been demonstrated to be a poor predictor of rank in foals.[7]

Bands with more than one stallion are not uncommon. Subject to the above, stallions within these groups establish a dominance hierarchy that helps to define roles. If there are several stallions associated with the family band, the dominant stallion copulates more than subordinate stallions.[3] Band cohesion is a task shared by stallions in multi-stallion bands but the subordinate males tend to herd and occasionally mate with the lower-ranking females. One study noted that mares are more likely to leave single-stallion harems and that therefore harems with several stallions are generally more stable.[8]

Linklater[9] defines a natal band as a stable association of mares, their pre-dispersal offspring and one or more stallions who defend and maintain the mare group, and their mating opportunities, from other males year round. For example, in New Zealand's Kaimanawa ranges, the horse population has a social structure like that of other feral horse populations, with an even adult sex

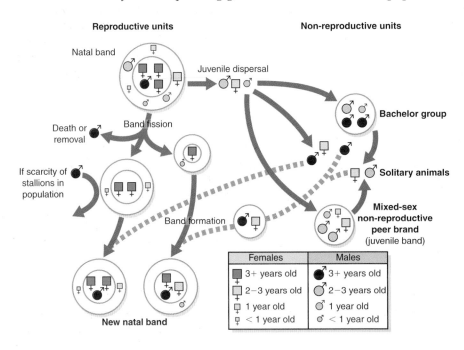

Figure 5.1 Social groupings of free-ranging horses. (After Waring.[16])

ratio, year-round breeding groups (bands) with stable adult membership consisting of 1 to 11 mares, 1 to 4 stallions, and their predispersal offspring, and bachelor groups with unstable membership.[2] Changes in the adult composition of natal bands are rare (e.g. Miller[10] suggests 0.75 adult changes per year). However, harems may split into smaller groups based on social attachment, when grass becomes scarce.[11]

Found in all free-ranging horse populations, the bachelor group comprises males that have dispersed from natal bands. Although most colts leave the natal band at around the birth of a sibling, or when there is a shortage of playmates or food, some remain.[12] However, as they mature and begin to represent a threat to a resident stallion's mating rights, pubescent males may occasionally be ostracized from their natal band. More generally, colts gravitate to bachelor groups because that is where they find many potential play partners. Bachelor groups also provide sanctuary to older stallions, including some that have been unsuccessful in defending their bands from other stallions.[13] Bachelors live in their groups adjacent to natal bands, waiting for opportunities to capture dispersing mares, perform sneak matings, herd away mares and to challenge natal band leaders. For this reason, membership of the bachelor band is subject to the greatest flux during the breeding season. Despite the companionship it offers, bachelor groups are literally full of competitors that engage in agonistic encounters that may persist over several months and may end in dispersal.[14] It is therefore perhaps predictable that young stallions usually spend some time alone before forming their own harems.[12] The bachelor group provides valuable physical and social learning opportunities for its transient members. In juveniles there is a relationship between time spent in the bachelor group and latency to form a harem.[12]

Role of stallions in natal band cohesion

The main roles of a resident stallion involve monitoring and maintaining the integrity of the group and protecting his band from predators and other stallions that may attempt to steal or perform sneak matings with mares and fillies. The reproductive success of a harem stallion is limited not least by his ability to prevent such matings.[15] Harem stability is not affected by the size of the harem nor by the age of the stallion, but is thought to be compromised by the presence of subordinate stallions attached to the harem.[8] Depending on the terrain the stallion will protect his band by patrolling a radius of 10–15 meters around the group as they move through the home range.[5] For this reason natal band stallions are less likely than mares, juveniles or bachelors to form pair bonds. The relationships they form tend to be heterosexual (usually with all adult females in the natal band) or paternal.[16]

Being less timid than mares and fillies,[17] stallions and colts usually take the initiative when the band encounters a potential threat. Having said that, the stallion's response to a challenge depends on whether the cause of the threat is a predator or another stallion.

If a predator threatens, the stallion will herd his group together and lead or drive them away from the threat using snaking gestures (Fig. 5.2). Feist[18] noted that in 77% of band movements, the stallion was either driving or leading the group. Stallions sometimes herd wandering foals back to the band and protect them from danger.[19]

By placing himself between the band and a predator the stallion can reduce the fragmenting effects such stimuli can have on the group. The

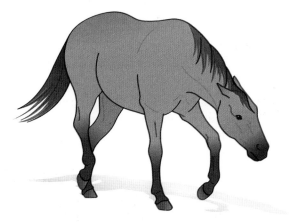

Figure 5.2 Snaking behavior used by a stallion to move other horses, especially members of his natal band.

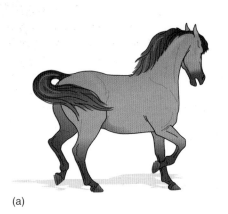

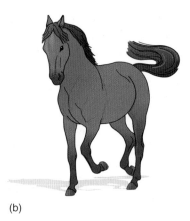

(a)   (b)

Figure 5.3 Stallions (a) and (b) approaching one another spend time assessing each other's fitness and readiness to fight.

role of the stallion in responding to potential predators is illustrated by the report that Camargue foals born into bands in which two stallions have an alliance are 20% more likely to survive than those in single-stallion bands because of reduced predation.[20]

If the threat is from another stallion, the initial response by the band's stallion will be to attempt to chase the challenger away. Agonistic behaviors are discussed later, but the resident stallion's motivation to fight depends on a number of variables summarized in a notional equation that forms the central tenet of game theory (Fig. 5.3).[21] Whenever two horses dispute access to any resource, both must weigh up the value of the resource, the cost of defending it and their ability to retain it (also known as their resource-holding potential).

Without performing any calculations as such, the would-be protagonists (a and b) compare

$$\frac{V_a + RHP_a}{C_a} \quad \text{with} \quad \frac{V_b + RHP_b}{C_b}$$

where: V is the value of the resource to that individual; RHP is the resource-holding potential of that individual; C is the cost of a fight to that individual. Factors on which these variables depend are given in Table 5.1.

This theory helps to explain why interactions between the resident stallions of two interfacing bands are less intense than those between a resident stallion and an interloping bachelor. The latter has a lower cost to pay for fighting more intensely since he is already outside a core group.

Table 5.1 Game theory variables predicting conflict between horses, and factors on which the variables depend

Variable	Factors include
Value	Experience of the resource, investment in the resource, short-term and long-term future needs
Resource-holding potential	Size, physical fitness (as evidenced by display used when the challenge is detected), ability to deceive observers, fighting experience and number of individuals involved in the dispute
Cost	Risks of being injured (with consequent risk of infection at the site), killed or displaced from natal band

The value of the home range is greater for the resident than the intruder so the resident may be more likely to persist in combat. This helps to explain why the forays of bachelors into the home range of natal bands are only rarely successful.

Snaking and herding are most likely to be seen in domestic contexts when the stallion is introduced to a group or when an existing family group is moved to a new pasture.[22] After either of these interventions the stallion's response generally returns to baseline levels by the third day.[22] The addition of new mares to an established natal band does not induce herding of the original mares. However, primarily because they are chased by the stallion for up to 3 days, the introduced mares are kept at a distance (of approximately 8–12 mare lengths) from the original mares.[22] Band integrity is further enhanced by a harem stallion when he facilitates bonding between mares and their neo-natal foals by keeping other conspecifics away from them. Again, snaking and herding may be used for this purpose.

Despite the benefits of having the company of a stallion, band members lose some of their freedom. In the absence of a stallion, mares mutually groom more, form more stable pair bonds and have better developed hierarchy.[23]

Role of mares in natal band cohesion

The chances of inbreeding between stallions and their daughters is reduced by the experience of having lived together before the filly's maturity, a factor thought to prompt migration of fillies from their natal band.[24] While 75% of the fillies disperse to other bands, the females that remain are the most fixed and stable members of most natal bands, often taking leadership roles in governing the band's daily activities. Although regarded as the resident core of the equine family group, mares will disperse from natal bands notably when resources are scarce: e.g. up to 30% of adult females have been observed changing harems during the winter.[8]

Affiliative behavior between females is important because mares of an established band remain together even in the absence of a stallion.[25] We should never underestimate the strength of social bonds among mares. Indeed there are anecdotal reports of mares abandoning their own foals to reach the comfort of their herd mates. These affiliations may have their origins in foal associations since fillies tend to spend more time with other fillies than with colts.[26] Daughters also tend to remain closely associated with their dams.[16,27]

The rank of a mare has a predictive effect on her role in band cohesion. For example, as a reflection of the investment they have made in the group, dominant mares are more likely to defend the area around the group. Although territorial behavior is an irregular feature of the equine ethogram,[28] in some free-ranging populations, such as those in Shackleford Banks on the eastern coast of the United States, that show defense of a territory

rather than simply maintenance of the integrity of the band,[29] higher-ranking mares within the natal band are more often involved in mutual grooming with the resident stallion, while lower-ranking mares are the chief recipients of his snaking and herding attention when he rounds up the band. Most adult mares in a natal band will contribute to band cohesion by responding to the sound of the resident stallion's call.[30]

Role of juveniles in natal band cohesion

In a natal band, the juveniles issue the least amount of aggressive behavior and conduct the most non-agonistic behavior.[6] One of the main behaviors of foals is play that is very important for them to learn how to interact with one another and for the establishment of pair bonds (see Ch. 10).

Play in foals is unrelated to rank. So, the play-rank order of foals, as measured by the number of times a foal left a bout of play, is not significantly correlated with rank order determined by agonistic interactions.[31] Yearlings continue to be involved in play activity but are also seen nipping each other as they consolidate their social hierarchy and as they practice herding or fighting for adulthood.

GROUP SIZE AND HOME RANGES

Herds of horses may be as large as 600 (Machteld van Dierendonck, personal communication 2002). Bands within herds form relatively stable nuclei[32–34] that are often at their most discrete when resting but may graze in close proximity to one another and usually unite when fleeing from a predatory threat. Band size tends to vary with population density. For example it can range from 12.3 in Shackleford Banks,[29] with a population density of 11 individuals/km² to 3.3 in Wassuk Ridge, in the Nevada Desert, with a population density of 0.1.[35] Because of the terrain and its resources, horse density in a given ecological sector can vary: e.g. while the population density in the Auahitotara of New Zealand averaged 3.6 horses/km², it ranged from 0.9 to 5.2 horses/km² within different zones.[2] Group size therefore is

Table 5.2 Demographic data for feral horse groups in North America

	Range	Mean	SD
Population size	78–703	266.8	206.9
Population density/km²	0.2–6.3	3.5	3.9
% Adults	53–77	63.2	7.5
% Juveniles	14–29	22.8	5.2
% Foals	9–19	14.2	3.6
Home range area (km²)	3–52	17.8	16.6

After Fraser[36] and Waring.[16]

dependent on the density and pattern of distribution of resources, and this is why, when external resources are provided, groups can become larger than those observed in the free-ranging state. For example, in working ponies that are seasonally managed on a free-living basis, groups of 30 or more can exist.[36] Island populations, such as those on Sable Islands and Shackleford Banks, have higher population densities than those with fewer limitations on their ability to spread.[29,37] Demographic data on feral horse groups in North America are given in Table 5.2.

Home ranges incorporate grazing sites, water-holes, rolling sites, shade, windbreaks and refuges from insects and can vary in area from 0.9 to 52 km².[38] Exploitation of the home range depends on numerous variables including the climate, the season, predation risk and the prevalence of biting insects. For example, Auahitotara horses generally avoid high altitudes, southern aspects, steeper slopes, bare ground and forest remnants.[2] Instead they tend to occupy north facing slopes (because they have warmer aspects) with short vegetation and zones with well-nourished swards. In spring and summer when subsistence is less of a challenge and there is less need to forage in hostile terrain, they tend to be found on gentler slopes.[2]

Horse populations do not use all parts of their home range equally since the grazing is rarely of uniform value and the emergence of latrine areas is normal (see Chs 8 and 9). Thus bands tend to spend much of their time in relatively small focal areas within the home range.[16] Natal bands often shift with the season such that in spring they gravitate to river basin and stream valley floors for the beginning of foaling and mating and, when there is a chance of frost, to higher altitudes in autumn and winter.[2] The appeal of certain areas changes with the season. For example, whereas during the winter months they may avoid standing in water, horses may be driven into surf or shallow bays by biting insects during the summer months. Having said this, in some groups of horses no pattern of cyclical use of areas has emerged.[16] Since the use of terrain seems to be initiated by leading members of the group and since a change of leader may bring a change in a band's use of resources, this finding may have arisen because behavioral observations were coincidentally made at a time of flux in the band's composition or hierarchy.

Social behavior in feral horse populations is more common than territorial behavior, in that if one band of horses encounters another, any defensiveness shown usually appears to be an attempt to maintain the integrity of the band rather than to defend a site.[16] Although the home range of one natal band often overlaps entirely with the home ranges of others, natal bands and bachelor groups are loyal to undefended home ranges with central core use areas.[2]

In cases where home ranges overlap, a hierarchy of groups can be observed that allows the displacement of subordinate (usually smaller) bands and individuals from shared resources such as watering-holes. Although linked to the size of the group, its relative rank compared with others is not a function of the number of males it contains.[33] This is illustrated by the deference exhibited by bachelor groups to natal bands and by the way in which the rank of a bachelor is enhanced once he has acquired a mare.[33] Disputes between bands are generally resolved by interaction between one or occasionally two high-ranking representatives from each. The remainder of both bands typically look on and await the outcome before accessing resources in an order determined by their representatives.[33]

SOCIAL HIERARCHY

The establishment of defined social status within any group of equids promotes stability within the

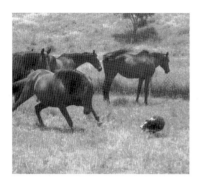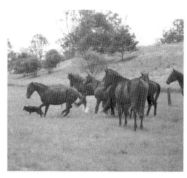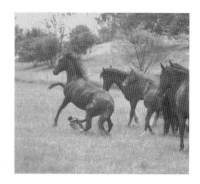

Figure 5.4 A mare moves forward to defend her group by attacking an approaching dog. (Photographs courtesy of Michael Jervis-Chaston.)

band. A stable social hierarchy within the band decreases the accumulative amount of injury by allowing *threats* of kicks and, perhaps more importantly, bites to replace the aggressive responses themselves.[6]

Each horse's position within the band is held through a blend of aggression and appeasement behavior. Aggressive behavior can be biting, kicking, circling and displacement, but the most common response to a competitor is a threat to kick or bite. Rank is determined not only by threats issued but also deference to threats received. Such submission may involve the lowering of the head and aversion of gaze.

Houpt et al[39] found that although individual rank order is unidirectional it may not be linear throughout the group. Thus A may dominate B who may dominate C, but C may dominate A.[39] This facilitates the formation of so-called social triangles. While rank orders are generally linear in the top and bottom of a band's hierarchy, most triangles occur in the middle.[40]

Also one must consider the role of protected threats that allow individuals to enhance their rank by associating with a higher ranking band member – for example as seen in foals that attain rank enhancement when with their dams. Because of the possible influence of the dam this may help to explain why Iceland yearlings often have a higher rank than their 2-year-old siblings (Machteld van Dierendonck, personal communication 2002).

If a hierarchy were not developed and maintained, each horse would need to affirm its rank by increasing levels of aggression during every dispute with a conspecific over a resource. Without a hierarchy, injury and distress associated with social flux may have reproductive costs, e.g. the rate of conception is decreased and there is an increase in the rate of fetal and foal mortality.[41] In general, a social structure is important for organization, especially during times of emergency such as when a predator approaches (Fig. 5.4). A defined social structure based on affiliative relationships allows the band to mount an appropriate response, be it fight or flight, as the lead animal rises to the defense of the group or herds it together to escape.

The determination of rank is complex and not easily predicted. Height or weight or both have been found to correlate with rank in many studies[42–44] but not all.[4,40] Age more usually shows a correlation with rank in studies of feral *E. caballus*[5,42,45] and *E. przewalski*[46] but again this is not always the case.[41] Where age contributes to social status, this is appropriate since it is likely to reflect experience in dealing with local challenges and a wealth of knowledge about how best to exploit the resources in the home range.[6] Having said that, in their dotage the oldest mares may relinquish leadership but occupy a beta position, much more elevated than their body condition would suggest. Perhaps this reflects some sort of respect earned earlier in life (Machteld van Dierendonck, personal communication 2002). In managed herds, the length of residency within a band also contributes to the determination of rank.[40,47] In geldings, rank seems strongly influenced by an individual's position in the social hierarchy at the time of castration (see Ch. 11).

Either sex can out-rank the other because there is little sexual dimorphism in the sizes of hooves and teeth, which are a horse's main weapons.[5] Stallions' ranks are very much context dependent. They may not truly dominate, as they have less contact with the band than female peers because of their need to patrol around rather than within the band. Furthermore they do not participate in many aggressive encounters if they enter the band only during sexual situations.[5] Therefore when a youthful stallion secures mating rights in a band containing mares older than himself, the oldest yet healthiest mare will tend to prevail in a leadership role. Although over 80% of threats are directed down the dominance hierarchy,[31] the use of the term 'dominance' is somewhat controversial since some authors highlight avoidance behavior on the part of subordinates as being the main activity necessary for the maintenance of the order. In view of this, it has been argued[36] that avoidance order is a better measure of the social system than the 'aggression order'.

In the process of learning to recognize their place in the hierarchy, yearlings receive the largest number of attacks (46% according to Keiper & Receveur[6]). Significant positive correlations have been found between rank of mares and foals and the rate at which they directed aggression to other herd members.[7]

As suckling foals play away from their dams, they establish a hierarchy based largely on birth order such that there is a linear relationship between age and social position.[6,7] Although weaning tends to have a disruptive effect on the ranks of foals (so that birth order no longer correlates with rank), significant correlations have been found between mare rank and the rank of foals both before and after weaning.[7,31] This would suggest that the influence of the dam is relatively constant over time.[7]

Since the adult offspring of a high-ranking mother does not *necessarily* become high-ranking, it cannot be said that dominance is purely genetic.[5] Status is a learned relationship between two individuals, and learning plays a role in the development of effective dominating strategies, which can include deceptive responses such as bluffing. Additionally there may be heritable behavioral predispositions in the high-ranking dynasties within a herd. Although offspring may learn aggressive behavior from their mothers this is challenged in part by evidence of inverse correlations between aggression rates and rank in foals.[31] Perhaps they have only to learn *how* to impose their rank rather than doing so frequently. One alternative is that status is bestowed upon the foals of high-ranking mares simply by association with their dams, since mares may assist their foals in agonistic encounters with other foals.[7] It is acknowledged that foals share their mother's rank while she is in close proximity[16] but that they are more likely to show deferential displays such as snapping (tooth-clapping, yawing, champing, yamming; Fig. 5.5) to adults when beyond her protection.[42] Furthermore the rates of aggression towards foals rise with weaning as the mare's support is withdrawn.[7] The relative contribution of environmental and genetic factors will be better understood when the influence of non-biological mothers can be measured from studies of foals that have been transferred as embryos or cross-fostered after birth.

Although mares may undergo significant changes in social behavior at the time of foaling,[48] no coincident changes in social status have been reported with foaling,[42] so mares with foals at foot do not necessarily rank higher in the social hierarchy than a mare without a foal.

THE EFFECT OF RANK ON BEHAVIOR

With higher rank comes priority access to most resources. In every dispute the rank of protagonists correlates with their resource-holding potential and contributes to the prediction of the outcome. However, rank alone is not a simple, absolute predictor, since game theory applies too. Therefore the outcome must also remain a function of the value of the resource (i.e. the motivation to acquire the resource) and the cost of any fight to possess it. For these reasons rank is also context-dependent, especially in stallions.

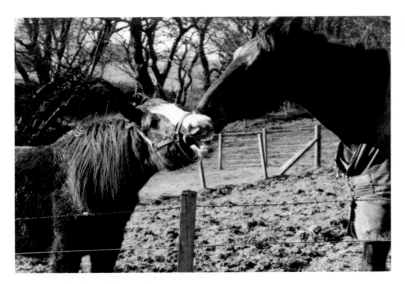

Figure 5.5 Youngster showing snapping response to an older horse. (Photograph courtesy of Francis Burton.)

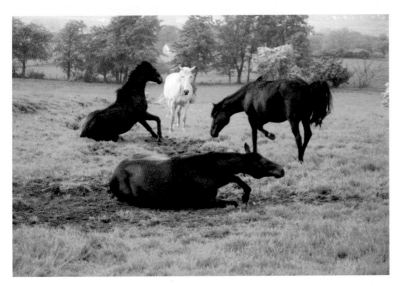

Figure 5.6 Horses in a group usually take turns rolling with the highest-ranking animal tending to roll last. (Photograph courtesy of Francis Burton.)

Rank has been correlated with the priority bestowed on those horses that gain first access to maintenance resources such as resting sites and watering holes,[33] unless they have been distracted by having to repel another band. Conversely, rank dictates the order in which bachelors eliminate on one another's excrement,[23] and all bands use rolling sites[49] (Fig. 5.6) such that the highest-ranking animal often marks last so that its scent prevails. Rank influences social dynamics within a band, including the selection of nearest neighbors and mutual grooming partners.[45]

The rank of an individual horse does not influence its sociability rate in any group.[7] However, the debate continues about the role of the higher-ranking partner in mutual grooming pairs, with evidence that high status animals may be both more likely[45] and less likely[42] to start a bout when grooming started asynchronously.

Despite the relationship between age and rank, difference in the ages of band members influences social networks. Bonded pairs with less difference in age that demonstrate frequent grooming, usually remain in close proximity to one another, beyond the effects of rank and kinship.[50] Additionally, middle-ranking horses tend to be more frequently in the close vicinity of another horse than high-ranking or low-ranking horses.[40]

There are a number of ways in which social rank affects reproductive behavior. Just as stallions can reject maiden mares, they have been reported to select high-ranking estrous mares for mating when offered a choice.[51] Males outside the natal band and low-ranking (juvenile) males within it are seldom able to mate with mature mares unless by sneak matings, because the resident stallion consorts with these mares when they are in estrus. The peripheral and subordinate stallions can therefore usually mate only with lower-ranking mares with reduced biological fitness. The trade-off for these males is that they have not invested time in protecting these females. For mares, elevated rank means they are less likely to be harassed by these males seeking sneak matings. As they solicit the attentions of the dominant stallion they may also be seen chasing away subordinate females that would otherwise divert his attention.[49]

The benefits of high rank in terms of biological fitness are clear. For example, since the foals of high-ranking mares may grow bigger and faster than other foals in the natal band, they may breed earlier and the colts among them may be more likely to gain a harem.[7,52] Other, less favorable associations with high rank are becoming better understood, with studies in wild dogs indicating that rank is positively correlated with cortisol concentrations.[53] In horses, one might predict this to be the case in herd leaders because of the associated burden of having to maintain band integrity and investigate potentially dangerous stimuli. Similarly, recent data demonstrate that the foals of higher-ranking mares are more likely to develop oral stereotypies than foals of middle- or low-ranking dams.[54] It is speculated that this may reflect the influence of mares' behavior towards foals prior to weaning or may relate to the nature of the mare–foal bond and effects of severance at weaning.

Certainly this is an area that merits more study. The role of rank in competitive success of race and sports horses continues to fascinate both ethologists and punters alike. It is possible that high-ranking animals in a race allow others to take the lead and with it the potential risks of what may lie ahead. This, however, may be offset by the reluctance of subordinate animals to overtake them, an abiding argument for the use of blinkers that may reduce the ability of horses to detect threatening behaviors from conspecifics as they overtake them in a race.

MEASURING RANK

Perhaps because there are fewer complexities such as social triangles and because of the complete absence of mare-foal dyads, measuring rank is easier in all-male groups than in natal bands.[23] Just as the factors that influence rank are complex, so is the determination of rank within a group of horses. The absence of an established protocol for the measurement of social hierarchies in horses accounts for the lack of consensus between studies. Instead of establishing hierarchy solely on the basis of threats given,[6] the trend is towards including submissive gestures[31,44] and calculating rank only from submission data[7] because the importance of deference displays by subordinate horses when retiring from disputes over resources has become recognized.

It is generally true that one can see best the dominance relations between individuals at the site of limited resources: water holes, saltlicks, sandy places to roll, shelter, etc. It is natural for horses to attempt to displace each other as they compete for mates, food, salt or water. For this reason, some studies of hierarchy tend to record all occurrences of agonistic behavior between pairs of subjects during feeding of supplemental grain.[7] However, the desire to acquire or defend food pellets in competitive situations is not necessarily the same for all individuals involved. Additionally, dominance in an isolated dyad is not necessarily a true reflection of what applies in an unmanipulated group that may feature coalitions, social triangles, leadership and defense.

Because simply recording the outcome of a bout is an inelegant measure of rank, submissive and aggressive behaviors should be analyzed in detail. This approach has shown that agonistic responses involving the head are related to offensive behaviors, while the hindquarters are used both offensively and defensively.[40] So, when scoring a dispute between two horses to determine rank, it is advisable to summate bites and bite threats separately from kicks and threats to kick because the latter are not so useful for determination of hierarchy.[40]

PAIR BONDS

Under free-range conditions, even where the territory is extensive, group bonding is important to the extent that horses maintain continual visual and, to an extent olfactory, contact with each other.[36] A central mechanism of band cohesion is the establishment of pair bonds and mare-foal bonds.[55] Pair bonds in bachelor groups are generally weaker than those observed in natal bands and become more tenuous as bachelors mature and are driven to establish reproductive relationships.[16]

While domestic horses generally group together according to certain sex or sex–age classes – adult mares, adult geldings, foals, juveniles – mares sometimes socialize according to their reproductive state: pregnant, postpartum and barren (Machteld van Dierendock, personal communication 2002). Most horses have one or more preferred associates with whom they maintain closer proximity than with other herd members.[45] The resilient bonds between such paired affiliates are of particular importance among equids and are demonstrated by reciprocal following, mutual grooming and standing together (Table 5.3).[56] The cardinal signs of stability among groups of horses include group activities such as rolling and trekking and mutual maintenance behaviors including insect control and grooming.

Although one recent study showed that a foal's sex had no significant effect on the choice of preferred associate,[7] others have found that foals tend to preferentially associate with other foals of the same sex.[31,57] Both before and after

Table 5.3 Features of the ethogram (as described for bachelor bands[14]) characteristic of stable groups

Response	Description
Trekking	Two or more animals moving together, typically following one another
Mutual grooming	Two horses standing beside one another, usually head-to-shoulder or head-to-tail, grooming each other's neck, mane, rump or tail by gentle nipping, nuzzling or rubbing

weaning, foals associated preferentially with the foal of their dam's most preferred associate.[7] As further confirmation of the influence of the mare on the social behavior of the foal, it has been reported that the sociability rates of mares and their foals are correlated prior to weaning but not after.[7]

Horses tend to bond with conspecifics of similar age and rank.[44,45] This means that in biological terms they associate with their closest competitors, and this may account for ongoing disputes over resources. Preferred associates receive more total aggression than do other herd members, but proportionately more of the aggression directed against preferred associates is mild, such as laying back of the ears, when compared with more severe aggressions, such as kicking.[44] This is supported by a study that compared 2-year-old colts that were group-reared and single reared for 9 months.[58] Whereas group-reared colts tended to make more use of subtle agonistic interactions (displacements, submissive behavior), more aggressive behaviors, i.e. bite threats, were recorded in the group of singly reared colts.[58] Increasingly, therefore the concept of a hierarchy based on dominance and subordination has been challenged by one based on tolerance and attachment.[56]

Social groupings have evolved for individual protection against predators, and cohesion is maintained by a variety of mutually beneficial behaviors such as mutual grooming and tail-to-tail

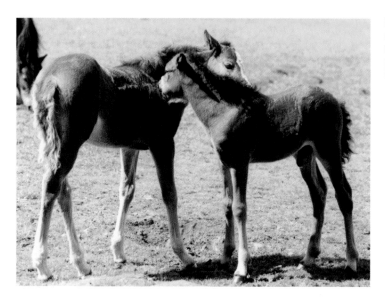

Figure 5.7 Pair-bonded foals can often be seen mutually grooming. Of all horses, foals seem to find being scratched in hard-to-reach places most gratifying. (Photograph courtesy of Francis Burton.)

fly-swatting. More than half (51%) of allogrooming contacts occur at the preferred site in front of the shoulder blade and include the cranial aspect of the withers.[59] This behavior (Fig. 5.7) has been reported in foals as young as 1 day old.[42]

Attachment between foals increases after the first 2 or 3 weeks of life, as the initial protectiveness of mares and the intensity of the foal–mare bond subsides.[16] As confidence with an affiliate increases, so do the boldness of play and the strength of the bond with a given peer, as shown by the frequency of mutual grooming bouts. Mutual grooming characterizes the relationship in filly–filly and colt–filly partnerships. This is regularly interspersed with sustained episodes of playfighting if the partners are both colts.[42] Since natal bands are largely female, the bonds formed between fillies at this stage can be lifelong, other partnerships tending to dissolve at the time of juvenile dispersal (see below).[16] Exceptions to these generalizations include the occasional formation of trios and the dispersal of juveniles in pairs.[16] As testament to the robust memory horses boast, pair-bonds can withstand extended periods of separation (e.g. 6 months in the case of two New Forest pony mares[42] and 5 years in the case of some Icelandic mares (Machteld van Dierendock, personal communication 2002).

Pair-bonded horses sometimes defend their affiliates from other band members (e.g. by intervening in mutual grooming that involves their preferred partner) as though they are possessive of the resource they represent.[16] Similarly, mares sometimes attack stallions found courting their female affiliates.

Pair-bonded individuals conduct most of their daily activities together. Penetration of the personal space tends to cause avoidance more often than defense on the part of the subordinate horse. This means that while affiliative behaviors are active, affirmatory actions shown by pair-bonded horses, in many cases proximity reflects simple passive acceptance of conspecifics.

The social distance of horses is defined as the spatial limit companions will occupy, and beyond which they will either return to their affiliates or await their arrival.[16] Social distance is shortest in mare–foal dyads but begins to increase after only 1 week of life.[42] Depending on the scarcity of forage the social distance may extend to 50 meters.[30] However, it is rapidly reduced as a transient response to alarming stimuli. On the other hand, even affiliated horses can be too close for comfort when they encroach on one another's personal space, usually within a radius of 1.5 meters of the forequarters.[23]

DISPERSAL

The proximate causes of dispersal from the natal band vary with the youngster's sex.[60]

The resident stallion plays a cardinal role in the dispersal of colts and only rarely allows a member that has been driven away to rejoin the natal band. If the stallion is not active in causing the departure of a surplus member, he may passively facilitate dispersal by simply allowing a member to drift away (i.e. in contrast to his usual band maintenance activities). Lead mares may also take a role in driving away colts that are beginning to make sexual overtures.

Because they reach puberty earlier, colts tend to leave before fillies. However, the age of departure from the natal band also varies with the experience of the departee and demographics (e.g. colts leave if they have no playmates) and social pressure in the natal band.[16] Most juveniles will eventually leave the natal band, with most having done so by the age of 4 years.[42]

When she matures sexually a filly will solicit attention from males. Since this is rarely effective with resident stallions in natal bands, the filly will consort with immature males in the natal band or males at the periphery of the group. Such behavior is rarely tolerated by the resident stallion, who precipitates dispersal by driving the couple away. Occasionally a stallion may drive away a female with whom he has failed to form a sociosexual bond.[16] Sometimes the birth of a sibling is a catalyst for the departure of a filly.[24] Once they have emigrated, females are usually quick to find established reproductive groups or form new ones. Most fillies leave the natal band during an estrous period[61] between the ages of 1.5 and 2.5 years and rapidly find companions, usually males.[62] Sometimes they join with colts with whom they have previously affiliated as members of the original natal band.[63] Exiled males, on the other hand, may remain solitary for months or sometimes years.[16]

The home ranges of neighboring bands often overlap, and freshly dispersed youngsters regularly consort with adjacent groups since the value of their home range is enhanced by its familiarity compared with a completely novel area. Some juveniles leave their natal bands with a companion and consort with another group as a bonded pair or provide the nidus of a new group after encountering a small bachelor group or a similar mixed-sex juvenile band.[16] Sometimes aged horses drift between bands.[23] As their rank slips, agonistic encounters escalate until they become untenably frequent and cause dispersal.

AGONISTIC BEHAVIOR

Agonistic behavior describes a whole suite of behaviors associated with aggression, protest, threat appeasement, defence and avoidance between conspecifics.[64] From the everyday alerts and flight responses of stable groups to the drama of stallions in combat, these behaviors are of tremendous significance to humans working with horses. They provide the cardinal signs of behavioral conflict that establish thresholds of spatial infringement.[65] Moreover, when ignored they form the basis of potentially lethal responses.

The frequency and character of agonistic displays depend on herd size, since triangular and more complicated relationships, such as reversals, are more likely to occur in large herds.[48] Agonistic encounters within a band are often repeated in a series that eventually diminishes to leave the protagonists grazing alongside one another.[14] As a dominance hierarchy becomes established, the intensity of repeated encounters declines and aggression can become ritualized.[14] Non-agonistic interactions outnumber agonistic for all horses except adult males that have yet to secure a natal band, i.e. bachelors.[6] The agonistic ethogram of the bachelor group has been described in detail and includes a total of 49 elemental behaviors, three complex behavioral sequences and five distinct vocalizations.[14]

RESPONSES TO POTENTIAL DANGER

One advantage of social living is the increased surveillance afforded by the group members' eyes and ears as they scan for potentially dangerous stimuli. In grazing animals it is important for all members of the group to remain alert since, with their heads to the ground, the bodies of other horses can block some of the views around them.

The chief alert response in horses is an elevated head and neck and intense orientation of the eyes (facilitating binocular vision) and ears. This tends to evoke similar responses in other members of the group, and false alarms can amount to a cost of social living. As a means of reducing this risk, natal bands tend to take their cue from the stallion and will soon calm down, despite having been originally alarmed, if the stallion remains calm.[23]

After alert responses come flight and investigation that is usually conducted by the dominant member of the group (Table 5.4). The advantage

Table 5.4   Features of the ethogram (as described for bachelor groups[14]) employed in investigation of a potential threat

Response	Description
Alert	Rigid stance with neck elevated and head oriented toward the object or animal of focus. The ears are held stiffly upright and forward and the nostrils may be slightly dilated. The whinny may accompany this response
Approach	Forward movement at any gait or speed toward the potential threat via a straight or curving path. The head may be elevated and ears forward or the head may be lowered and the ears pinned back
Arched neck threat 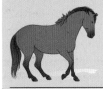	Neck tightly flexed with the muzzle drawn toward the chest. Especially characteristic of stallions, arched neck threats are observed during close aggressive encounters and ritualized interactions and may complement or coincide with other responses such as olfactory investigation, parallel prance, posturing, pawing and strike threat
Avoidance/retreat 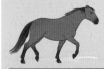	Movement that maintains or increases an individual's distance from an approaching threat. The head is usually held low and the ears turned back. The retreat can be at any gait but typically occurs at the trot
Balk 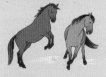	Abrupt halt or reversal of direction with movement of the head and neck in a rapid sweeping dorsolateral motion away from an apparent threat, while the hindlegs remain stationary. The forelegs lift off the ground. Typically associated with an approach or lunge of another horse
Olfactory investigation 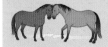	As part of interaction between conspecifics, this investigation of the head and/or body is seen after horses have approached one another nose-to-nose. After mutually sniffing face to face, typically one horse works its way along the other's body length, sniffing any or all of the following: neck, withers, flank, genitals, and tail or perineal region. During the investigation, it is common for one or both to squeal, snort, kick threat, strike threat or bite threat

of investigation over constant fleeing is that it may allow the group to continue grazing in an otherwise ideal part of their home range. Species that lack this response pay a heavy price because they are obliged to spend a great deal of time and energy in flight. Horses tend to investigate potential threats by wheeling round and adopting a circuitous approach. Depending on the novelty of the stimulus, the horse may trot as it conducts a visual appraisal of the situation. This may have the advantage of preparing its muscles for a possible flight response. The circuitous approach may be deployed in both directions before the horse gets any closer to the stimulus, thus increasing the information gained without a related increase in danger. Dilation of the nares and blowing of air accompany visual examination of the stimulus, and the noise made by this blowing often alerts band members that have not picked up on the visual indications of their peers' concern. Snorting may have the added advantage of causing some approaching animals to flee or simply disperse either because they did not intend to prey or, if they did, because they appreciate that they have been detected.

Often a horse has to get quite close to the threatening stimulus to sniff it thoroughly. For this reason it may make a series of false starts before getting close. While increasing the approaching horse's confidence, these false approaches may invite a naïve predator to launch a premature attack. When approaching a conspecific, dominant horses may be accompanied by one or two affiliates to form assemblies.[14] Solitary horses confronted with any potential threat tend to make more cautious approaches than when accompanied.

If the auditory or olfactory investigation confirms the presence of a potential predator the horse takes flight. Intriguingly humans evoke a swifter flight response by naïve unhandled horses when they assume a quadrupedal stance.[67] The putative role of human actions in round-pen work (see Ch. 13) solely as analogues of predatory responses should be considered conjecture in the light of this finding. Possibly because it is the most economical (see Ch. 7), the trot is the gait adult horses tend to use for withdrawal from a threat; while the gallop is often employed by foals. Postural tonus increases with arousal and brings the horse into a state of readiness for flight and alerts conspecifics to the possible need for escape. This response is regularly accompanied by defecation and occasional pawing at the ground.

AGGRESSION

As we have seen, aggression is generally associated with head threats and bites whereas defense involves responses by the hindquarters. Since horses are primarily in the company of affiliated band members, more demonstrations of aggression are exchanged between pair-bonded individuals than between other members of the group. Gestures used differ in their frequency depending on the sex and age of the horse making them, e.g. mares have been shown to make more kick threats than stallions and juveniles.[67]

The most common form of aggression among all horses is the head threat, which involves the extension of the aggressor's head and neck towards another individual while flattening the ears against the head. Head threats are economical and can achieve results without the aggressive animal having to move away from the resource it is seeking to protect. If the mouth is open and biting motions are included but no contact is made with the recipient, the response is labeled a bite threat. Such a response may or may not be used before an actual bite. Similar gestures are seen when horses respond to other annoyances such as flying insects and abdominal pain.[16] Bites delivered to the hindquarters of conspecifics may be used to drive other horses forward, and bite threats have the same effect. This is most notable in the snaking gestures offered by stallions when herding and driving his band. Here lateral swinging of the lowered head and neck is accompanied by the ubiquitous pinning of the ears to repel band members. Another sort of threat a horse can give using its forequarter is the threat to strike which again is accompanied by ear-pinning but is characterized by movement of one or both forelimbs outward and forward in the direction of the recipient.[7]

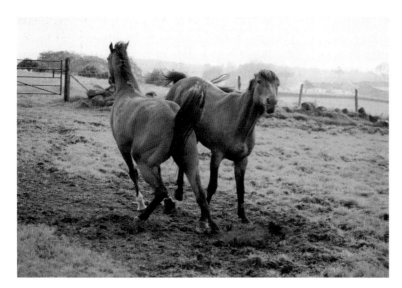

Figure 5.8 Two horses exchanging threats. Aggression between horses is accompanied by liberal signaling, i.e. threats that are used primarily to repel protagonists in a bid to avoid physical combat. (Photograph courtesy of Francis Burton.)

If the object of a horse's displeasure is closer to its hindquarters than its forequarters then kick threats and kicks are the more likely response (Fig. 5.8).[16] The hindlegs can be especially effective in aggression, and threats to use them involve simply moving the hindquarters near another animal, or lifting, occasionally hopping and ultimately kicking with the hindlegs. As with other threats, the ears are laid back as a cardinal element of these responses and the more the ears are flattened the more serious is the threat (and with it the more likely will be the emergence of physical contact). Tail-swishing and squealing often accompany kick threats. Horses are remarkably accurate when they choose to strike with their hindlegs,[68] and this is why kicks that do not engage on the protagonist are described as threats rather than misses. If threats given with the fore or hindquarters are ineffective, the aggressor may give chase.

To discipline a herd member, for example a colt that is jostling for status, the highest ranking adult may transiently exile him from the band by aggressive signaling, such as facing him squarely and staring him in the eye, chasing him away only if this is ineffective (Fig. 5.9). When the dominant animal is prepared to let the horse back into the band, having seen some signs of deference and submission (see below), the staring will abate

and the dominant animal may turn to show him part of its body's long axis.[69]

Where there is a lack of deference, for example when two band members are virtually level in the hierarchy or when an interloping bachelor makes a bid to displace a resident stallion, fights typically ensue. Mares tend to engage in kicking fights whereas stallions are more likely to rear. The specific ritualized displays stallions offer in a bid to offset the need for combat are described in Chapters 6, 9 and 11.

Posturing describes a suite of responses that are not ritualized but often seen together before combat.[14] It includes generalized muscular stiffening of the limbs, olfactory investigation, stomping, prancing and head-bowing and arched head threatening. If displays are ineffective in dispelling aggression between stallions, fights of tremendous intensity and violence may arise. These may include circling or rearing and striking. Biting is very common and serves to impair the balance or nerve of the combatant. If one of the protagonists is knocked to the ground his chances of defeat and serious injury are increased. Broken bones are a not uncommon result of fights between feral and, for that matter, domestic stallions. The repertoire of behaviors associated with aggression is summarized in Table 5.5.

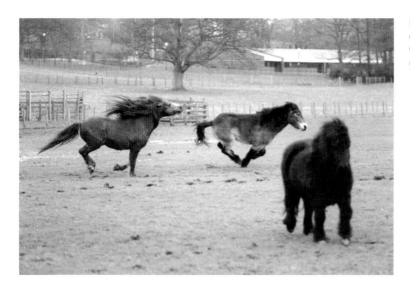

Figure 5.9 Chasing by band members is costly in terms of energy so it occurs only when threats have not been heeded. (Photograph courtesy of Francis Burton.)

Table 5.5 Features of the ethogram (as described for bachelor groups[14]) employed in aggression

Response	Description
Bite 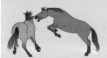	Opening and rapid closing of the jaws with the teeth grasping the flesh of another horse. The ears are pinned and lips retracted
Bite threat 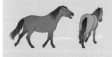	Similar to a bite except that no contact is made. The neck is stretched and ears pinned back as the head swings towards the target. The miss appears deliberate, as opposed to accidental or successfully evaded by the target, thus giving the appearance of a warning to maintain distance. Bite threats are typically directed towards the other horse's head, shoulder, chest or legs and may be performed during an aggressive forward movement such as a lunge or toward the hind end of an animal being chased or herded
Chase 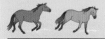	One horse pursuing another usually at the gallop in an apparent attempt to overtake, direct the movement of or catch the other. The chaser typically pins the ears, exposes the teeth and bites at the rump and tail of the pursued horse who may kick out defensively with both rear legs. Chasing is usually a part of fight sequences
Ears laid back/pinned 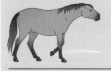	Ears pressed caudally against the head and neck. Typically associated with intense aggressive interaction
Grasp 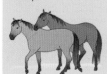	Similar to a bite but a hold that is maintained with the jaws and teeth usually on the crest of the neck or on a foreleg above the knee or hindleg above the hock

(contd.)

Table 5.5 *(Contd.)*

Response	Description
Head threat 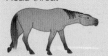	Head lowered with the ears pinned, neck stretched or extended toward the target and the lips often pursed
Interference 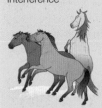	One or more horses may simultaneously interfere with an ongoing agonistic encounter between conspecifics. Disruption of combat occurs by moving between the fighting individuals, pushing, attacking or simply approaching the combatants
Kick	One or both hindlegs lift off the ground and rapidly extend backwards towards another animal with apparent intent to make contact (in contrast to the kick threat described below). The forelegs support the weight of the body and the neck is often lowered. It is common for two horses to simultaneously kick at each other's hindquarters, often associated with pushing each other's hindquarters
Kick threat	Similar to a kick, but without sufficient extension or force to make contact with the target. The hindleg(s) lift slightly off the ground and under the body in tense 'readiness', usually without subsequent backward extension. The horse may turn its rump and may back up toward the target. The tail may lash in accompaniment and/or the horse may issue a harsh squeal. This action is often indistinguishable from the preparation for an actual kick
Lunge	A swift forward thrust or charge from close range toward another horse (usually towards its forebody), most often displayed concurrently with a bite threat, with ears pinned
Nip 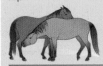	Similar to a bite but with the mouth less widely opened and the teeth closing only on a small piece of flesh, nipping is seen during play-fighting, courtship, mutual grooming and moderate to serious aggressive interactions
Pawing 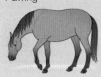	One front leg is lifted off the ground slightly, then extended quickly in a forward direction, followed by movement backward dragging the toe against the ground in a digging motion. Most commonly, this action is repeated several times in succession. The horse's nose may be oriented towards the substrate at which he is pawing or, if the activity is exhibited as a direct apparent threat (usually only between stallions) the head will remain elevated and the neck arched. Pawing is frequently seen in aggressive encounters between stallions. It is also seen near fecal piles or dusty rolling sites, either as a solitary activity or during pair or group interactive encounters

Table 5.5 *(Contd.)*

Response	Description
Push 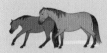	Pressing of the head, neck, shoulder, chest, body or rump against another in an apparent attempt to displace or pin the target horse against an object
Rear 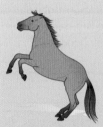	The forequarters are raised high into the air while the hindlegs remain on the ground, resulting in a near-vertical position. As a part of inter-male combat (see also boxing, dancing in stallions), two stallions will rear in close proximity and attempt to bite one another on the head and neck or strike with the forelegs
Rump presentation 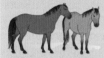	One horse positions its rump squarely in front of another horse's head, lifting the tail in a way slightly reminiscent of estrous presentation of mares. If the horse to which the rump is presented is a stallion, he usually sniffs the perineal region and may push his shoulders against the hindquarters, and/or rest his chin or head on the rump and may mount
Stomp 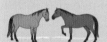	One foreleg is raised and lowered sharply and firmly against the ground, usually repeatedly. Stomping differs from pawing in that it is a vertical rather than horizontal movement of the leg. Stomping is most commonly seen during posturing and ritualized interactive sequences
Strike 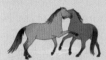	One or both forelegs are rapidly extended forward to contact another horse, while the hindlegs remain in place. The strike is typically associated with arched neck threat and posturing. A horse may also strike when rearing. The strike is often accompanied by a snort or squeal
Strike threat 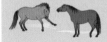	An abbreviated strike in which the foot is lifted off the ground in a gesture that mimics the preparation for an actual strike. However, no forward motion with the leg or contact with a target is actually made. The strike threat is often part of ritualized interactions between stallions and is frequently accompanied by a loud squeal or snort

SUBMISSION

Submission is the cement of equine social integrity but, perhaps because it involves signaling that is less obvious to human observers than that of aggression, it is often overlooked and its importance underestimated.[14,56] It allows subordinate animals to avoid injury and is similarly helpful to dominant individuals since it can conserve energy and thus reduce the cost of holding a resource. The same principle applies or inter-band aggression, with fewer than 25% of interactions between bands of horses over resources such as water and winter grazing ending in physical contact.[30,43]

When in close proximity with their aggressors, submissive horses often simply have to turn their heads away from their protagonists to switch off the aggression. If this fails, then they must give ground. If the subordinate horse finds that it is unable to get out of the way of an aggressor to the fore, it may throw its head with a rapid swing and roll its eyes thus exposing their sclera. The presence of an ongoing threat from the rear will usually cause the horse to tuck its tail and drop its croup as it tries to shuffle out of the way.

Other signals of deference may be given when horses are at a greater distance from one another. Signs of submission in a colt transiently exiled from the band (as described by Roberts[69]) are said to include lowering of his head to the ground, chewing, and licking his lips. Having said that, head-lowering or licking-and-chewing may be displacement responses. Their presence in free-ranging horses is the subject of ongoing discussion.[56] These oral responses are slightly reminiscent of the snapping (tooth-clapping, champing, yawing, yamming) gestures illustrated in Figure 5.5 and the jaw movements of estrous mares, especially maidens[42] and Standardbreds.[71] An alternative explanation is that such oral movements are the behavioral manifestation of a physiological response. As part of the plasma response to the distress of being in the pen with a potential predator, circulating adrenaline will rise and lead to a relatively dry mouth. This prompts licking which may elicit saliva secretion when the balance of sympathetic and parasympathetic discharges returns to normal (Francis Burton, personal communication 2002).

The true snapping display involves extending the head, often while splaying the ears laterally and drawing the corners of the mouth back. It is characteristic of horses 3 years of age and younger. The mouth is opened and closed but without any true biting, i.e. the teeth usually fail to meet. Usually performed while approaching the head of another horse at an angle, the snapping display exposes the incisors. A sucking sound may be made as the tongue is drawn against the roof of the mouth. Typically the head and neck are extended, with the ears relaxed and oriented back or laterally.

There is some debate surrounding the communication intended by animals performing these gestures, the frequency of which declines with age. For example, it has been suggested that this response has its origins in allogrooming[70] and that the performer is trying to placate the recipient by demonstrating an intention to consolidate a putative pair-bond.[23] Foals that have become displaced

from their dams snap as they approach adults in the band and continue to do so until they have recognized their dams.[42] It is interesting to note that stallions evoke more of this response than do other adults, and that male foals offer it more often than females.[67] However, studies have shown that snapping fails to inhibit aggression and in some cases may even precipitate it.[7,26] This breadth of circumstance and consequence has led some to suggest that the interpretation of snapping may be context-dependent or alternatively a displacement response derived from a suckling behavior.[26,56]

HOMING

Being less opportunistic than other species, the horse has evolved to be able to find its way back to its home range – for instance, after being pursued by a predator.[72] In addition to the promise of finding its companions there, the value of the home range to its occupant reflects the comfort of knowing tracks and escape routes within the area as well as the topographical location of resources such as food and water and shelter. The role of olfaction (and the detection of familiar fecal material) in homing is likely to be significant.[73] Horses have been recorded homing over distances of more than 15 kilometers, and Icelandic horses seem to be especially good at finding their way home.[66]

The tendency to increase speed when turned for home, shared by most horses, speaks of the motivation to remain in the home range. Bolting is far more often in the direction of home than in any other direction, and riders of horses not intended for high-speed performance do well to avoid reinforcing this tendency, e.g. by never racing in the direction of home. Horses are generally more wary of novel stimuli away from their home range, and this is one of the reasons why schooling at home is often easier than at a competition.

SOCIAL ORGANIZATION IN DONKEYS

The social structure adopted by donkeys in any particular area is dependent on the availability of resources such as food and water. In bountiful environments, donkeys use a natal band system, similar to those of horses and ponies, with complex hierarchies within the groups, in which rank is not a simple function of age, sex, aggression or weight (Jane French, personal communication). In arid and semi-arid regions, a loose social structure (also typical of African asses and Grevy's zebras) exists with temporary groups of males, or females, or males and females predominating while some jacks become solitary. Small aggregations in this system rarely last more than a few days – membership is very fluid with mixing and splitting of groups occurring when animals congregate, for example at watering sources. There is no aggression between groups. Dominant jacks do not maintain a harem but dominate breeding activity within a large area, called a lek. The only permanent association is between a female and her foal, who travel together unassociated with others. This behavioral characteristic has a profound effect on the frequency of interactive behaviors, e.g. social play is rare in donkeys when compared with harem equids.[74]

The characteristic flexibility of hemionine social structure has practical implications for the management of grazing and the housing of donkeys with horses. Since donkeys are good mixers they are used as companion animals for performance horses. Being familiar and calm, they are considered particularly valuable as travel companions when reactive sports horses leave their home yard for competitions and shows.

Although separation-related distress expressed with the drama of bolting back to the herd is less common in donkeys than in horses, some donkeys show some signs of extreme separation-related distress, such as braying, pacing and general pining, most notably when the individual is one of a bonded pair. These coping strategies do not become stereotypic. If one of a bonded pair dies, allowing the companion contact with the body for about 30 minutes seems sufficient to prevent the onset of overt separation-related distress.

Aggression toward people is very rare among donkeys (Jane French, personal communication 2001). In contrast, aggression toward other species, such as dogs and sheep, is more common in donkeys than aggression toward other equids. Indeed, along with llamas, donkeys are recognized as an effective guardian species.[75]

APPLYING THE DATA FROM FREE-RANGING HORSES TO DOMESTIC CONTEXTS

When considering the effect of domestication on the social behavior of the horse, it is appropriate to compare the social structure of domestic groups with Przewalski horses and those that have had an opportunity to revert to type. The organization of social structure in wild, feral and domestic horses is similar enough to suggest that domestication has not had an effect on this facet of horse behavior. Perhaps because of artificial selection of passivity in *E. caballus* over the past six thousand years, *E. przewalskii* in captive environments were said to have a higher level of aggression than domesticated and feral horses.[6] Having said that, it is worth noting that reintroduced *E. przewalskii* stallions do not show the high aggression recorded in confined populations. Furthermore, we should be cautious about making inferences about behavior of male *E. przewalskii*, because the extant population has only one Y chromosome since a single-stallion cohort was originally salvaged from the wild. So, presumed aggressiveness may not be a case of a characteristic of the species, but an individual variation on that chromosome (Machteld van Dierendock, personal communication 2002).

Horses naturally defend a space around them, and this accounts for the reluctance of many horses to stand close to one another when being ridden. Notwithstanding the need to maintain such a distance between horses, there are excellent reasons for riding naïve horses in the company of calmer, more experienced animals. Just as free-ranging horses after being alarmed soon calm down if the stallion remains calm,[23] so do domestic horses take their cues from companions. It is advisable to capitalize on this tendency as often as possible when introducing naïve horses to novel stimuli. It is likely that, in the process of domestication, while we have found innate reactivity desirable in racing breeds, we have selected some breeds to be less reactive than their wild forebears. This is especially so for draft work that requires animals to be docile. Cold-blooded types are therefore generally preferred as exemplars and propagators of desirable behavior in potentially fearful situations such as heavy traffic.[68]

Since it is natural for horses to develop bonds and hierarchies, managers and owners must understand that, once relationships have formed, the introduction of new horses increases the risk of injury and stress in the group. Youngsters receive the largest number of attacks in any group of horses as they are naïve and may be less responsive to threats. Just as horses in free-ranging groups tend to bond with conspecifics of similar age, so when establishing long-term groups it is appropriate to provide companions of similar ages and sufficient space for bonded pairs in a paddock to avoid one another. It has been suggested that the restrictions associated with human management may precipitate higher rates of aggression than may be seen in the free-ranging state.[4,7] This should be borne in mind when horse-holding facilities are designed: e.g. paddocks should have rounded corners to prevent subordinate animals becoming trapped and kicked by dominant 'bullies'.[68] Structures in paddocks that provide a visual screening or baffling effect may be used for sanctuary by subordinate field-mates.

Since most aggression occurs near resources it is best to place water, feeding stations and even gates away from corners. The extent to which an individual can monopolize a resource can be limited by providing one more portion of that resource than there are horses in the enclosure. To avoid low-ranking individuals failing completely to access concentrates, it is worth providing them with feeding havens or removing them from the group for supplementary feeding. Even pair-bonded affiliates may maintain a personal space of 1.5 meters when feeding, and so this should be used as the approximate minimum distance between individual feeding bays. Wire partitions along a feeding trough have been shown to reduce aggression by allowing subordinate horses to eat alongside dominant individuals.[76]

Horses adapt poorly to the constant introduction of newcomers to a social group. Indeed, equine physiologists have used social instability to induce chronic stress as indicated by elevated free plasma cortisol concentrations (i.e. a reduction in corticosteroid-binding globulin).[77] It can take 3 weeks for a new hierarchy to be established.[78]

Fighting can lead to severe injuries especially when animals are crowded or continuously grouped or regrouped.[14] Where there is a continuous flux in the complexion of a domestic group such as on a livery yard, placing mares and geldings in separate groups helps to reduce agonistic encounters that are reproductive in origin. The adoption of single-sex groups provides an analogue of the social dynamics that prevail in natal bands without a stallion (in which mare–mare bonds are successful) and bachelor groups that offer a model for male-only groupings. Providing an even number of horses in all groups facilitates pair-bonding and, if the space is available, large groups seem to be associated with less aggression than small groups, perhaps because the increased choice of preferred partners reduces the need to defend key field-mates.

In some domestic contexts mixed groups can work well, but they are more often avoided because of over-bonding between individuals of the opposite sex. Most commonly, this manifests when geldings become difficult to ride away from mares with which they have bonded. Such animals often demonstrate signs of considerable anxiety, and in their hurried return to the group they show little consideration for their own safety, let alone that of their riders. Sometimes a gelding may entirely monopolize one mare in a group to the extent that she is prevented from socializing with any other horses. Equally, one gelding may harass another for the monopoly of a given mare.

Before placing new horses in a group, it is preferable to introduce horses to one another individually so that they have the opportunity to form pair bonds. The first meeting of two strangers can be facilitated if both are sufficiently hungry to be distracted by food sources placed a safe distance apart. To facilitate the establishment of social hierarchies in very small groups, horses of disparate predicted rank (e.g. old and young horses) can be mixed. Conversely, placing horses of similar ages in the same paddock has the potential to

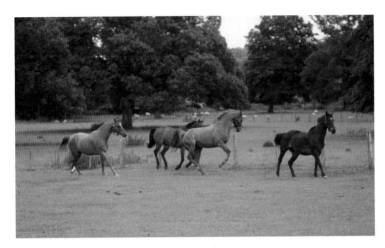

Figure 5.10 Horses that have very recently been introduced to one another posture and jostle to form a hierarchy. (Reproduced by permission of the University of Bristol, Dept of Clinical Veterinary Science.)

extend the period of flux (Fig. 5.10) during which peers challenge each other repeatedly until a hierarchy emerges. It is therefore not the preferred blend for transient groupings.

Allowing horses to meet for the first time with a fence between them has its merits but only if the barrier is safe and solid. Injuries, especially to the legs, should be expected if the fence is of wire or barbed wire. If there is no choice but to mix a new horse directly with an established group, it is best to first turn out the newcomer alone so that it can explore the paddock before it has to cope with the intensity of the whole group at once with their 'home ground advantage'. With particularly reactive animals that are likely to run rather than graze when turned out, it is advisable to walk them around the fenceline before release since this may reduce the chances of them running into the fence. This is most likely to work if other horses that may distract new arrivals are out of sight.

The overall effect of isolation of mares from an established group with or without a companion for short periods has been described as minimal.[79] Its behavioral effects include increased whinnying, urination and rolling.[79] In contrast, the effects of long-term isolation on youngsters are profound. The complete isolation of foals and juveniles is particularly inadvisable since it can lead to mal-imprinting in foals[80] and compromise social skills in juveniles.[68] Animals that have undergone such isolation as youngsters regularly

offer undesirable social behaviors upon being introduced to other horses.[13] The same animals can learn to be assertive with humans, and this seems to have the capacity to foster aggression. By way of an example, young horses that have been inadvertently reinforced for pushing humans bearing supplementary feed, can ultimately defend the resource with frank aggression.[68] Providing foals with conspecific peers is the best way to channel play-fighting in an appropriate direction and reduce the extent to which dangerous coltish responses such as rearing are directed towards humans. As the colts mature, fights become less playful when estrous mares are detected, and separation of males is advisable. This management decision should not mean that colts have to be isolated completely, as this can result in undesirable and maladaptive responses such as self-mutilation. Two-year-old colts have been shown to be sensitive to social deprivation in that stabling in isolation has long-term effects, lasting 6 weeks at least, on their social behavior.[58] Stallions can be successfully pastured together if the paddock is spacious and several watering holes are available.[14]

The companionship of an older horse can help to teach youngsters 'manners'. Meanwhile providing colts intended for breeding with a mature female companion may even help them learn mounting techniques.

Wherever possible, horses should be kept in social groups. The horse responds poorly to isolation and is likely to show physiological and behavioral distress responses including stereotypies if deprived of contact with conspecifics.[81] Horses without conspecific company have been shown to spend 10% less time eating and are three times more active than those that could make auditory, visual and tactile contact with other horses.[82] There is also evidence of physiological stress reactions with increasing time spent confined in stalls and in isolation.[83] Affiliations cannot be imposed on horses by simply housing them beside one another. This is borne out by comparisons of 2-year-old colts that were group-reared and single reared for 9 months.[58] Once released together, group-reared colts frequently had a former group mate as their nearest neighbor, whereas singly reared colts did not associate more with their former neighbors with whom they had limited physical contact via bars between stalls.[58] Instead of guessing which horses will enjoy being neighbors, stable managers should take care to stable beside one another horses that have demonstrated some affiliation in the paddock. This may serve to reduce the distressing effects of confinement. There is evidence that mirrors can provide some of the stimuli that isolated horses need (Fig. 5.11).[68] Horses do not appear to recognize the mirror images as their own, since they will sometimes show transient aggression towards

them.[68] For this reason, feed should be provided at a safe distance from the mirror, especially when the mirror has only recently been introduced.

Housing horses together in the long term allows stress reduction activities (such as mutual grooming) to take place.[65] Furthermore it is possible for managed herds to be more stable and therefore involve less risk of injury than free-ranging groups, since most changes in the social hierarchy are due to changes in the younger age classes.[67,84]

Although housing horses together is better than isolating them, care must be taken to avoid unwelcome analogues of herd responses. Social facilitation can cause hysteria to spread through a group of horses, and this is why stabling should be designed to facilitate visual and auditory contact between close neighbors but not between large numbers of horses.

Homing tendencies can be put to good use as in the case of most racecourses that have the stabling beyond the finishing line (being the site of some food and company, the stables are likely to represent the horses' temporary home range). Similarly desirable responses can be reinforced when providing horses with access to their band or affiliates, e.g. when jumping novice horses it is best to ride them over obstacles towards rather than away from other horses.

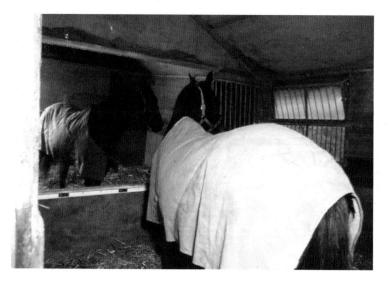

Figure 5.11 When given mirrors, isolated horses often stand beside their own image. Mirrors used in this way should have rubber backing that prevents dispersal of shards should any damage occur. (Reproduced by permission of the University of Bristol, Dept of Clinical Veterinary Science.)

SOCIAL BEHAVIOR PROBLEMS

MAL-IMPRINTING AND OVER-BONDING

Hand-reared foals often show evidence of mal-imprinting, when they prefer human company to that of other horses.[80,85] The first suspicion that a foal is adopting an individual human caregiver as a surrogate mother may be when it offers the snapping response to humans.[85] This rule of thumb should be used with caution since naturally reared foals occasionally offer the same greeting to humans. Mal-imprinting is less likely if the foal is housed in visual contact with its own kind (any non-aggressive conspecific will serve the purpose) during the sensitive period that has been estimated to end at approximately 48 hours of age.[16] While this so-called window period remains ill-defined, it is worth noting that the vocalization rate of foals experimentally separated from their dams peaks just before 4 weeks of age. This implies that their needs are maximal during this time, and therefore the possibility of

bonding on a surrogate caregiver can also be considerable at this time. So there is a strong argument for fostering such orphans or, failing that, rearing them within a group of conspecifics.

Over-bonding is recognized in horses that fail to behave normally in the absence of an attachment figure – usually an affiliated horse, rather than a member of another species. Prevention involves habituating the pair to separation during the early stages of bond formation.

Vocalization and locomotion which is often frenzied are the most common features of the affected horse's response to separation. Anorexia and failure to drink are also seen in horses distressed by separation, thus contributing to transit stress (see Ch. 14). Signs of separation-related distress can persist for several months.[16] Affected horses often attempt to escape from their enclosure, thus compromising their safety. Similarly, concerns are raised for the welfare of horses that work a trough into the ground in front of the critical piece of fence-line that separates them from the companion or where it was last seen or heard (Fig. 5.12).

Treatment should be based on the provision of an appropriate new companion or, if this is

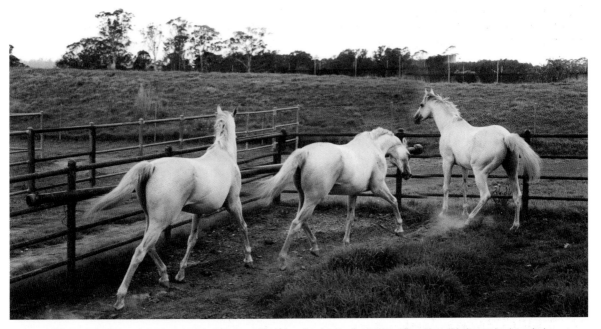

Figure 5.12 Composite image from three stills of a stallion showing barrier frustration. Over time this horse had eroded a 1 meter deep track beside the fenceline.

impractical, a mirror may have desirable effects. Not least because anxiolytics take longer to work than most horses take to form a bond with conspecifics, they are often less desirable than the provision of a companion. It should be noted that horses do not always crave company for its own sake, e.g. once a stallion's behavioral needs for female companions are met, he will not generally continue to seek others.

AGGRESSION TO HUMANS

Aggression towards humans is a common problem behavior seen in fearful horses but also in those that have learned to defend the resources within their enclosures from humans. These horses may charge or simply stand their ground to prevent humans getting past. It is thought that others may become 'socially dominant' to humans, but this is highly contentious since it may prompt some humans to perceive a need to prevail over their horses and this can lead to breakdown in the human–horse relationship. The learned aspect of this response should not be underestimated. The unwelcome behavior is reinforced by the departure of the human. Therefore, notwithstanding safety considerations, personnel should be warned that capitulating to horses that show aggressive responses in the paddock is an effective means of exacerbating the problem.

Houpt[86] describes a gelding aggressively guarding a mare to which he had bonded. Other horses may have learned to defend food, water or even their liberty (especially in the case of horses that have grown to associate ridden work with pain). Resolution of this problem requires the handler to identify which resource the horse is defending. If the horse resents the human approaching affiliates, the key members of the group or the whole group should be brought in using supplementary feed as necessary. By controlling the group, handlers can retain control while extinguishing the defensive response.

If the horse is defending resources within the paddock, moving the group into a new paddock usually disorients the animal long enough for a fresh regimen to be instituted. Provision of multiple feeding and watering spots helps to dispel

defensive aggression. The diagnosis of dominance has been controversial not least because it has been suggested that the relationship between humans and horses is profoundly different from relationships between horses.[25]

While operant conditioning techniques are often successful in shaping safe, neutral or deferential responses in aggressive horses[25] (see Fig. 5.13), the use of muscle relaxants such as succinylcholine, followed by comprehensive handling, has been advocated to induce learned helplessness in extremely aggressive horses.[87] The ethical problems with such an approach are manifold.

Trainers who hit horses for displaying aggression demonstrate poor consideration of the effects of contiguity (see Ch. 4). It is rare indeed to find someone hitting a horse in a field, because most humans can work out that this will simply drive the horse away. Instead, one tends to find whips being used punitively in stables from which there is no escape for the horse. This must increase the horse's fear and the likelihood of it using agonistic responses towards humans when trapped. If the desired response is a calm, passive approach to humans, trainers who are aware of the effects of contingency and contiguity would not expect this to be offered readily if humans have freshly been associated with aversive stimuli. When threatened by horses, personnel should remove themselves from danger and then plan a strategic program of learning opportunities that allows the horse to develop safe alternative responses to the eliciting stimuli. Examples of such programs are offered in the case studies of Chapters 11 and 15. For horses that habitually turn their hindquarters towards people as they enter the stable, shaping techniques can be very helpful in teaching the horse to turn and face humans (Fig. 5.13). If there is no time for behavior modification, the tactful use of chemical restraint for dangerous horses is vastly preferable to physical restraint or punishment (see Ch. 14).

The use of mirrors seems to reduce aggression in stabled horses (Daniel Mills, personal communication 2002). This indicates that at least some instances of aggression towards humans (e.g. as they pass the stable door) are related to social frustration.

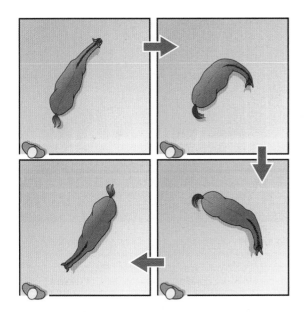

Figure 5.13 For horses that habitually turn their hindquarters towards people as they enter the stable, shaping techniques can be very helpful in teaching the horse to turn to face humans. Food should not be used as a lure. As with all shaping, the reward is withheld until the horse has shown some improvement on previous responses. In this case the shaped response is turning of the forequarters towards the human.

VOLUNTARY ISOLATION

Horses are so very social that one can regard individuals (other than peri-parturient mares) that habitually avoid other horses as abnormal. Locoweed poisoning[88] is associated with a tendency to seek isolation, and any deficit in perception may affect the individual's ability to locate and remain with its affiliates or the group. Just as old free-ranging horses begin to wander between bands, so do domestic horses tend to withdraw from group activities and ultimately the group itself in their dotage.

WEAVING AND BOX-WALKING

Two locomotory behaviors are described as stereotypic: weaving and box-walking. They are very similar in causation and their strong association with social needs indicates that this chapter

is an appropriate home for them in the current text. Weaving is the lateral swaying of the head, usually over the stable door or in the face of some other barrier.[89] The activity may include swaying of the rest of the body, notably the shoulders, and picking up the front, and sometimes the hind, legs. Box-walking is the pacing of a fixed route around the stable.[27] Typically, a circular route is traced but, in larger stables or in the field, horses may trace a 'figure of eight' shaped route.

Concern exists for the ongoing soundness of the weaving horse, as it is likely to cause excessive wear and tear on the hooves and the musculoskeletal system. Similarly box-walking in a single direction is likely to cause lateralized atrophy and hypertrophy of the lumbar musculature.

TIMING

Locomotory stereotypies and similar repetitive activities such as pawing the ground are commonly seen in stabled horses prior to feeding or other arousing daily events such as when other horses arrive at or leave the stable-yard.[27,89,90] Therefore it seems unlikely that they are caused by understimulation (or what might be labeled 'boredom') but rather they may arise when horses' motivation to move (e.g. to be with other members of the group or to reach to food) is thwarted.

RISK FACTORS

In a prospective study of a population of foals, locomotory stereotypies tended to arise at a median age of 60 weeks for weaving (i.e. after the foals have been sold from the stud to new homes) and 64 weeks for box-walking, compared with 20 weeks for crib-biting and 30 weeks for wood-chewing.[54] Therefore weaving does not appear to be related to weaning practice. Instead it seems to be related to environmental social disturbances. So research efforts should focus on reducing the impact of management interventions during this high-risk period, e.g. by examining the effects of anxiolytics and antidepressants.

Although weaving has been reported as both more[91] and less prevalent[92] in standing stalls than in loose boxes, it is seen at pasture only when horses have encountered a barrier. If being in a stable is frustrating for a horse, it is possible that the lack of free exercise plays a role in the motivation to stereotype. However, the evidence for a relationship between exercise routine and stereotypy is equivocal. For example, exercise routine was not identified as a risk factor in epidemiological studies[81] and there was little evidence that exercise routine has a consistent effect on incidence of stereotypy in the stable.[92] However, there is evidence to suggest that turning out acts as a focus for the expression of locomotory stereotypies.[90] Many owners report that preparatory cues prior to the event of turning out seem to initiate the performance of weaving and nodding.[90] So locomotory activity may either be the expression of an unusual form of species-typical anticipatory behaviors such as attempts to socially interact with other horses being led away, or a learned response to a desirable outcome such as leaving confinement.[90,93] It is interesting to speculate how some horses evolved to have these responses in the absence of domestication.

Allowing close tactile and visual contact with the neighboring horse, directly through a grille or open space between stables rather than over the stable door, significantly reduces weaving and nodding when compared with the traditional solid-walled box.[90] Indeed, in short-term studies, the incidence of weaving dropped to zero when the horses had opportunities for social interaction with their neighbors on all four sides of their enclosure.[90] Therefore weaving and, by inference, box-walking can be regarded as frustrated escape responses.[27]

PHYSICAL PREVENTION

Anti-weaving bars that provide a V-shaped aperture through which horses can put their heads and necks but which limits lateral movement are the most common response to, or prophylactic for, weaving (Fig. 5.14).[94] Their use is reported in approximately 70% of establishments.[94] Other attempts to prevent weaving include suspending a heavy object or fixing an upright bar to occupy the space above the door, both of which aim to

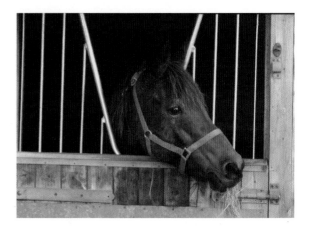

Figure 5.14 Anti-weaving bars thwart the performance of weaving, but they are unlikely to be effective in reducing the emergence of weaving in young horses. (Reproduced by permission of the University of Bristol, Dept. of Clinical Veterinary Science.)

interrupt the weaving motion, or preventing the horse from putting its head over the stable door.[95] In response to all of these physical barriers, most weavers simply move to a different area of the box and weave without having their head and neck over the door.[67,95] In stables with weaving grilles a stereotypic activity labeled treading[27] may be observed. This involves swaying of the body or alternative lifting of the forelegs, without the swaying of the head and neck.[27] Box-walking may be less easily accomplished if obstacles such as straw bales are arranged on the stable floor or if the horse is tied up, but these crude approaches are largely impractical.[96]

The use of physical impediments to locomotory stereotypies has to be questioned since they reduce the utility of the spaces occupied by affected horses and their overall effect may be to increase total frustration with the environment.[97]

MANAGING LOCOMOTOR STEREOTYPIES

Changing the cues that precede feeding or changing the time of feeding reduces pre-feeding stereotypy but not post-feeding stereotypy (Jonathan Cooper, personal communication 2002). This and the involvement of certain stimuli that reliably elicit locomotory stereotypies suggest that the role of learning in the emergence of stereotypies is significant.[97] Therefore changing the husbandry routine may be an effective treatment of such stereotypies but it is unlikely to be permanent, because the horses will most likely learn new associations that predict feeding in novel routines. Therefore, unless the husbandry routine is continually changed to maintain the novelty effect the stereotypy would return to its original level. Additionally, flux in routine is generally considered to be harmful to horses, not least in terms of gastrointestinal motility and health.

Empirical studies indicate that if stereotypic or normal horses must be stabled it is advisable to provide them with visual and tactile contact with conspecifics. The provision of close contact with conspecifics may help to explain the low incidence of stereotypies reported in some stall-tied horses,[92] but even close contact between neighboring horses does not stop weaving completely.[98] Giving stabled horses a wall to look at rather than other horses and activity in the service passage may reduce arousal and therefore the perceived prevalence of stereotypies but it provides little of the environmental enrichment we know to be of tremendous value. Although husbandry systems are being developed to facilitate social housing,[58] they may remain unattractive to some owners because of undesirable social interactions, risk of infection, or financial outlay required to maintain additional horses. Exercise may help reduce time spent stereotyping by inducing fatigue and therefore rest which is an appropriate activity for stabled horses. Additionally a practical band-aid measure may be to provide stabled horses with mirrors.[68] In both short-[99] and long-term[100] studies, mirrors appear to have a similar effect to social contact. With long-term use of mirrors, fewer repetitive head threats are reported.[100] Although the effects are impressive, it is not clear whether horses are simply distracted by reflected visual stimuli or whether they 'see' another horse. The latter seems more likely since unpublished data show similar effects with posters of horses but not when these images were pixelated (i.e. when they had the same content but the equine form

was scrambled) (Daniel Mills, personal communication 2002).

As interest grows in weaving a model of human behavioral disorders,[101] we may well see the development of pharmaceutical approaches to horses that show barrier frustration. However, we should avoid becoming reliant on such approaches, especially if they are used in the absence of appropriate environmental enrichment.

SUMMARY OF KEY POINTS

- Free-ranging horses form social hierarchies that are complex and rarely linear.
- Under natural conditions, equids seldom have the equivalent of an alpha individual, because the social roles of leadership and defense are more critical than domination.
- Domesticated horses have similar social organization to groups of free-ranging horses but often show more aggression as a product of various artificial impositions, including social flux.
- Social hierarchies increase stability in the band and decrease aggression, injury and distress.
- Individual attachment, most notably in the form of pair bonds, is the fabric of social groups.
- Housed horses benefit from social contact with conspecifics.
- Social status determines the order in which members of a group access resources.
- Horses are not usually territorial but work to maintain the integrity of their group.
- Matrilineal dynasties can be observed in many bands of horses.
- Social rank is not determined by weight, height or sex, but by age and length of residency.
- The hierarchical position of geldings reflects their rank at the time of castration.
- Stallions are not always the leaders of their natal bands. Their rank is context dependent.
- Stallions tend to form weaker pair bonds than mares, juveniles or bachelors, but this does not justify isolating them from conspecifics.

REFERENCES

1. Goodwin D, Hughes CF. Horse play. Havemeyer Workshop on Horse Behavior and Welfare, Holar, Iceland, 2002.
2. Linklater WL, Cameron EZ, Stafford KJ, Veltman CJ. Social and spatial structure and range use by Kaimanawa wild horses (Equus caballus: Equidae). NZ J Ecol 2000; 24(2):139–152.
3. Keiper RR, Houpt KA. Reproduction in feral horses; an eight-year study. Am J Vet Res 1984; 45:991–995.

4. Houpt KA, Keiper R. The position of the stallion in the equine hierarchy of feral and domestic ponies. J Anim Sci 1982; 54:945–950.

5. Keiper RR, Sambraus HH. The stability of equine dominance hierarchies and the effects of kinship, proximity and foaling status on hierarchy status. Appl Anim Behav Sci 1986; 16:121–130.

6. Keiper RR, Receveur H. Social interactions of free-ranging Przewalski horses in semi-reserves in the Netherlands. Appl Anim Behav Sci 1992; 33:303–318.

7. Weeks JW, Crowell-Davis SL, Caudle AB, Heusner GL. Aggression and social spacing in light horse (Equus caballus) mares and foals. Appl Anim Behav Sci 2000; 68(4):319–337.

8. Stevens EF. Instability of harems of feral horses in relation to season and presence of subordinate stallions. Behaviour 1990; 112(3–4):149–161.

9. Linklater WL. Adaptive explanation in socio-ecology: lessons from the Equidae. Biol Rev 2000; 75:1–20.

10. Miller R. Band organisation and stability in Red Desert feral horses. In: R.H. Denniston, ed. Symposium on the ecology and behavior of wild and feral equids. 6–8 September 1979. Laramie: University of Wyoming; 1980:113–128.

11. Kaseda Y. Seasonal changes in the home range and the size of harem groups of Misaki horses. Jpn J Zootech Sci 1983; 54:254–262.

12. Khalil AM, Kaseda Y. Early experience affects developmental behaviour and timing of harem formation in Misaki horses. Appl Anim Behav Sci 1998; 59(4):253–263.

13. Cox JE. Behaviour of the false rig: causes and treatment. Vet Rec 1986; 118:353–356

14. McDonnell SM, Haviland JCS. Agonistic ethogram of the equid bachelor band. Appl Anim Behav Sci 1995; 43:147–188.

15. Kaseda Y, Khalil AM. Harem size and reproductive success in Misaki feral horses. Appl Anim Behav Sci 1996; 47:163–173.

16. Waring GH. Horse behavior: the behavioral traits and adaptations of domestic and wild horses including ponies. Park Ridge, NJ: Noyes; 1983.

17. Budzynski M, Slomka Z, Soltys L, et al. Characteristics of nervous activity in Arab horses. Annales Universitatis Mariae Curie-Slodowska 1997; 15:165–175.

18. Feist JD. Behavior of feral horses in the Pryor Mountain Wild Horse Range. Thesis, University of Michigan, Ann Arbor, 1971.

19. Boyd LE. The natality, foal survivorship and mare–foal behavior of feral horses in Wyoming's Red Desert. Thesis, University of Wyoming, Laramie, 1980.

20. Feh C. Alliances and reproductive success in Camargue stallions. Anim Behav 1999; 57:705–713.

21. Maynard-Smith J. Evolution and the theory of games. Cambridge: Cambridge University Press; 1982.

22. Ginther OJ, Lara A, Leoni M, Bergfelt DR. Herding and snaking by the harem stallion in domestic herds. Theriogenology 2002; 57(8):2139–2146.

23. Feist JD, McCullough DR. Behaviour patterns and communication in feral horses. Zietschrift für Tierpsychologie 1976; 41:337–376.

24. Kaseda Y, Nozawa K. Father–daughter mating and its avoidance in Misaki feral horses [Japanese]. Anim Sci Technol 1996; 67(11):996–1002.

25. Crowell-Davis SL. Social behaviour of the horse and its consequences for domestic management. Equine Vet Educ 1993; 5:148–150.

26. Crowell-Davis SL, Houpt KA, Burnham JS. Snapping by foals. Zietschrift für Tierpsychologie 1985; 69: 42–54.

27. Kiley-Worthington M. The behaviour of horses: in relation to management and training. London: J Allen; 1987.

28. Duncan P. Determinants of the use of habitat by horses in a Mediterranean wetland. J Anim Ecol 1983; 52(1):93–109.

29. Rubenstein DI. Behavioural ecology in island feral horses. Equine Vet J 1981; 13:27–34.

30. Baskin LM. [Distribution of animals on pastures as a function of group behaviour (sheep, camel, reindeer, horse)] [Russian]. Sel'skokhozaistvennaya Biologiya 1975; 10(3):407–411.

31. Araba BD, Crowell-Davis SL. Dominance relationships and aggression of foals (Equus caballus). Appl Anim Behav Sci 1994; 41:1–25.

32. Klingel H. Social organisation of feral horses. J Reprod Fertil Suppl 1975; 23:7–11.

33. Miller R, Denniston RH. Interband dominance in feral horses. Zietschrift für Tierpsychologie 1979; 57:340–351.

34. Salter RE, Hudson RJ. Social organization of feral horses in Western Canada. Appl Anim Ethol 1979; 8:207–223.

35. Pelligrini S. Home range, territoriality and movement patterns of wild horses in the Wassuk Range of western Nevada. Thesis, University of Nevada, Reno, 1971.

36. Fraser AF. The behaviour of the horse. London: CAB International; 1992:214–216.

37. Welsh DA. The life of Sable Island's wild horses. Nat Canada 1973; 2(2):7–14.

38. Keiper RR. Social structure. Vet Clin North Am Equine Pract Behav 1986; 2:465–484.

39. Houpt KA, Law K, Martinisi V. The position of the stallion in the equine dominance hierarchy of feral and domesticated horses. J Anim Sci 1978; 54:945–950.

40. Van Dierendonck MC, Devries H, Schilder MBH. An analysis of dominance, its behavioural parameters and possible determinants in a herd of Icelandic horses in captivity. Neth J Zool 1995; 45(3–4): 362–385.

41. Cameron EZ. Maternal investment in Kaimanawa horses. PhD thesis, Massey University, Palmerston North, NZ, 1998.

42. Tyler SJ. The behaviour and social organization of the New Forest ponies. Anim Behav Monogr 1972; 5:85–196.

43. Berger J. Organizational systems and dominance in feral horses in the Grand Canyon. Behav Ecol Sociol 1977; 2:131–146.

44. Ellard ME, Crowell-Davis SL. Evaluating equine dominance in draft mares. Appl Anim Behav Sci 1989; 24:55–75.

45. Clutton-Brock TH, Greenwood PJ, Powell RP. Ranks and relationships in Highland ponies and Highland cows. Zietschrift für Tierpsychologie 1976; 41: 207–216.

46. Feh C. Social behaviour and relationships of Przewalski horses in Dutch semi-reserves. Appl Anim Behav Sci 1988; 21:71–87.

47. Monard AM, Duncan P. Consequences of natal dispersal in female horses. Anim Behav 1996; 52(3):565–579.

48. Estep DO, Crowell-Davis SL, Earl-Costello SA, Beatey SA. Changes in the social behaviour of draft horse (Equus caballus) mares coincident with foaling. Appl Anim Behav Sci 1993; 35(3):199–213.

49. Stebbins MC. Social organization in free-ranging Appaloosa horses. Thesis, Idaho State University, Pocatello, 1974.

50. Roberts JM, Browning BA. Proximity and threats in highland ponies. Social Networks 1998; 20(3):227–238.

51. Asa CS, Goldfoot DA, Ginther OJ. Sociosexual behavior and the ovulatory cycle of ponies (Equus caballus) observed in harem groups. Hormones Behav 1979; 13:49–65.

52. Feh C. Long term paternity data in relation to different aspects of rank for Camargue stallions. Anim Behav 1990; 40:995–996.

53. Creel S, Creel NM, Montfort SL. Social stress and dominance. Nature 1996; 379:212.

54. Waters AJ, Nicol CJ, French NP. Factors influencing the development of stereotypic and redirected behaviours in young horses: findings of a four year prospective epidemiological study. Equine Vet J 2002; 34(6):572–579.

55. Goodwin D. The importance of ethology in understanding the behaviour of the horse. The role of the horse in Europe. Equine Vet J Suppl 1999; 28:15–19.

56. Kolter L. Social relationships between horses and its influence on feeding activity in loose housing. In: Unshelm J, van Putten G, Zeeb K, eds. Proceedings of the International Congress of Applied Ethology in Farm Animals, KTBL Darmstadt, Kiel 1984:151–155.

57. Crowell-Davis SL, Houpt KA, Carini CM. Mutual grooming and nearest neighbor relationships among foals of Equus caballus. Appl Anim Behav Sci 1986; 15:113–123.

58. Christensen JW, Ladewig J, Sondergaard E, Malmkvist J. Effects of individual versus group stabling on social behaviour in domestic stallions. Appl Anim Behav Sci 2002; 75(3):233–248.

59. Feh C, De Mazieres J. Grooming at a preferred site reduces heart rate in horses. Anim Behav 1993; 46:1191–1194.

60. Rutberg A, Keiper R. Proximate causes of natal dispersal in feral ponies: some sex differences. Anim Behav 1993; 46:969–975.

61. Berger J. Wild horses of the Great Basin. Chicago: University of Chicago Press; 1986.

62. Monard AM, Duncan P, Boy V. The proximate mechanisms of natal dispersal in female horses. Behaviour 1996; 133:1095–1124.

63. Salter RE. Ecology of feral horses in western Alberta. Thesis, University of Alberta, Edmonton, 1978.

64. McFarland D. The Oxford companion to animal behaviour. Oxford: Oxford University Press; 1987.

65. Pollock J. Welfare lessons of equine social behaviour. Equine Vet J 1987; 19(2):86–88.

66. Zeeb K. Equus caballus (Equidae)—Erkundungs—und Meideverhalten. Encyclopaedia. Film no E506. Gottingen: Inst Wiss Film; 1963.

67. Wells SM, von Goldschmidt-Rothschild B. Social behaviour and relationships in a herd of Camargue horses. Z Tierpsychol 1979; 49:363–380.

68. McGreevy PD. Why does my horse …? London: Souvenir Press; 1996.

69. Roberts M. The man who listens to horses. London: Arrow Books; 1997.

70. Houpt KA, Kusunose R. Genetics of behaviour. In: The genetics of the horse. Wallingford, UK: CAB International; 2000:281–306.

71. Zeeb K. Das Verhalten des Pferedes bei der Ausienandersetzung mit dem Menschen. Säugetierk Mitt 1959; 7:142–192.

72. Williams M. Horse psychology. London: JA Allen; 1976.

73. Janzen D. How do horses find their way home? Biotropica 1979; 10(3):240.

74. McDonnell SM, Poulin A. Equid play ethogram. Appl Anim Behav Sci 2001; 78(2–4):263–295.

75. Smith ME, Linnell JDC, Odden J, Swenson JE. Review of methods to reduce livestock depredation, I: Guardian animals. Acta Agric Scand A: Anim Sci 2000; 50(4):279–290.

76. Holmes LN, Song GK, Price EO. Head partitions facilitate feeding by subordinate horses in the presence of dominant pen-mates. Appl Anim Behav Sci 1987; 19:179–182.

77. Alexander SL, Irvine CHG. The effect of social stress on adrenal axis activity on horses: the importance of monitoring corticosteroids-binding globulin capacity. J Endocrinol 1998; 157:425–432.

78. Rees L. The horse's mind. London: Stanley Paul; 1984:199.

79. Strand SC, Tiefenbacher S, Haskell M, et al. Behavior and physiologic responses of mares to short-term isolation. Appl Anim Behav Sci 2002; 78(2–4):145–157.

80. Grzimek B. Ein Fohlen, des kein Pferd kannte. Z Tierpsychol 1949; 6:391–405.

81. McGreevy PD, Cripps PJ, French NP, et al. Management factors associated with stereotypic and redirected behaviour in the Thoroughbred horse. Equine Vet J 1995; 27:86–91.

82. Houpt KA, Houpt TR. Social and illumination preferences of mares. J Anim Sci 1989; 66: 2159–2164.

83. Mal ME, Friend TH, Lay DC, et al. Physiological responses of mares to short-term confinement and social isolation. J Equine Vet Sci 1991; 11(2):96–102.

84. Houpt KA, Wolski TR. Stability of equine dominance hierarchies and the prevention of dominance related aggression. Equine Vet J 1980; 12:18–24.

85. Williams M. Effect of artificial rearing on social behaviour of foals. Equine Vet J 1974; 6:17–18.

86. Houpt KA. Aggression and intolerance of separation from a mare by an aged gelding. Equine Vet Educ 1993; 5(3):140–141.

87. Houpt KA. Domestic animal behavior for veterinarians and animal scientists. 2nd edn. Ames: Iowa State University Press; 1998.

88. McBarron EJ. Poisonous plants: handbook for farmers and graziers. Department of Agriculture, New South Wales, Australia: Inkata Press; 1983.

89. Mills DS, Nankervis K. Equine behaviour: principles and practice. Oxford: Blackwell Science; 1999.

90. Cooper JJ, McDonald L, Mills DS. The effect of increasing visual horizons on stereotypic weaving: implications for the social housing of stabled horses. Appl Anim Behav Sci 2000; 69:67–83.

91. Schafer M. The language of the horse. London: Kaye & Ward; 1975.

92. Marsden MD. Feeding practices have greater effect than housing practices on the behaviour and welfare of the horse. In: Collins E, Boon C, eds. Proceedings of the 4th International Symposium on Livestock Environment. American Society of Agricultural Engineers. Coventry: University of Warwick; 1993:314–318.

93. Nicol CJ. Understanding equine stereotypies. Equine Vet J Suppl 1999; 28:20–25.

94. McBride SD, Long L. Management of horses showing stereotypic behaviour, owner perception and the implications for welfare. Vet Rec 2001; 148(26):799–802.

95. McBride SD, Cuddeford D. The putative welfare-reducing effects of preventing equine stereotypic behaviour. Anim Welfare 2001; 10:173–189.

96. Bush K. The problem horse – an owner's guide. Marlborough: Crowood Press; 1992.

97. Cooper JJ, McGreevy PD. Stereotypic behaviour in the stabled horse: causes, effects and prevention without compromising horse welfare. In: Waran N, ed. The welfare of horses. Dordrecht: Kluwer; 2002.

98. Flannigan G, Stookey JM. Day-time time budgets of pregnant mares housed in tie stalls: a comparison of draft versus light mares. Appl Anim Behav Sci 2002; 78(2–4):125–143.

99. Mills DS, Davenport K. The effect of a neighbouring conspecific versus the use of a mirror for the control of stereotypic weaving behaviour in the stabled horse. Anim Sci 2002; 74:95–101.

100. McAfee LM, Mills DS, Cooper JJ. The use of mirrors for the control of stereotypic weaving behaviour in the stabled horse. Appl Anim Behav Sci 2002; 78(2/4):159–173.

101. Nurnberg HG, Keith SJ, Paxton DM. Consideration of the relevance of ethological animal models for human repetitive behavioral spectrum disorders. Biol Psychiatry 1997; 41(2):226–229.

6

Communication

BODY LANGUAGE

Monitoring of Przewalski horses has shown that a band's behavior can be synchronized between 50% and 98% of the time.[1] Communication between members of a social group of horses facilitates this synchrony. Horses most often communicate without using their voices. This is because they are social prey animals that must organize themselves as a group but without attracting predators. Used to scan for responses after vocalization, the ears are the most important body part in equine non-vocal communication. When flattened, they qualify all concurrent interactions as agonistic, and the extent to which they are pinned back correlates with the gravity of a threat.[2] An important feature of bite threats, ear pinning may have evolved simply as a means of avoiding ear injury during fighting, but it has taken on an additional signaling function. Rather than being pinned back, ears are simply turned to point backwards during avoidance responses as horses retreat as a display of submission.[3]

The positions of horses' ears in a moving band seems to be predicated on the positions of the bearers in the group. Horses at the front of a moving group tend to have their ears forward while those to the rear orientate their ears backwards. This suggests that, in this instance, ears are used chiefly for surveillance rather than for signaling.

Ears are not central to expressions of threatened aggression alone. Indeed they are focal to a series of expressions elegantly described by Waring & Dark.[4] Neck posture changes significantly during agonistic encounters between

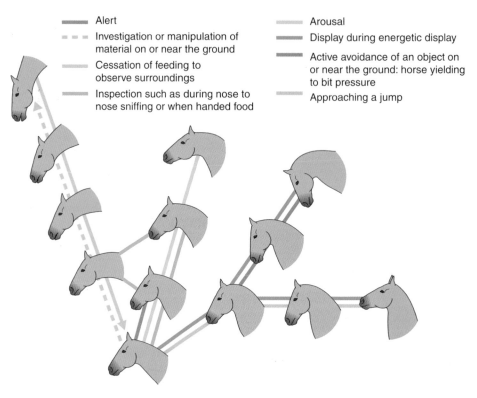

Alert

Investigation or manipulation of material on or near the ground

Cessation of feeding to observe surroundings

Inspection such as during nose to nose sniffing or when handed food

Arousal

Display during energetic display

Active avoidance of an object on or near the ground: horse yielding to bit pressure

Approaching a jump

Figure 6.1 Expressions of forward attention. (Redrawn from Waring[2], after Waring & Dark[4], with permission.)

horses, being flexed during approach responses and often arched in response to threats, especially by stallions.[3] Head bowing that involves rhythmic exaggerated flexing of the neck to the extent that the muzzle may touch the pectoral region is seen as a synchronous display by two stallions as they approach one another head to head.[3]

The series of illustrations in this chapter examine the importance in communication of various features of the equine head, including the nostrils or nares. The nares dilate and constrict with changes in mood. For example, during forward attention, as a horse sniffs the ground, they are moderately dilated whereas during aggression they become drawn back to form wrinkles on their aboral edge. In combination with head position, the ears and nares contribute to expressions of forward attention (Fig. 6.1), lateral attention (Fig. 6.2), backward attention, alarm, aggression, submission and pleasure.

When ears are pointing forward the horse is, as one might expect, attending to a stimulus in front of it. Horses are sometimes seen pointing their ears in two directions (see, for example, Fig. 2.13 on p. 49). Swiveling of the ears is associated with pain: e.g. a horse with colic may swivel its ears back in the direction of its abdomen before it gets to the stage of kicking at its belly.

In a group of horses, those that are not leading tend to focus their aural surveillance on stimuli from the rear and are therefore usually seen with their ears pointing back (Fig. 6.3.). This strategy makes sense for the safety of the group since it allows the leaders to concentrate on hazards ahead of the group.

When horses are frightened by or simply suspicious of a stimulus, their alarm is often indicated by switching the direction of the ears and by a tense mouth and dilated nostrils. Alarmed horses tend to withdraw from such stimuli with rather jerky movements that contribute as a survival strategy because they confound a predator's ability to predict the horse's intended route of escape. The same unpredictable responses can

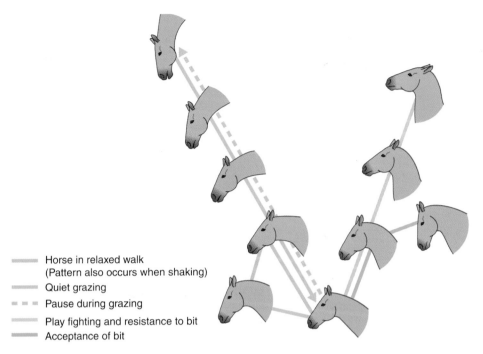

Horse in relaxed walk
(Pattern also occurs when shaking)

Quiet grazing

Pause during grazing

Play fighting and resistance to bit

Acceptance of bit

Figure 6.2 Expressions of lateral attention. (Redrawn from Waring[2], after Waring & Dark[4], with permission.)

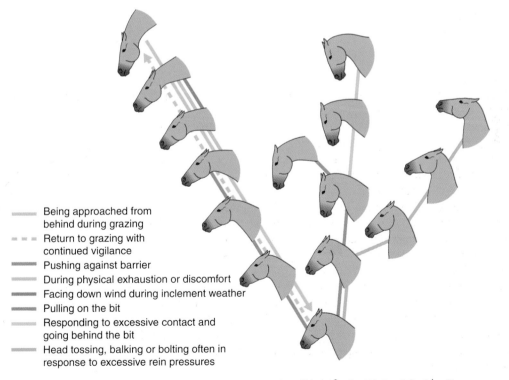

Being approached from
behind during grazing

Return to grazing with
continued vigilance

Pushing against barrier

During physical exhaustion or discomfort

Facing down wind during inclement weather

Pulling on the bit

Responding to excessive contact and
going behind the bit

Head tossing, balking or bolting often in
response to excessive rein pressures

Figure 6.3 Expressions of backward attention. (Redrawn from Waring[2], after Waring & Dark[4], with permission.)

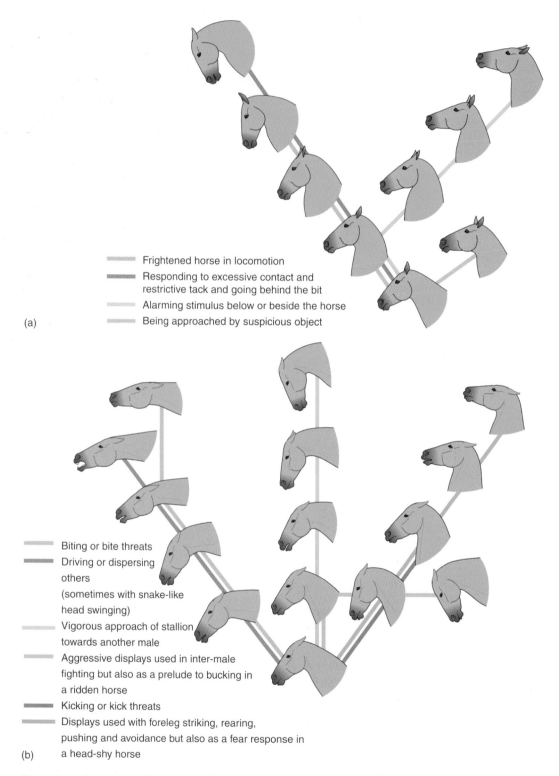

(a)

Frightened horse in locomotion

Responding to excessive contact and restrictive tack and going behind the bit

Alarming stimulus below or beside the horse

Being approached by suspicious object

Biting or bite threats

Driving or dispersing others (sometimes with snake-like head swinging)

Vigorous approach of stallion towards another male

Aggressive displays used in inter-male fighting but also as a prelude to bucking in a ridden horse

Kicking or kick threats

Displays used with foreleg striking, rearing, pushing and avoidance but also as a fear response in a head-shy horse

(b)

Figure 6.4 Expressions of (a) alarm and (b) aggression. (Redrawn from Waring[2], after Waring & Dark[4], with permission.)

make frightened horses dangerous to lead and ride (see Ch. 15).

Aggressive horses look similar to alarmed horses (Fig. 6.4). Indeed, one expression can give rise to the other, except that aggressive horses tend to pin their ears back and wrinkle the aboral edge of their nares, sometimes to the extent that their teeth are exposed. When driving his mares (see Ch. 11), a stallion feigns snapping[2] and drops his head below the horizontal with additional nodding and swinging movements. These embellishments to the posturing of regular aggression represent expressive movements that qualify the signal as a driving cue rather than direct aggression.

The reasons for horses to signal submission have been dealt with in the previous chapter but it is worth emphasizing that, in the midst of a conflict between horses, it is often the appeasement signals that determine the outcome. These may be very subtle. Mindful of the example offered by Clever Hans (see Ch. 4), we would do well to remember that, with their excellent vision, horses are able to detect minute cues in animals around them. When submitting, a horse will look away from the threat and try to shuffle away, often with its croup and tail lowered. If trapped in a melée, submissive horses raise their heads and often show the whites of their eyes.

Head nodding forms part of the greeting a stallion makes when he approaches a new mare or a mare which may be in estrus. Head lowering and lip-licking have been identified as signs of submission in round-pen exercises and indeed they tend to precede movement of the horse towards the trainer. Because these responses have not been recorded in scientific literature on studies of free-ranging horses, it remains difficult to interpret them. Therefore there is a need for studies of physiological responses that coincide with such behaviors. It may be that these behaviors are not so much signals as signs of conflict. Regardless of their intention, the trainer can capitalize on these warning signals by withdrawing to reinforce appropriate responses. For example, when the horse slows down or looks towards the trainer after showing these responses, the trainer can reward the horse by retreating and reducing the threats offered by his posture.

Although still the source of some controversy, the snapping action of youngsters is regarded as an attempt to communicate (Fig. 6.5). The extent to which it is successful remains unclear. Since prevalence is inversely correlated with the age of the performer, it may be that its relevance wanes as its refinement peaks. It is not offered exclusively to horses, having been observed being offered to cows, humans and horse-rider pairs. Although sometimes accompanied by sucking and tongue clicking sounds, it is chiefly a visual signal that is marked by the assumption of a characteristically extended neck and exposure of the teeth.[2] The performer often lolls its ears laterally but maintains visual focus on its target.

While the lips are usually drawn back to expose the incisors during snapping displays, they are often pursed as part of a head threat display.[3] The teeth and masseter muscles may be clenched during pain even though the lips may appear loose. The same loose lipped appearance has been noted in some sexually receptive mares and many older animals.

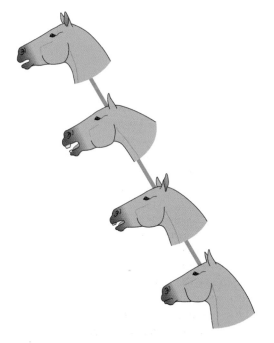

Figure 6.5 Juvenile greeting used on adults. (Redrawn from Waring[2], after Waring & Dark[4], with permission.)

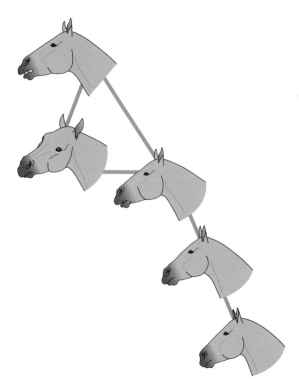

Figure 6.6 During pleasurable stimulation the upper lip may extend and twitch and on some occasions the head may turn. (Redrawn from Waring[2], after Waring & Dark[4], with permission.)

During mutual grooming, horses often extend the upper lip (Fig. 6.6) and move it from side to side and sometimes tilt their head and swivel their eyes laterally. With the panoramic quality of equine vision, it is possible that a grooming partner is able to detect this response as a signal that it has located a seat of irritation. This response, also seen when a solitary horse uses a scratching post, is sometimes accompanied by deep respiratory excursions and some luxuriant groaning.

Although rarely used in isolation from other forms of body language, the tail, or more especially its position, is an important indicator of mood or intention (Fig. 6.7). Horses are likely to be able to see the tail of another herd member if they cannot see its ears. So the tail plays a key role when horses are sorting out social spacing while at rest or while grazing in close formation. Tail movements form a characteristic element in kick threats and as such are most commonly seen

in play and courtship rather than in disputes over resources such as food or shelter.

As a characteristic of anti-insect responses, swishing movements of the tail are a sign of irritation. Riders often report this response when a horse resists or enters behavioral conflict (see Ch. 13). The significance of tail-swishing in dressage competitions is recognized by the rules which stipulate that such signs of resistance should attract penalties. Tail-raising is generally associated with the high postural tonus of arousal and an intention to move forward, while tail-lowering signals to observing horses that the bearer is intending to decelerate.[5] The tail is also lowered in horses as they withdraw from threatening stimuli. It is unfortunate that, in recognizing the importance of tail carriage in articulating demeanor, humans have chosen to interfere with it for the sake of supposed competitive success in the show ring. For example, in a bid to mask excitement, horses shown as Western pleasure horses, which are judged partly on an absence of reactivity to stimuli, may have their tails deadened by local anesthetic or even neurectomy.[6] Conversely, Arabian show horses are expected to have an elevated tail carriage as a measure of their reactivity and therefore, to raise the tail of some unfortunate individuals, irritants such as ginger are inserted per rectum.[6] Unfortunately, in contrast to tail deadening, which can be detected by an electromyogram, 'gingering' is difficult to detect.[6]

These abuses, along with 'soring' (the application of caustic material to the pasterns) to accentuate the extension of the forelimbs of Tennessee Walkers[6] are more likely to be controlled if veterinarians remain aware of them and prioritize the welfare of the animals in their care. Legislation may have outlawed many such interventions, but policing the emergent rules relies on the cooperation of the profession.

Other movements of the tail accompany urination and defecation. Clitoral winking and the increased frequency of urination of mares during estrus serve as visual signals that attract stallions to investigate the performer. Meanwhile the characteristic flagging of the stallion's tail during coitus is used by stud managers as evidence of ejaculation.

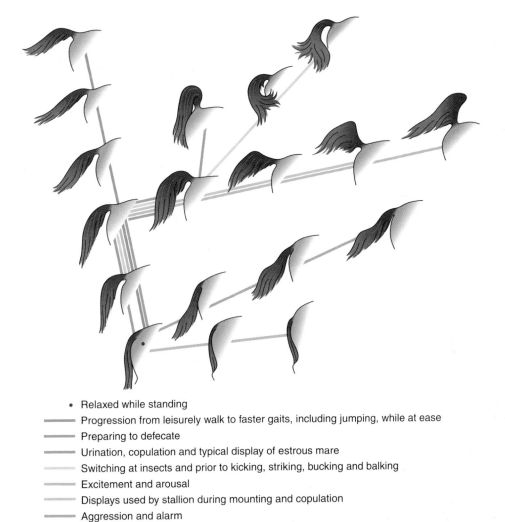

- Relaxed while standing
——— Progression from leisurely walk to faster gaits, including jumping, while at ease
——— Preparing to defecate
——— Urination, copulation and typical display of estrous mare
——— Switching at insects and prior to kicking, striking, bucking and balking
——— Excitement and arousal
——— Displays used by stallion during mounting and copulation
——— Aggression and alarm
——— Used during extreme fear, submission or prolonged pain as well as when facing downwind during inclement weather

Figure 6.7   Tail positions during various displays. (After Kiley-Worthington.[5])

Lifting of the fore- or hindlegs is used as part of striking or kicking threats, respectively. Pawing is recorded in free-ranging horses as they attempt to unearth hidden water soaks or remove snow from forage. A similar feet-stamping response is seen as a sign of frustration in domestic contexts. This is because it is often seen in combination with restraint, especially when a ridden horse is held back from joining the rest of the group, when a horse is denied access to food, or when a stallion is required to wait before approaching a mare in a service area.[7] The response can be reinforced if it occurs at the time of feeding[8] and can readily be trained as a trick.[2]

RITUALIZED DISPLAYS BETWEEN STALLIONS

There are generally thought to be five possible steps in the display sequence exchanged by stallions before they get as far as actually fighting.[2]

Table 6.1 Five stages that occur in recurring sequences when stallions meet

Core response	Additional movements	Vocalization
Standing and staring at one another while separated	• Tail switching • Pawing • Scanning for other bands • Ears forward	Whinnying
Posturing and mobile displays with elevated trotting action	• Arching of neck • Flexing of the poll • Nodding • Tail elevated • Ears forward • Pawing of fecal piles • Sniffing of fecal piles	Snorting
Advance towards one another and conduct olfactory investigation during close encounter	Start by sniffing the nostrils and muzzle then often moving over neck, withers, flank, groin, rump and perineum	Snorting followed by sudden squealing
Threats and pushing	• Bite threats • Strike threats • Biting • Striking • Circling and occasional hindleg kicking	Squealing
Defecating on a fecal pile either one after the other or simultaneously (see Fig. 9.2)	Smelling the pile usually before and after defecation	

After Waring.[2]

Partially driven by the need to prevent mixing of natal bands, these displays are performed at a distance and allow demonstrations of resource holding potential without combat as a reflection of the possible cost of fighting between stallions. While it should be noted that any element may be omitted, the five steps in the characteristic interactions between stallions are described in Table 6.1.

After any stage in the sequence of responses a pair of stallions may separate. After the fecal pile display, the sequence either as a whole or in parts may be revisited. With each sequence, one element may be accentuated and the threats tend to escalate.[2]

SOUNDS

Noises produced by the larynx are considered more important in communication between horses than the non-laryngeal noises such as groaning which are, to an extent, byproducts of the expiratory effort as it passes through the upper airways. For example, groaning is often made by swimming horses, chiefly because the respiratory excursions are made very difficult when the thorax is immersed (David Evans, personal communication 2002). Coughing and sneezing are other sounds linked to upper-airway maintenance. Kiley-Worthington[5] notes that waves of sneezing may occur in groups of horses in stables and at exercise. This may be a result of an irritant common to all affected members of the group or may even represent social facilitation.

When they use their voices, horses capitalize on their voluminous sinuses to produce sounds that travel well. Indeed in the case of a stallion, snorts and nickers can be heard from 30 and 50 meters, respectively, while his neigh can be heard by humans 1 kilometer away.[2] Depending on the sound that is being produced, the mouth may be opened or closed during vocal communication. For example, squeals are usually emitted through a closed mouth whereas whinnies are generally produced with the mouth slightly open.[3] Laryngeal and non-laryngeal vocalizations are considered in Table 6.2.

Table 6.2 Laryngeal and non-laryngeal vocalizations

Name	Context	Mean duration (ms) ± SD	Sonographic form[a]
Laryngeal vocalizations			
Squeal	Associated with both defense and aggression in agonistic interactions and with frustration on the part of mares when touched in sexual encounters and when resentful of having their udder palpated. Particularly loud and long squeals are sometimes referred to as screams[3]	870 ± 340	
Neigh (Whinny)	Used to maintain or regain contact with affiliates or offspring. A confident greeting,[6] usually followed by playful or friendly interaction[3]	1500 ± 530	
General greeting nicker	Generally associated with the arrival of food or the return of an affiliate	870 ± 370	
Mare nicker	Used by dam when she affirms the maternal-infant bond as her foal returns to her side. Can be successfully mimicked by humans when working with foals	870 ± 370	
Stallion nicker	Part of early courtship	870 ± 370	
Groans and grunts	Associated with pain, the strain of rising and swimming but also with relaxation when standing. Grunting is associated with combat (including boxing, rearing, circling and kneeling) and olfactory investigation	450 ± 380	

(contd.)

Table 6.2   (*Contd.*)

Name	Context	Mean duration (ms) ± SD	Sonographic form[a]
Non-laryngeal vocalizations			
Snort	Used defensively and aggressively,[6] especially by stallions as part of a display to alien conspecifics and in equestrian contexts in association with exercise and conflict during restraint. Also associated with startle, pain and fear responses,[3] olfactory investigation (e.g. after rolling) and upper airway maintenance	900 ± 410	
Snore	Associated with recumbent sleep	1380 ± 270	
Blow	Associated with arousal as part of an exploratory sniffing response	390 ± 50	

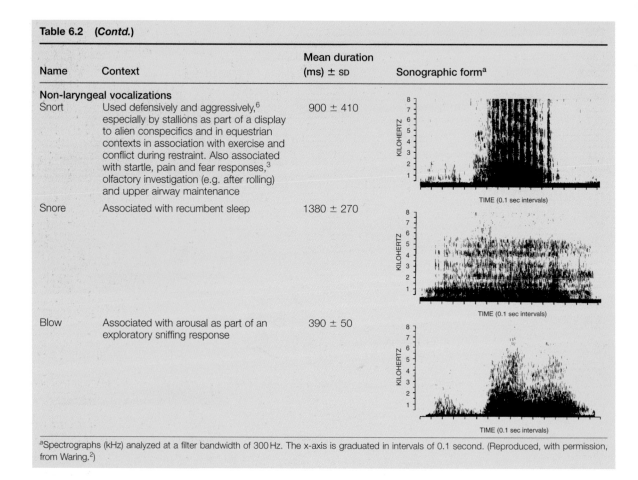

[a]Spectrographs (kHz) analyzed at a filter bandwidth of 300 Hz. The x-axis is graduated in intervals of 0.1 second. (Reproduced, with permission, from Waring.[2])

Other noises made by horses without involvement of the larynx include the rhythmic sloshing sound made by the sheath during trotting and the footfalls that other horses use to help locate conspecifics. The sound of footfalls, especially the characteristic pattern emitted when a horse investigates a novel stimulus,[2] can communicate the possible need for flight.

RECOGNITION OF SOUNDS

Field studies suggest that, by 3 weeks of age, foals can recognize their dam's neighs.[9] Other interesting observations imply that band members may respond only to the calls of affiliates that have been absent from the group for some time.[9] The importance of the neigh as a means of connecting affiliates is demonstrated by its increased frequency when one places a horse in unfamiliar company. The sight of another horse often prompts neighing, presumably in a bid to ascertain whether the conspecific is familiar.

By playing back recordings of equine vocalizations, we can begin to measure the extent to which individual calls can be recognized by their intended recipients. Compared with recorded squeals and nickers, neighs elicit more attention.[10] There is evidence that mares are better at recognizing recordings of their foal's calls than vice versa.[11]

TACTILE COMMUNICATION

As social creatures, horses have a behavioral need for tactile communication. Foals are first licked (immediately post-partum), and nuzzled (during suckling) by their dams. In return, mares are regularly nibbled by their offspring in attempts to initiate mutual grooming and play. This sets the pattern for interactions between the pair and with other horses in general. Tactile contact with the conspecific's flank and groin forms a pivotal stage when two horses greet.[2] Unfortunately, stable managers often find that meeting the need for tactile contact is made unattractive by the risk of neighbors fighting and causing injuries as they become familiar with one another. The traditional design of standing stalls in coach houses prevented contact by the inclusion of high sides at the head end of the partitions between horses. Abnormal behaviors are commonly associated with stable designs that deny tactile communication between neighbors.[12]

COMMUNICATION BY ODORS

Although they very often squeal and strike afterwards, horses sniff each other and each other's breath as part of greeting and recognition (Fig. 6.8). This had led some authors[5] to advocate blowing up the noses of horses as a means of saying 'hello'. Until we more fully understand the function of the squeal-and-strike epilogue to sniffing, this practice remains appropriate only for experienced personnel, since novices may misread the signals that the horse sends back to this overture and injuries may result.

As demonstrated by the accuracy with which mares can recognize the odor of their own foals, horses use odor to identify group members. Similarly they are sensitive to the odors of alien conspecifics, and this is why they investigate excrement carefully when given the opportunity. By leaving a sample of urine, mares are able to communicate their proximity to estrus. Stallions investigate mares' urine using the characteristic flehmen response that is thought to facilitate sampling of pheromones (see Ch. 2).[13] Typically the flehmen response includes rolling back of the upper lip, rotation of the ears to the side and extension of the neck while the head is elevated.[3]

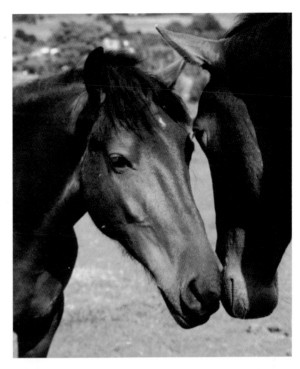

Figure 6.8 Horses sniffing one another's breath. (Photograph courtesy of Francis Burton.)

Estrous urine does not elicit more of a flehmen response than non-estrous urine, so it seems that visual displays including an increased rate of urination in estrous mares and their clitoral winking help to prompt the stallion's interest in their deposits.[14,15] Approximately 50% of female urinations may be inspected by the natal band stallion.[16] His usual response after sampling the volatile odors from the urine is to walk forward slightly, urinate on top of the mare's urine and then turn to sample the composite odor that remains. The composition of stallion urine varies in its fatty acid, phenol, alcohol, aldehyde, amine and alkane content according to maturity, sex and stage in the breeding season.[17] Because of the high concentration of cresols in the urine of stallion urine during the breeding season it has been suggested that one role of urinating on top of a mare's feces is to mask their odor and presumably thus thwart other stallions' attempts to locate potential breeding partners.[17]

Olfactory communication between stabled stallions and mares that are expected to breed can be enhanced by personnel delivering samples of both urine and feces from the stallion to the mare and vice versa. There are anecdotal reports that this practice reduces injuries when partners are brought together for mating.

MARKING STRATEGIES

Marking, especially with feces, enables horses to communicate their presence and status and to be able to know the whereabouts of other groups of horses. Because rank dictates the order in which bachelors eliminate onto one another's excrement, the highest-ranking member of the group may try to ensure that his scent, be it from rolling, urine or feces, prevails. This is why highest-ranking members of a group tend to be the last to roll in a given site (see Ch. 10). Regular marking by the natal band stallion is an effective means of avoiding fighting and confrontation between neighboring stallions. The significance of stallion piles lies in their utility as sources of both visual and olfactory signals. They do not occur only at the periphery of a stallion's range but rather are throughout the area he patrols. This makes sense given their role in inter-stallion displays, which are by no means limited to home range boundaries.

DONKEY COMMUNICATION

Donkeys have a more limited repertoire of vocalizations than horses. Five types of vocalizations have been described: grunts, growls, sorts, whuffles and brays.[18] While many calls are similar to those of horses, the most obviously different is the bray. Brays can carry over several kilometers and as a result they allow donkeys to stay in touch across sparsely populated areas. Braying choruses are a feature of social communication, but donkeys other than harem leaders usually reserve braying for attracting other donkeys when isolated, anticipating food or searching for a mate (Jane French, personal communication 2001).

In the free-ranging state, breeding donkey stallions bray most often. Unless part of a braying chorus, subordinate males rarely bray in the presence of higher-ranking males. The bray is used to affirm the stallion's status and advertise the group's presence in and possession of the area. Free-ranging jennies and foals usually bray only in response to the braying of a stray group male or when separated from the group. In domestic conditions, they often bray in response to other brays, when expecting food, or when they or their companions are in estrus (see Chs 11 and 12). When braying, the donkey's message is qualified by the position of its ears. During greeting rituals, usually prior to tactile contact, the ears are held back slightly. Whereas they are flattened further back during agonistic challenges, the ears point forwards during courtship.

SUMMARY OF KEY POINTS

- Because horses have excellent vision, the nuances of equine body language can be very subtle.
- Ear position and head posture are the most important variables in non-vocal communication.
- Tail positions can help to coordinate the movements of a group of horses.
- The olfactory cues in urine and the visual stimuli offered by characteristic estrous urination postures are used by mares to communicate their readiness to mate.
- Dung-piles and the rituals attached to them are effective means of avoidance of aggressive interactions between stallions.

REFERENCES

1. van Dierendonck MC, Bandi N, Batdorj D, et al. Behavioral observations of re-introduced Takhi or Przewalski horses in Mongolia. Appl Anim Behav Sci 1996; 50:95–114.
2. Waring GH. Horse behavior: the behavioral traits and adaptations of domestic and wild horses including ponies. Park Ridge, NJ: Noyes; 1983.
3. McDonnell SM, Haviland JCS. Agonistic ethogram of the equid bachelor band. Appl Anim Behav Sci 1995; 43:147–188.
4. Waring GH, Dark GS. Expressive movements of horses. Paper presented at Animal Behavior Society Annual Meeting, University of Washington, Seattle, 1978.
5. Kiley-Worthington M. The behavior of horses: in relation to management and training. London: JA Allen; 1987:265.
6. Houpt KA. Equine welfare. In: Recent advances in companion animal behavior problems. Ithaca,

NY: International Veterinary Information Services; 2001. A0810. 1201.

7. Ödberg FO. An interpretation of pawing by the horse (Equus caballus Linnaeus), displacement activity and original functions. Säugetierk Mitt 1973; 21:1–12.

8. McGreevy PD. Why does my horse …? London: Souvenir Press; 1996.

9. Tyler SJ. The behavior and social organisation of New Forest ponies. Anim Behav Monogr 1972; 5:85–196.

10. Ödberg FO. Bijdrage tot de studie der gedragingen van het paard (Equus caballus Linnaeus). Thesis, State University Ghent, Belgium, 1969.

11. Munaretto KR. Reciprocal voice recognition from auditory cues by a mare and her foal (Equus caballus). Unpublished Research Report, Southern Illinois University, Carbondale, 1980. Cited in Reference 2.

12. McGreevy PD, Cripps PJ, French NP, Green LE, Nicol CJ. Management factors associated with stereotypic and redirected behavior in the Thoroughbred horse. Equine Vet J 1995; 27:86–91.

13. Lindsay FEF, Burton FL. Observational study of 'urine testing' in the horse and donkey stallion. Equine Vet J 1983; 15:330–336.

14. Marinier SL, Alexander AJ, Waring GH. Flehmen behavior in the domestic horse: discrimination of conspecific odours. Appl Anim Behav Sci 1988; 19:227–237.

15. Stahlbaum CC, Houpt KA. The role of the flehmen response in the behavioral repertoire of the stallion. Physiol Behav 1989; 45:1207–1214.

16. Feist JD, McCullough DR. Behavior patterns and communication in feral horses. Z Tierpsychol 1976; 41:337–371.

17. Kimura R. Volatile substances in feces, of feral urine and urine-marked feces horses. Can J Anim Sci 2001; 81(3):411–420.

18. Moehlman PD. Feral asses (Equus africanus): intraspecific variation in social organization in arid and mesic habitats. Appl Anim Behav Sci 1998; 60(2–3):171–195.

7

Locomotory behavior

FETAL MOVEMENTS

The movements of the equine fetus have been studied with ultrasonography in a bid to explore the extent of normal locomotion in utero and its roles in optimizing presentation before labor and preparing the musculoskeletal system for work immediately post-partum. In addition, ultrasonography has demonstrated that sucking and swallowing is common in fetal foals, a finding that explains the development and strength of the sucking reflex at birth.[1]

Simple movements, such as the extension or flexion of a limb or the spinal column, can be detected from the third month of gestation.[1] As the fetus matures, these combine and become repeated to form complex movements that eventually appear coordinated.[1] The hooves are tipped with collagenous eponychia, which prevents damage to the amnion and beyond. Most of the coordinated kinetic activity of the foal, including extension of the forelimbs and head toward the maternal pelvis, occurs well in advance of uterine contractions, sometimes as much as 12 days earlier.[1] These final adjustments are considered critical in the avoidance of dystocia.[2]

While simple movements may occur 55 times per hour from the fifth to the ninth month of gestation,[1] complex movements as frequent as 84 times per hour have been recorded in the 3 days pre-partum.[1] The frequency of the final complex movements that ultimately change the fetal position from supine to prone and occasionally from posterior to anterior[1] is illustrated in Figure 7.1.

INFANT GROWTH AND MOVEMENTS

An appreciation of the normal development of foals is useful for practitioners, since deviations from the typical developmental pattern can

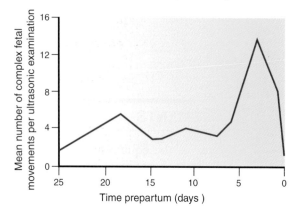

Figure 7.1 Frequency of the final complex movements in the terminal stages of gestation. Complex movements of the equine fetus become more frequent until a position suitable for engagement in the maternal pelvis is achieved. (After Fraser.[1])

indicate abnormal progression in a neonatal foal.[3] Fraser[1] suggests that five steps can be identified in the development of the primary mobility required of a foal before it takes its first mouthful of milk and the self-reinforcement of feeding can take place (Table 7.1).

The order in which features of the ethogram emerge is described in Figure 7.2. Foals that accomplish one phase quicker than the mean often show similar precociousness in other domains.[1] Perhaps because they have shorter long bones and therefore require less leverage to stand, pony foals are usually stable on their feet within half an hour,[1] much earlier than neonatal Thoroughbreds. The time taken to stand depends on the sex of the foal (average for Thoroughbred fillies being 56.3 minutes and for colts 70.6 minutes, n = 127)[4] – a difference attributed to the lighter bodyweight of fillies, who therefore require relatively less strength to rise. Unsurprisingly, fillies are the first to feed, generally having their first drink 1.5 hours after birth while colts take an average of 2 hours before feeding.[1]

Table 7.1   The steps involved in achieving primary mobility in the equine neonate

Step	Foal's responses	Dam's responses
Recumbent coordination	• Elevation of the head and neck • Head shaking • Movement of the ears • Flexion of the forelimbs • Defecation of meconium • Arranging limbs before first attempt to rise • Body-shaking between attempts	• Completing third-stage labor • Licking dorsum of foal
Rising and quadrupedal stability	• Maintenance of a half-up posture as a prelude to successful standing • Extension of the neck and forelimbs • Standing in stable position on all four feet • Gradual adduction of limbs	• Demonstrable concern for unstable offspring
Ambulation	• Four-step walking	• Demonstrable concern for unstable offspring
Maternal orientation	• Attraction to the underside of large solid objects • Attraction to junctions between the legs and trunk of the mare • Tactile exploration with muzzle • Nibbling and mouthing of objects • Location of the mammary glands • Development of dam as focus of all activity	• Minor positional changes • Sniffing and licking the foal • Nickering vocalization that helps bring the foal back to the dam and teaches avoidance
Teat-seeking and sucking	• Tactile identification of the teat • Tilting of the head • Drinking	• Pelvic tilting – often shown before milk-letdown

After Fraser.[1]

After the first drink, a melange of rest and sleep occupy most of the foal's first week but, along with locomotory play, this is punctuated by feeding every 15–30 minutes.[1]

A daily tally of motor activities in the equine neonate is given in Table 7.2. The prevalence of vigorous stretching from the first day of life suggests that it is not only pleasurable as a comfort behavior, but also that it occurs as a result of uterine confinement.[1] Stretching may occur when the foal is recumbent or upright (Fig. 7.3). The importance of stretching (or pandiculation) is dealt with elegantly elsewhere[1] but can be summarized in terms of its role in athletic development, growth and joint correctness. By the third day of life, estimates of 80 or so stretches per day have been recorded.[1] Some support for the putative orthopedic benefits of stretching comes from the coincidental peak in the frequency of stretching on day 3

of life, the age by which marginally contracted tendons have self-corrected. It would be interesting to investigate the effect of post-foaling thoracic trauma[5] on the frequency of holistic stretching.

In the first 6 weeks of a foal's life, most vigorous exercise takes the form of play,[6] but the

Table 7.2 Frequency of motor patterns in the equine neonate

Activity	Daily frequency
Defecation	2–4
Urination	4–10
Walking	8–14
Sleeping	20–25
Sucking	18–24
Stretching (recumbent and upright)	40–60

After Fraser.[1]

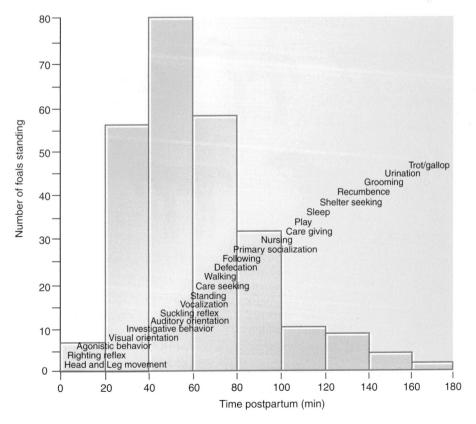

Figure 7.2 The distribution of time taken to stand, and the progressive appearance of novel responses, in the equine neonate. (After Waring[3] and Fraser.[1])

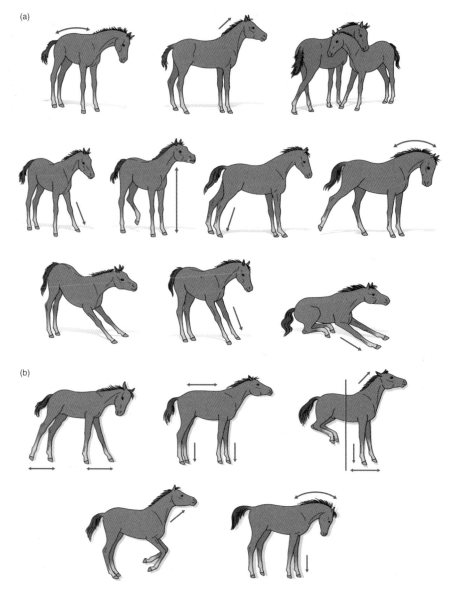

Figure 7.3 Stretching can be observed before and after locomotory activity and may occur when the foal is (a) upright or (b) recumbent. (Redrawn, with permission, from Fraser.[1])

motivation to rest, play and feed changes with age. Crowell-Davis[7] identifies three periods of behavioral development in foals, all of which involve different proportions of locomotory activity:

1. dependence (first month)
   – maximal dependence on dam
   – minimal contact with other conspecifics

2. socialization (second and third month)
   – rapidly increasing contact with non-dam conspecifics, especially peers
   – peak frequencies for mutual grooming and snapping are reached

3. stabilization and developing independence (fourth month and beyond)
   – gradually increasing independence from all conspecifics.

ADULT KINETICS

Horses have been shown to travel on open ranges (for example, to water) up to 65–80 km daily. For pastured horses, movement during grazing is the main initiator of locomotion, and an estimated daily figure for kinetic behavior in this context is 20 km.[1] The distance that grazing horses travel depends on the location of water, the availability of food and the time that has been spent foraging.

As a means of returning horses to their home range and indeed their social group, homing can occur over distances of more than 15 km.[3] The stimuli used to guide this locomotion probably involve olfaction, but they remain the subject of some debate,[8,9] especially since homing may even be conducted through water.[3]

While incessant walking has been reported as a presenting sign in serum hepatitis,[3] route-tracing in the form of box-walking (stall-walking in the USA) is far more common and emerges as a stereotypic behavior in animals that fail to cope with social isolation (see Ch. 5). Conversely, stereotypies are reported less frequently as exercise is increased.[10] Locomotion is useful as an indicator of distress, especially when conducted at the expense of feeding; for example, solitary horses walk and trot three times more often than those that can make auditory, visual and physical contacts with other horses.[11] Furthermore, locomotion's role in recreation is considerable, with 75% of the kinetic activity of foals, for example, being in the form of play.[12]

While locomotion is an integral part of equine anti-predator strategy and ingestive behavior, it is also used in communication and courtship. Exercise tends to affect other behaviors. For example, exercised horses spend more time drinking and lying but urinate less than unexercised controls.[13] Tantalizing insights into the effect of training on behavior have been offered by studies showing that horses that proceed to lose races tend to be more aroused and require greater control in the parade ring/mounting yard than winners.[14] Some of the more important dependent variables are summarized in Table 7.3. For a more comprehensive list and detailed consideration

Table 7.3 Some of the features of a racehorse's behavior and presentation that can be used to predict poor performance (not winning)

Location	Variable	Extent to which this variable predicts poor performance
Birdcage[a]	Weaving and repetitive head movements	********
	Kicking	*****
	Pawing	**
Parade ring	Crossover (figure-of eight or grackle) noseband	********
	Gaping mouth	****
	Twisting neck	***
	Nose roll (sheepskin noseband)	***
	3rd metacarpal bandages	***
	Other bandages	**************
	Pacifiers (meshed eye protection)	**
Mounting yard	Slow gait	********
	Fast gait or circling	*****
	Bucking	*****
	Balking	****
	Courtship behaviors	***
	Ears pointing laterally or aborally	**
	Defecating	**
	Flicking ears	*
Track	Late	********
	Conflict behaviors	****

Adapted from *Watching Racehorses*[14] with kind permission of Geoffrey Hutson.
[a] In Australia, racehorses can be observed in a gallery of open-front standing stalls called the birdcage, prior to being paraded (Fig. 7.4).

of the likely reasons for these variables being of significance to performance, readers are commended to an informative and entertaining book, *Watching Racehorses*.[14]

SIDEDNESS AND SYMMETRY

Even in symmetrical gaits, such as the trot and the pace, asymmetries often become evident at high speeds. In pacers, temporal gait variables, including suspension times, may differ between the left and right couplets, while in trotters high speeds have been used to expose left-right asymmetries that are particularly apparent in the hindlimbs.[15] This is not necessarily an effect of training to

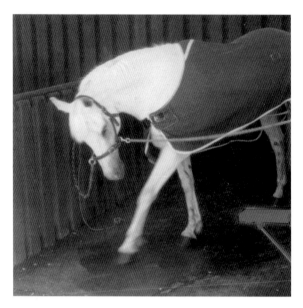

Figure 7.4 Horse in cross ties pawing in the standing stalls of a birdcage gallery at a racecourse. (Reproduced, with permission, from Hutson.[14]).

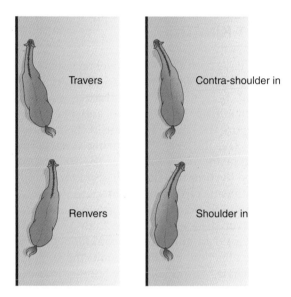

Figure 7.5 The labels for lateral movements depend on the lateral flexion of the horse's vertebral column and the direction of movement relative to the side of the school.

work in one direction. Slight individual tendencies toward either left or right laterality in general responses, such as in lying down,[1] and in foraging, have been reported by others.[16,17] Kinematic differences between the left and right limbs have also been reported in 8-month-old Standardbreds that have yet to be trained.[18]

It is reported that, when jumping, most horses seem to lead with and land with the right leg.[1] However, other workers have shown this preference only when horses are jumping on a right-handed turn.[19]

LATERAL FLEXION

If by design or by default a horse fails to use its hindlimbs in the same path as its forelimbs, it is said to be traveling in two tracks (or two-tracking). Horses can perform a number of lateral movements, most but not all of which require some flexion of the vertebral column.

In the leg yield, the neck and vertebral column are straight except for a slight flexion at the atlanto-occipital joint that flexes the head away from the direction of motion. For the movements in which the vertebral column is flexed, it is easiest

to consider the horse moving relative to an imaginary straight line. In some of the movements the neck and forequarters align with the line and the hindquarters deviate to the side (travers, renvers). In other movements the hindlegs follow the line while the forequarters deviate from it (shoulder-in, contra shoulder-in) (Fig. 7.5).

The naming of lateral movements depends on the direction in which the horse's body is bent relative to the direction of movement around the arena – clockwise (on the right rein) or counterclockwise (on the left rein). When the convex curve of the body forms the leading edge of the horse as it travels forward, the maneuver is called shoulder-in. For the reverse maneuver, in which the direction of flexion is the direction of locomotion, the terms travers or renvers are used. Half pass (Fig. 7.6) is the same as travers except that it is performed on a diagonal line across the arena.

SIMPLE TURNS AND PIROUETTES

Turns on the forehand and turns on the quarters are achieved by the rider signalling for more movement by the quarters and forehand respectively. In their elementary forms they are conducted

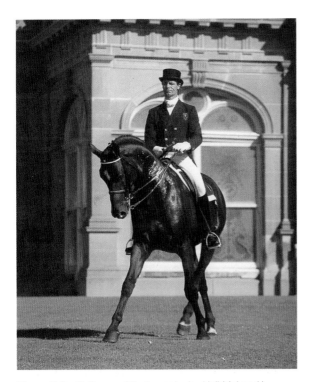

Figure 7.6 Half-pass. (Photography by Neil McLeod.)

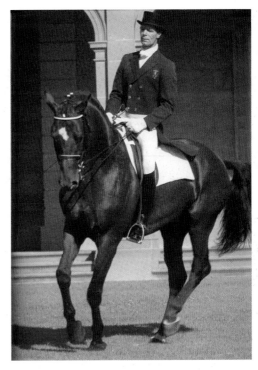

Figure 7.7 Canter pirouette to the left. (Photography by Neil McLeod.)

at the rhythm of a collected walk, but when the same principles are applied in advanced horses, elaborate balancing maneuvers, such as canter pirouettes (Fig. 7.7), are the result. However, despite the theoretical requirement that a good canter pirouette be conducted with the same tempo and rhythm as the collected canter, this is rarely the case. Analysis of individual medal finalists at the Barcelona Olympics showed that pirouettes were performed at about two-thirds of the tempo of a collected canter, had no suspension phase, and were dissociated to the extent that they could be considered to have a four-beat rhythm.[20]

This chapter will consider the gaits and maneuvers of ridden horses and those at liberty.

GAITS

By measuring oxygen consumption in trained ponies that change gait on command, Hoyt & Taylor[21] demonstrated that walking is the gait that needs least energy at low speeds, trotting at

intermediate speeds, and galloping at high speeds. This accounts for the evolution of gaits as adaptations for economical locomotion within a range of speeds.

It is argued that, in many ways, the physics of equine locomotion have evolved to their limits in that, for example, if the horse's legs were any longer, its hindlegs would be repeatedly interfering with its forelegs, as happens when the hurried (so-called butcher's boy) trot leads to forging. Budiansky[22] points out that this is the reason species such as the giraffe, with its relatively longer legs, cannot trot.

The care with which horses place their feet at speed is remarkable. With only one toe upon which to land there is little margin for error. Balance is matched by the tremendous care horses take over their hooves. This book would not be a book for hippophiles without the oft-quoted adage 'no foot – no horse'. This appears here to remind us that horses seem to live by the very same dictum. Their motivation to avoid getting their feet trapped accounts for the reluctance of some horses to accept hoof-care. Considerable neural circuitry is required for any animal to plot a safe course for four limbs, especially one that disappears once it is under the animal's nose. To perform this at the speeds horses reach and through the terrain they can traverse helps to explain why so much of the brain has to be devoted to the coordination of limbs and the control of locomotion (see Ch. 3).

Much has been said about the need for good gaits, since they give horses a head-start in training for jumping and dressage. The term kinematics describes the scientific measurement of gait. Gifted horse breeders using a visual impression, and indeed scientists using kinematic data, can predict future gait performance of foals by the age of about 4 months.[23,24] This is because the kinematic indicators of gait quality (swing duration, the maximal protraction-retraction angle and the maximal flexion of the hock joint)[25,26] show a good correlation between foals of this age and adults. A horse's conformation affects the way it moves, the extent to which its rider is displaced and the work it can successfully perform. For example, although their relative stance durations are similar, ponies make shorter strides than horses, evidenced by a shorter stance and swing duration.[26] By way of a further example, although there are occasional exceptions, Arabian horses are not generally suited to dressage because of their conformation: they frequently have disunited canters, and the hips are rotated, which has the effect of raising the tuber ishii so that their hindlegs 'trail' out behind and abduct during lengthened strides. For this reason Arabians often have trouble collecting their hindquarters (Andrew McLean, personal communication 2002).

Gaits are either asymmetrical or symmetrical. If some legs appear to work together and others do not, the horse is doing an asymmetrical gait – either a canter or gallop. As shown in Table 7.4, all of the lateral, diagonal and square gaits are symmetrical, in that the legs on one side of the horse mirror the actions of those on the other. When the legs appear to move independently of one another, not moving forward as ipsilateral or diagonal pairs, the horse is doing a square gait which may be either a walk, flat walk, running walk or tölt.

Table 7.4 The footfalls and beats that characterize symmetrical equine gaits

Gait	Footfalls	Beat	Other names
Walk	Square	1–2–3–4	–
Flat walk	Square	1–2–3–4	–
Running walk	Square	1–2–3–4	*Paso llano* (Peruvians) *Tölt* (Icelandic)
Trot	Diagonal	1–2	–
Fox-walk	Diagonal	1–2– –3–4	–
Fox-trot	Diagonal	1–2– –3–4	*Trocha* (Paso Finos) *Pasitrote* (Peruvians)
Pace	Lateral	1–2	–
Stepping pace	Lateral	1–2– –3–4	*Broken pace* *Slow gait* *Amble* *Sobreandando* (Peruvians)
Rack	Lateral	1–2–3–4	*Hreina tölt* (Icelandic) *Trippel* (Boerperds) *Largo* (Paso Finos)

If the legs on one side appear to move in opposite directions, the horse is doing a diagonal gait which will be either a trot, fox walk or fox trot. If the legs on one side move forward at the same time, the horse is doing a lateral gait which may be a pace, stepping pace, or rack.

WALK

The normal equine walk is a four-beat gait in which the feet move individually and sequentially in diagonals as follows: right fore, left hind, left fore, right hind (Fig. 7.8). At any one time the horse is supported by two feet (about 60% of the time in elite dressage horses[27]) or three (about 40% of the time in elite dressage horses[27]).

Four types of walk are recognized by the FEI: collected, medium, extended and free. In the free, performed only in the lower levels of competitive dressage, the horse is allowed to stretch the neck. As can be seen from Table 7.5, differences in the kinematics of the medium and extended walks of dressage horses are not significant. This helps to explain why dressage performances will never be scored by machines.

As with all transitions in dressage, great importance is given to the maintenance of a given rhythm and tempo, so different gaits and variations within

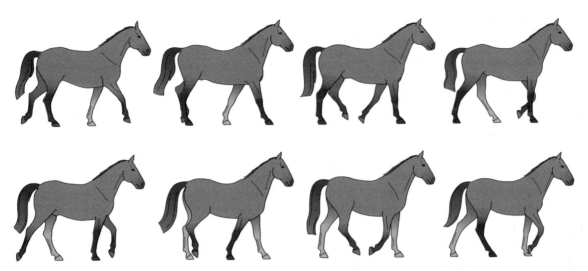

Figure 7.8   The cycle of movements at the walk. The weight-bearing limbs at each stride are indicated.

Table 7.5   Mean values for stride kinematics of the collected, medium and extended walk in dressage horses

	Speed (m/s)	Stride length (m)	Stride frequency (strides/min)	Lateral distance (cm)	Tracking distance (cm)
Collected walk	1.4[a]	1.57[a]	52[a]	158[a]	−7[a]
Medium walk	17[b]	1.87[b]	55[b]	167[a]	19[b]
Extended walk	1.8[b]	1.93[b]	56[b]	166[a]	27[b]

Data from Clayton.[28] Different superscripts indicate values that differ significantly, $p < 0.05$.

gaits are achieved by changes in stride length independent of stride frequency. Despite its being a rule of the FEI that the same stride frequency be maintained at all types of walk, this has proved difficult to demonstrate even in advanced horses.[28] Irregularities in rhythm arise because of the inclusion of lateral couplets.[28]

Stride-length is of interest to equestrians because the hindfoot should at least reach the impression made by the ipsilateral hoof (this is also known as tracking-up). If this is not the case in walks other than the collected walk, the horse is either being badly ridden or is in poor condition. In horses that have been educated for self-carriage

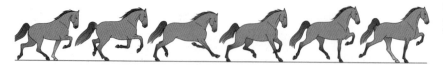

Figure 7.9 The running walk. (Redrawn, with permission, from Waring.[3])

(see Ch. 13), there is a longer stance duration (the time during which weight is borne) in the hindlimbs than the forelimbs at both the collected and extended walk.[28,29]

In the show ring, the ability of American gaited horses to demonstrate an exaggerated reach with the forelimbs and a substantial over-stride with the hindlimbs (the so-called 'big lick') is highly prized.[30] While it can be shaped behaviorally, this attribute can also be enhanced by abusive interventions. The practice of 'soring' to make horses' soles, heels or pasterns hypersensitive in a bid to emphasize their ability to lift their feet extravagantly has been subject to considerable scrutiny by the welfare lobby. Indeed it is the focus of legislation and industry self-regulation, but unhappily, as fast as the industry can agree on a protocol to identify cases of horses that are sore or have been sored, certain trainers develop new means of avoiding detection.[30]

FLAT AND RUNNING WALKS

The flat walk is the same as an ordinary walk, speeded up a little bit. A good running walk (Fig. 7.9) is the same as a flat walk, with more speed again. In Icelandics it is called a tölt and attracts different additional labels according to the speed with which it is performed (see hreina tölt, below). The fastest of the four-beat show gaits, the running walk, is characteristic of the Tennessee Walking Horse. Maximal stride frequencies are accompanied by tremendous stride lengths rather than the high foreleg action of the rack.[3]

DIAGONAL AND LATERAL WALKS

Horses can perform a diagonal walk in which the footfalls occur as diagonal couplets. The lateral walk (or fox-walk) is characterized by movement of the first foreleg being followed by movement of the ipsilateral hindleg, contralateral foreleg and contralateral hindleg. This gives rise to a lateral rocking action. An extreme example of this is the gait called the foxtrot, in which diagonal pairs of hooves lift off and move forward together, with the front landing noticeably before the hind of the pair.

TROT

The trot is a two-beat gait in which the diagonal pairs of limbs move in apparent synchrony and the footfalls of the diagonal limb pairs are evenly spaced in time (Fig. 7.10).[31] The four recognized types of trot (collected, working, medium and extended) are distinguished by their speed, stride length, stride frequency, lateral distance and tracking distance (Table 7.6).

The interval between the contacts of the fore- and hindlimb with the ground is termed the diagonal advanced displacement. This value is positive if the hindlimb contacts the ground before the forelimb and is negative if vice versa (and zero if both contact simultaneously). Although a positive diagonal advanced displacement is considered desirable for dressage, the extended trot variable that correlates closest with high scores in elite dressage competitions is stride length.[27]

At the trot, stride length depends on the distance between both diagonal pairs of hoofprints (diagonal distance) and lateral pairs (tracking distance). To increase stride length, the horse must increase the suspension phase of the trot by pushing off the ground with a greater vertical velocity (Fig. 7.11).[32] Ponies have a larger range of protraction and retraction, with a more protracted forelimb and a more retracted hindlimb, therefore they demonstrate a more extended trot.[26] However, they move with a stiffer trot than the supple trot of horses, which show a larger maximal fetlock extension during the stance phase.[26]

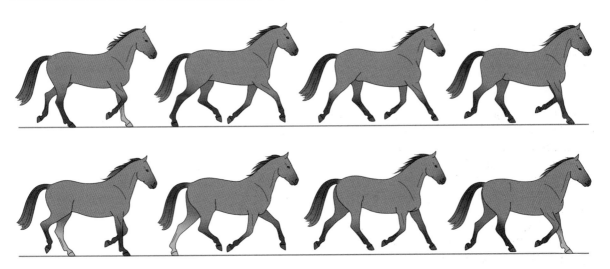

Figure 7.10   The cycle of movements at the trot. The weight-bearing limbs at each stride are indicated.

Table 7.6   Mean values for stride kinematics of the collected, working, medium and extended trot in FEI-level dressage horses

	Speed (m/s)	Stride length (m)	Stride frequency (strides/min)	Diagona distance (cm)	Tracking distance (cm)	Suspension (ms)
Collected trot	3.20[a]	2.50[a]	77[a]	132[a]	7[a]	16[a]
Working trot	3.61[b]	2.73[b]	79[a,b]	132[a,b]	4[b]	17[a]
Medium trot	4.47[c]	3.26[c]	82[a,b]	136[a,b]	27[c]	32[b]
Extended trot	4.93[d]	3.55[d]	83[b]	137[b]	39[d]	37[b]

Data from Clayton.[32] Different superscripts indicate values that differ significantly, $p < 0.05$.

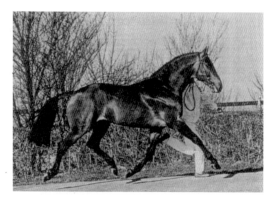

Figure 7.11 A good-quality trot is characterized by a long duration of both swing phases and suspension phases as a result of emphatic retraction and protraction of the forelimb and hindlimb, respectively. (Reproduced from Back W & Clayton HM, eds; *Equine Locomotion*; London: WB Saunders; 2001.)

PACE

The most lateral gait, the pace, is innate for some horses (e.g. Icelandics) but can be acquired by others. The progeny of pacers almost always pace, whereas only some 20% of the offspring of trotters are innate pacers.[33] As with the trot, there are two periods of suspension in each pace stride. Ipsilateral couplets are used almost synchronously so that the left fore is swung with the left hind, and the right fore with the right hind. The hindfoot makes contact with the ground before the ipsilateral foreleg (Fig. 7.12).[34] Although the pace is often described as a two-beat gait, there is sufficient dissociation between the footfalls at racing speed for it to be considered a four-beat gait.[31] A pacing horse tends to swing or 'wag' its hindquarters from side to side, while its whole body may appear to rise and fall in a motion similar to the trot.

STEPPING PACE

In five-gaited show horses, the stepping (or broken) pace is one of the acquired gaits characterized by lateral rather than diagonal couplets, and the return of the hindleg to the ground before the ipsilateral foreleg, which undergoes pronounced elevation (Fig. 7.13). The horse is supported by one, two or three legs at a time.

RACK

In five-gaited show horses, such as occur within the American Saddlebred to name but one of the numerous so-called gaited breeds, the foot-fall sequences of the lateral walk are applied in a variation called the rack. The beat is an even 1-2-3-4 (Fig. 7.14). With striking animation achieved largely through heightened foreleg action, the rack can be performed with considerable speed, stride frequencies reaching 120 per minute.[35] In the rack the horse is supported first by two, then by one hoof at a time, jumping forward between transverse pairs of legs (both front, both hind). There is a moment when the horse's weight is supported by first one hindhoof, then by one front hoof.

When Icelandics travel at the hreina (meaning clear) tölt, there is no 'jump' in the movement. The hreina tölt has the footfall sequences of the lateral walk, with an even 1-2-3-4 beat. Only one or two feet support the horse's weight, with never a moment of suspension or a moment of three-legged weight bearing. In the higher speeds the two-feet-weight-bearing phase becomes shorter while the one-foot-weight-bearing phase becomes longer. Since the horse never takes its weight from the ground, this gait is very comfortable for the rider, and allows the horse to be sure-footed in uneven terrain. Icelandic horses are the only breed in which individuals can innately show both pace and tölt from slow to gallop speed.

PASSAGE AND PIAFFE

With diagonal pairs of fore- and hindlimbs moving more or less in synchrony, the passage and its almost stationary analogue, the piaffe, are similar in footfall sequencing to the trot but differ from even a collected trot in terms of speed and stride length (Table 7.7). With two suspensions per stride and a characteristically long positive diagonal advanced displacement, the passage involves marked elevation of the limbs, which visibly pause for a moment before descending. It is seen in free-ranging horses as the prancing display characteristic of stallions (see Ch. 6).[3] Classically, the toe of the fore hoof should be elevated to the middle of the contralateral cannon, while the hindhoof

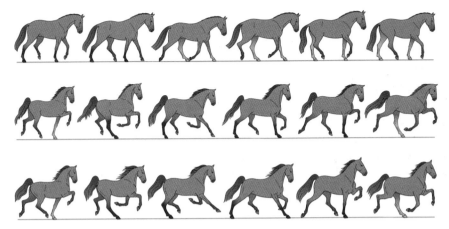

Figure 7.12 The pace. (Redrawn, with permission, from Waring.[3])

Figure 7.13 The stepping pace. (Redrawn, with permission, from Waring.[3])

Figure 7.14 The rack. (Redrawn, with permission, from Waring.[3])

Table 7.7 Mean values for stride kinematics of the collected trot, passage and piaffe in dressage horses in the individual medal finals of the Barcelona Olympics

	Speed (m/s)	Stride length (m)	Stride frequency (strides/min)
Collected trot 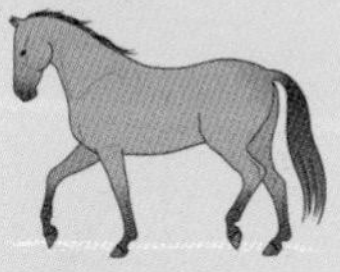	3.3[a]	2.50[a]	71[a]
Passage 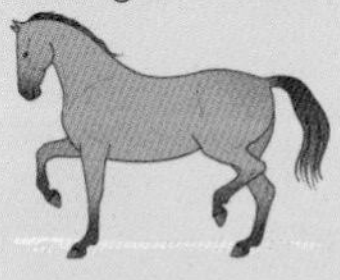	1.6[b]	1.75[b]	55[b]
Piaffe 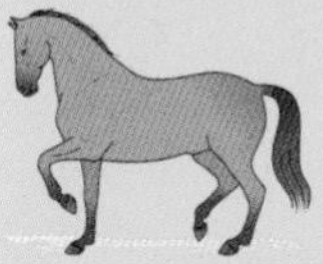	0.2[c]	0.20[c]	55[b]

Data from Clayton.[60] Different superscripts indicate values that differ significantly, $p < 0.05$.

should rise slightly above the contralateral fetlock. Notably, none of the individual medal finalists in the Barcelona Olympics demonstrated this degree of forelimb elevation.[36]

Studies of the ground reaction forces during passage demonstrate its similarity to the collected trot, in that the hindlimbs provide forward and upward propulsion while the forelimbs have the higher peak vertical force and elevate the forehand while providing longitudinal retardation.[31]

Conversely, the ground reaction forces from the piaffe show that the forelimb provides all there is of longitudinal propulsion, while the hindlimb has a retarding influence.[31] The piaffe shares a momentary pause at the peak of elevation in the swing phase, but can be readily distinguished from all other variants of the trot by having little, if any, forward movement and no suspension phase – there is always at least one hoof in contact with the ground.

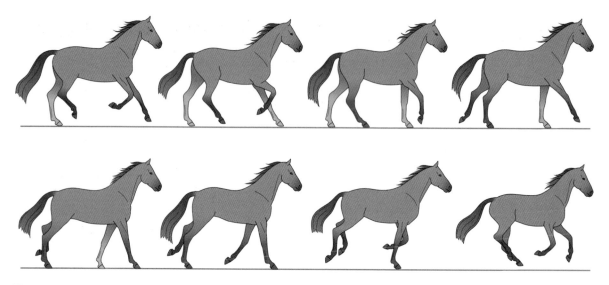

Figure 7.15   The cycle of movements at the canter (right-lead). The weight-bearing limbs at each stride are indicated.

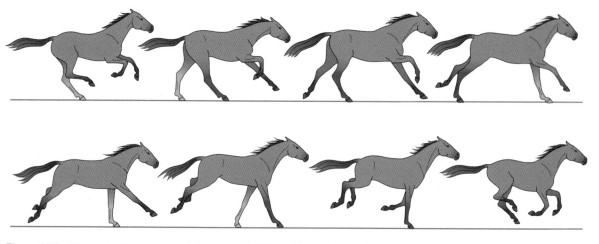

Figure 7.16   The cycle of movements at the gallop (right-lead). The weight-bearing limbs at each stride are indicated.

CANTER AND GALLOP

The canter, with three beats to the stride (Fig. 7.15), and the gallop (Fig. 7.16), with four, are asymmetrical gaits and are labeled left or right in reference to the leading foreleg and ipsilateral hindleg. The body pivots over the leading leg, which is the last leg to lift off the ground. As the horse leans toward or makes a turn to the right, it usually leads with its right leg, and vice versa. So, a right-lead canter footfall sequence is as follows: left hind, right hind/ left fore, right fore. Conversely, a left-lead canter footfall sequence is: right hind, left hind/right fore, left fore.

Speed can be used to distinguish the four types of canter recognized by the FEI (Table 7.8), with stride length being the cardinal marker of elite horses performing the extended canter.[27] In its slowest form, the canter may adopt a four-beat pattern as the second and third feet meet the ground separately. Paradoxically, as the speed increases, the four beats return with a diagonal or transverse

Table 7.8 Mean values for stride kinematics in the collected, working, medium and extended canters in FEI-level dressage horses

	Speed (m/s)	Stride length (m)	Stride frequency (strides/min)	Suspension (ms)
Collected canter 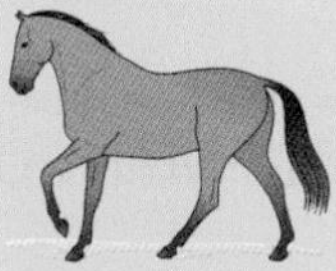	3.27[a]	2.00[a,b,c]	99[a]	0[a,b]
Working canter 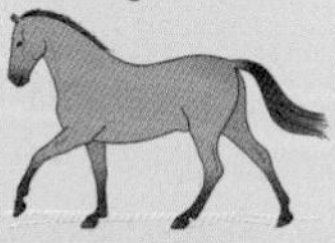	3.91[b]	2.35[a,d,e]	99[a]	5[c,d]
Medium canter 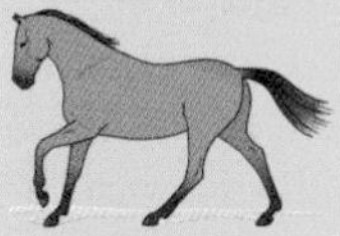	4.90[c]	2.94[b,d,f]	101[a]	54[a,c]
Extended canter 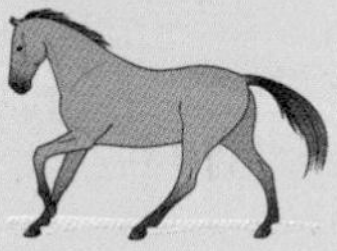	5.97[d]	3.47[c,e,f]	105[a]	87[b,d]

Data from Clayton.[61] Different superscripts indicate values that differ significantly, $p < 0.05$.

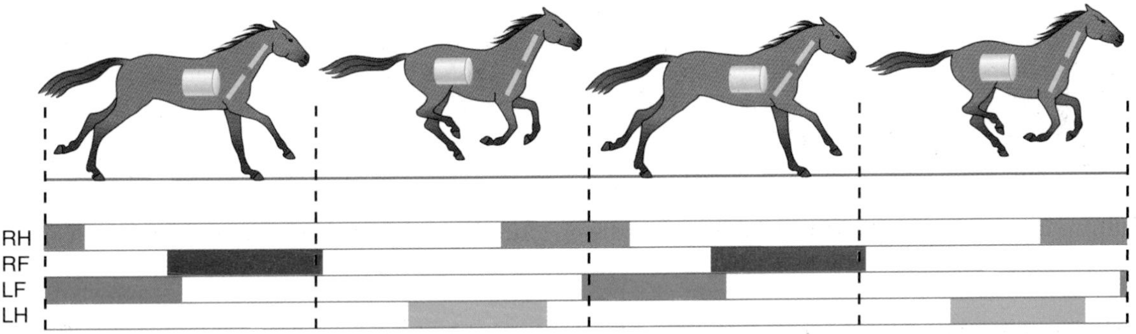

Figure 7.17 The pendular action of the head and neck are coordinated with the footfalls of the gallop stride, so that propulsion from each limb is optimized sequentially. (The barrel represents the centre of gravity.) (© Stephen Budiansky. Redrawn, with permission, from Budiansky.[22])

sequencing that distinguishes the equine gallop from the lateral or rotary gallop of the cheetah.

Although minimal dorsolateral flexion of the vertebral column is noted during galloping, systematic angular displacement of the neck occurs, presumably to assist balance. The angulation correlates with support periods of the individual legs so, effectively, the head is raised maximally shortly after the lead foreleg leaves the ground.[37] The rolling action of the neck gives the impression of the horse's cervical musculature lifting the body forward as it descends[3] (Fig. 7.17). This notion is further supported by evidence that the semispinalis capitis and splenius muscles differ in terms of their fiber type and histochemistry.[38]

Neck movement is not a feature of natural equine locomotion that is encouraged in dressage and the show ring, where maintenance of head carriage is considered desirable. Regardless of head restraint, the vertebral column, rather like the frame of a bellows, contributes to the forces of ventilation as it undergoes flexion and extension. For this reason each gallop stride is accompanied by a respiratory cycle with the horse exhaling as it lands on its leading foreleg.[39]

It is fascinating to note that, without prompting by riders, horses need considerable space to canter readily. It has been demonstrated that the tendency for horses to canter is restricted in fields of 1.5 ha or less.[40] Therefore, the dimensions of available paddocks should be borne in mind when turnout is advocated as an effective means of normalizing the behavior of a stabled horse.

AIRS ABOVE THE GROUND

A number of in-place leaps can be achieved with meticulous training (Fig. 7.18). Evocative as they are of the military origins of dressage, they are not performed in FEI competitions but instead form part of demonstrations of haute école training. All of these maneuvers involve the horse beginning by elevating its forehand. With the forelegs tightly flexed and the vertebral column inclined between 30° and 45° above the horizontal, this is called the *levade*. Maintenance of this posture requires balance, strength and the ability to flex the hindquarters profoundly. A series of levades joined together by the horse rocking smoothly forward and punctuated briefly by the forelegs contacting the ground is called *mezair*.

If the horse leaps off the ground from a levade and lands in virtually the same place, it is said to have performed a *croupade*. This is distinct from a *courbette*, which integrates deliberate forward movement within the leap. The *capriole* is a smooth sequence of movements in which the horse

emerges from levade to take off and then kick backwards with the hindlimbs while at the peak of the airborne phase. In the *ballotade* the horse leaves the ground in much the same fashion, but tucks its hindlegs underneath it.

OTHER LOCOMOTORY MANEUVERS

JUMPING

Unless trained to jump, horses generally avoid ditches and horizontal obstacles. Experienced horses approach fences in an active canter.[41] This makes sense because, in its simplest form, jumping can be viewed as an animated canter stride, except that at the moment of take-off a half-bound is inserted that aligns the hindlimbs so that both can be used to push off the ground together.[31] In 92 of 96 jumps analyzed (over oxers; see Glossary), the leading forelimb was the appendage closest to the fence at take-off.[42] In the remaining four jumps in this series, the leading hindleg was the appendage closest to the fence at take-off. The non-leading hindlimb is usually placed between the hoofprints of the two forelimbs at take-off.[42]

Although limb placements do not differ between a vertical fence and an oxer, more faults occur when horses jump the former,[31] suggesting that horses regularly get too close to fences. Forelimb errors, often forced by riders, are involved in the vast majority of jumping faults (e.g. 87% in one study of trunk accelerations[43]).

A study of 72 horses jumping in 609 rounds of competition produced some fascinating results that demonstrated that the number of faults at a particular obstacle depended on several major variables: the obstacle-type, height, color and arrangement.[44] Attempts to jump the third and fourth obstacles in the courses were faulty most often. Furthermore, while walls were the most often avoided by lateral run-outs, uprights and oxers were the most frequently knocked-down. The least number of faults was accrued at the second obstacle in a combination compared with the first and third.[44]

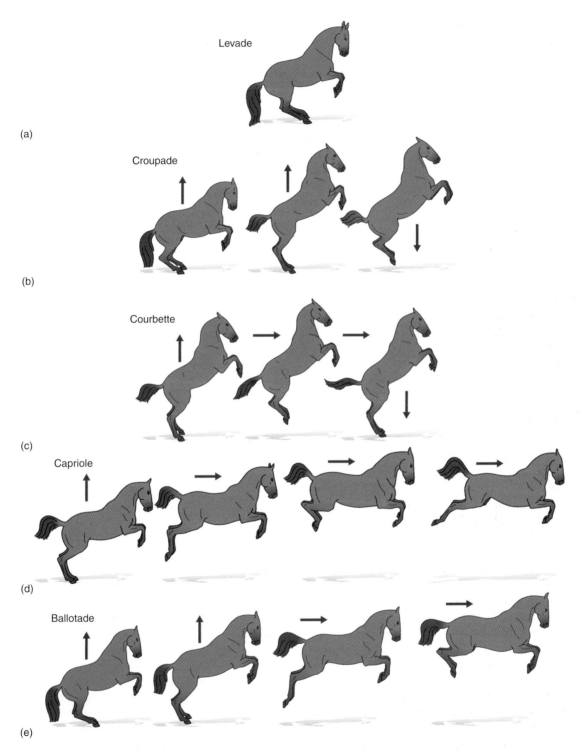

Figure 7.18 The airs above the ground: (a) levade; (b) croupade; (c) courbette; (d) Capriole; (e) Ballotade. (Redrawn, with permission, from Waring.[3])

A trajectory of 45° is implied by riding manuals that advocate the ideal take-off point for a simple vertical fence as a distance equal to its height. However, this dictum has been questioned in the light of data that demonstrate Grand Prix show-jumpers using reasonably consistent take-off distances over a variety of upright and spread fences.[22] In contrast to a standard show-jumping technique, steeplechasing is associated with the placing of both hindlimbs closer to the fence than the leading forelimb.[41]

When a horse lands after a jump, the non-leading forelimb is the first to meet the ground. It provides forward propulsion that carries the horse along, in contrast to the next limb to make contact, the leading forelimb, which has an effective braking action. The return of the trailing hindlimb, which provides more forward thrust, means that the horse has resumed a normal canter stride by the time the fourth foot falls. Good jumpers naturally tuck their forelegs more than average jumpers, and therefore, in untrained horses, this feature and the absence of excessive speed while approaching fences are considered the best predictors of later competitive success.[45]

BUCKING

Arching and humping of the vertebral column in combination with retrograde propulsion of the forehand ('pig-rooting') occur in play and as a resistance to forward movement in horses under saddle or on the lunge. Classically, the horse is said to be bucking when the hindlegs leave the ground. If the horse vaults into the air completely, it is described as buck-jumping. Although bucking is often interpreted as a demonstration of joie de vivre, it is worth remembering that in evolutionary terms it may have been a maneuver designed to dislodge a predator or, possibly, as a signal to predators that means 'don't bother with me, I'm in the very best of health'. It is important to eliminate pain, either from the saddle or in the horse's vertebral column, before assuming that a horse that starts to buck is simply being disobedient (see Ch. 15).

REARING

As part of the horse's agonistic repertoire and as a defensive maneuver used to evade aversive stimuli suddenly appearing to the fore, rearing is generally an unwelcome response in ridden horses. It is difficult to resolve because as an evasion it is often the result of conflicting rein pressure and leg pressure. For that reason, there is little left for the rider to do in the case of a rearing horse but to hang on. Since it can be difficult for horses to balance on their hindlegs the greatest danger is that the horse may fall to one side and crush the rider. For this reason many texts advise the rider to dismount from a rearing horse as soon as possible. However, to eliminate any reinforcing outcomes if the behavior has emerged as an evasion, it is important to drive the horse forward towards the stimulus that evokes the resistance. Therefore, many experienced riders choose to stay on-board to pursue the lesson.

Interestingly, in horses, such as circus animals, taught to rear, this maneuver is one of the first responses that proves difficult to achieve as the horse approaches old age. The strength a horse needs to support itself on its hindlegs and balance there is considerable and can prove limiting for these performers, as it does for geriatric stallions when required to mount mares.

SWIMMING

When swimming, the horse uses its hooves as paddles with a trotting action, but is required to keep the neck extended and the head relatively still. Despite the buoyancy afforded by displacing such a large volume of water, the effort required to move in the water with such small paddles, while inflating the lungs against the pressure of all the surrounding water, makes swimming very hard work (Fig. 7.19). This accounts for much of the grunting one hears from horses as they swim. The benefits of swimming in the conditioning of race horses and as a therapy for orthopedic injuries are well recognized but may be offset by the respiratory effort required from the horse, the coaxing required by personnel and the risk of injury associated with the activity.

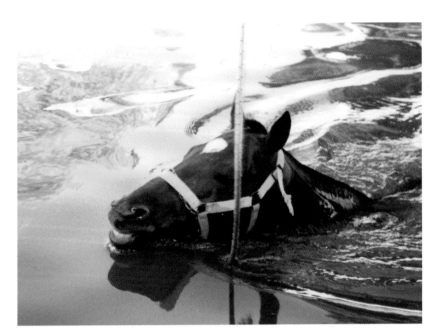

Figure 7.19 The collapse of the nostrils in a swimming horse helps to illustrate the inspiratory effort that this form of locomotion demands. (Photograph courtesy of David Evans.)

INFLUENCES ON LOCOMOTION

THE EFFECT OF CONDITIONING

Naïve riding animals may trip when ridden, simply because they are unused to supporting the weight of a rider. At the other end of the equine educational spectrum, highly trained dressage horses move in self-carriage, which implies lightness of the forehand and a greater reliance on the hindquarters for propulsion.[31] At the walk and the trot, trained horses have an increased ratio of swing to stride duration. This is achieved by a short stance duration and reduced flexion in the hindlimb, which combine so that maximal protraction occurs earlier in the stride. The action is characterized by increased fetlock extension, which is said to illustrate that more weight is being carried by the hindlimbs. This is what equestrians refer to as 'engagement of the hindquarters'. Most notable at the trot, the hindlimbs generate what is termed 'impulsion' by operating faster and with less limb flexion. Although these variables may seem of importance chiefly to dressage competitors, similar changes as a result of fitness-training are reported in young Standardbreds trained for

5 months. They show increased carpal and fetlock extension in the forelimb and increased tarsal and fetlock extension in the hindlimb.[46] The gait of pastured horses is characteristically more relaxed, with the forelimb acting as a passive strut and therefore giving the impression of movement on the forehand.[31]

THE EFFECT OF THE RIDER

Kinematics change when a horse carries a rider,[47] and the effects tend to be amplified as a function of the rider's weight. When first broken in and ridden under saddle, horses show movement that is described as being short in front.[31] This reflects the need to increase muscular strength and a new balance in order to support the rider. With training, most young horses find their balance and are therefore able to carry themselves 'on the bit' while being ridden (see Ch. 13).[31] The extent to which a rider can help a horse balance is the stuff of riding manuals rather than a horse behavior text. However, it is worth noting that, with experience, and as their balance improves, riders adopt a more upright position in the saddle and other characteristics of a good seat as illustrated in

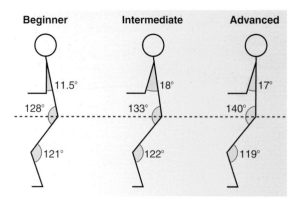

Figure 7.20 At a sitting trot, the angles of the arm, hip joint and knee joint of the beginner, intermediate and advanced riders show significant differences that can have an effect on the way in which the horse can carry itself. (Redrawn from Back W & Clayton HM, eds; *Equine Locomotion*; London: WB Saunders; 2001.)

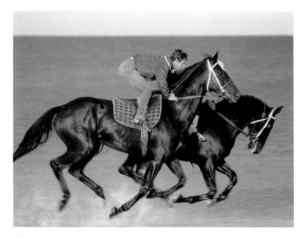

Figure 7.21 Flexion of the neck can compromise pulmonary ventilation. (Photography by Neil McLeod.)

Figure 7.20. Although this posture may make humans more effective as riders, because it makes them more stable in the saddle and increases the flexibility of the legs for delivering signals, it is not clear whether it makes the horse's task easier. With the rider in a more upright position, the centre of gravity shifts to the hindquarters, which, in an educated animal, are required to do proportionally more work than when at pasture.

During the rise phase of a rising trot, riders may set up a left–right asymmetry in ground reaction forces, but competent riders are able to compensate for this by shifting part of the weight to the hindlimbs.[48]

A great deal of effort on the part of riders goes into pursuit of a desirable outline in their horses, which involves the nasal planum being within 6° of the vertical. To the novice observer, this gives the illusion of the horse being in self carriage and therefore well-trained. Unfortunately, regardless of whether the horse has learned to carry itself that way or whether it has simply lost the battle with its rider to keep its head in a more natural position, the effect of head and neck flexion is variable upper airway obstruction (Fig. 7.21).[49]

It has been shown that in 87% of cases, faults attracted during jumping can be blamed on forelimb error,[43] and they are usually the result of inappropriate stimuli from the rider.[50] Interestingly, over-jumping occurs when horses are ridden by less competent riders. The effect of dead weight on a horse's ability to jump is seen chiefly in the clearance achieved by the leading forelimb and the extension of the fetlock and carpal joints on landing.[51] Because these indices are respectively precursors of falls over solid fences and strains of the suspensory ligament and the superficial digital flexor tendon,[31] these data led to the abolition of the minimum weight rule for eventers.

RESPONSES TO THE WHIP

In a study of Quarter Horses at the gallop, the use of a whip on the shoulder of the leading forelimb, in rhythm with the stride, did not increase speed but reduced stride length and increased stride frequency.[52] Analysis of racetrack patrol videos has shown that 38% of breakdown injuries occur after use of the whip.[53] (This may reflect the rider's response to the horse beginning to pull up with an acute lameness.)

RESPONSES TO CONFINEMENT AND REFUSAL TO LOAD

Many horses seem to find pleasure in exercise.[9] When mares were confined in standing stalls for

6 months, they showed no significant differences in baseline plasma cortisol levels or in cortisol responses to ACTH compared with exercised controls.[54] However, in the same way that cribbiters show more of the behavior after a period of deprivation, confined mares show a post-inhibitory rebound in locomotion, indicating a compensatory response to exercise deprivation. When, after 6 months of confinement, exercise was permitted, the confined group showed an increase in cortisol, whereas mares given 30 minutes of exercise per day showed a decrease in plasma cortisol levels.[54]

Unfortunately, because the motivation for movement and indeed general activity is greater in horses kept in confined and isolated environments,[55] turning-out can be associated with injury. Airs above the ground are not uncommon when confined horses are turned-out (Fig. 7.22). This can have harmful effects on the musculoskeletal system, which is generally in poor condition as a result of confinement.[56]

Confinement does not just bring reduced opportunities for exercise, but is often also associated with the absence of companions, a reduced ability to observe surroundings, and relative darkness. The enriching effects of being at pasture may help to account for data showing that training takes less time in pastured horses than stabled horses.[57] Horses in a dark stabled environment have demonstrated a preference for a lighted environment by learning to turn on lights by means of an operant device (trial-and-error conditioning).[11] Similarly, since stress responses are associated with confinement in stalls,[55] one would predict that horses would prefer to remain outside a trailer (a float in the USA and Australia) (see Fig. 2.7). There is generally very little reinforcement to be found in a confined space and, therefore, using the principles of learning theory, one would predict that the likelihood of the horse entering the trailer would naturally decline. This is often what happens when horses that naively load once or twice learn that it is a response that yields few rewards. If, when they balk and refuse to load, they are summarily punished, some learn to associate the presentation of the trailer with pain and back away from it.[58] The subsequent introduction of

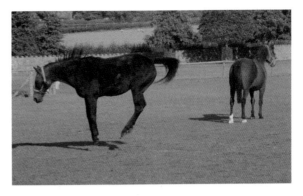

Figure 7.22   A 27-year-old horse frolicking enthusiastically after 3 months of box rest. (Reproduced by permission of the University of Bristol, Dept of Clinical Veterinary Science.)

ropes to drag the horse in, and various aversive stimuli to send the horse forward, do nothing to dissuade the horse of these associations. The learned fear abates only when time is taken to allow the horse to enter the confined space at its own pace and find reinforcement therein. Because of the horse's resistance to behavioral extinction,[9] this takes time and should be conducted at home under relaxed conditions.

Owners of horses that load without being reinforced are fortunate to have obliging, tolerant and adaptable animals. Owners of horses that associate no benefits with being loaded do well to approach this problem by reinstalling the leading signals (see Ch. 13) and by instituting a remedial reward system. Given the time such an approach takes to bring results, there is a strong argument for putting rewards in place for all novice horses until loading becomes a habit. The rewards used include premium food items and the opportunity to join a favored affiliate. Offering youngsters daily feeds in a stable (then in a horse-box and then a trailer) is a simple means of creating positive associations with confinement.

THE EFFECT OF WARMING UP

Routine exercises before competitive work help to warm up the muscles, establish rhythm and reacquaint the horse with the tasks currently required. The effects of such warm-up exercises on stride length are considerable. In endurance horses, stride length at the walk and at the trot, respectively, can increase to 115% and 151% of their pre-race values after 41 km.[59]

SUMMARY OF KEY POINTS

- Movements in utero are of tremendous importance in priming a foal for precocial existence.
- Horses have a behavioral need to stretch and locomote.
- Gaits have evolved for economical energy use at any given speed.
- Kinematic studies are useful for understanding the within-gait differences required in dressage.
- Riders, whips, conditioning and warming-up can influence locomotion in ridden horses.

REFERENCES

1. Fraser AF. The behavior of the horse. London: CAB International; 1992.
2. Rossdale PD, Ricketts SW. Equine stud farm medicine. 2nd edn. London: Baillière Tindall; 1980.
3. Waring GH. Horse behavior: the behavioral traits and adaptations of domestic and wild horses including ponies. Park Ridge, NJ: Noyes; 1983.
4. Campitelli S, Carenzi C, Verga M. Factors which influence parturition in the mare and development of the foal. Appl Anim Ethol 1982; 9(1):7–14.
5. Jean D, Laverty S, Halley J, et al. Thoracic trauma in newborn foals. Equine Vet J 1999; 31(2):149–152.
6. Fagen RM, George TK. Play behavior and exercise in young ponies (Equus caballus L). Behav Ecol Sociobiol 1977; 2:267–269.
7. Crowell-Davis SL. Developmental behavior. Vet Clin North Am Equine Pract: Behav 1986; 573–590.
8. Williams M. Horse psychology. London: JA Allen; 1976.
9. Kiley-Worthington M. The behavior of horses: in relation to management and training. London: JA Allen; 1987.
10. McBride SD, Long L. Management of horses showing stereotypic behavior, owner perception and the implications for welfare. Vet Rec 2001; 148(26):799–802.
11. Houpt KA, Houpt TR. Social and illumination preferences of mares. J Anim Sci 1989; 66:2159–2164.
12. Fraser AF. Ontogeny of behavior in the foal. Appl Anim Ethol 1980; 6:3,303.
13. Caanitz H, O'Leary L, Houpt K, et al. Effect of exercise on behavior. Appl Anim Behav Sci 1991; 31(1–2):1–12.
14. Hutson GD. Watching racehorses: a guide to betting on behavior. Melbourne: Clifton Press; 2002.
15. Drevemo S, Fredricson I, Dalin G, Bjorne K. Equine locomotion, 2: The analysis of coordination between limbs of trotting Standardbreds. Equine Vet J 1980; 12:66–70.
16. Grzimek B. Die Rechts- und Linkshandigkeit bei Pferden, Papageien und Affen. Z Tierpsychol 1949; 6:406–432.

17. McGreevy PD. The functional significance of stereotypies in the stabled horse. PhD thesis, University of Bristol, 1995.
18. Drevemo S, Fredricson I, Hjerten G, McMiken D. Early development of gait asymmetries in trotting Standardbred colts. Equine Vet J 1987; 19:189–191.
19. Leach DH, Ormrod K, Clayton HM. Stride characteristics of horses competing in Grand Prix jumping. Am J Vet Res 1984; 45(5):888–892.
20. Burns TE, Clayton HM. Comparison of the temporal kinematics of the canter pirouette and collected canter. Equine Vet J Suppl 1997; 23:58–61.
21. Hoyt DF, Taylor CR. Gait and the energetics of locomotion in horses. Nature 1981; 292:23–24.
22. Budiansky S. The nature of horses – exploring equine evolution, intelligence and behavior. New York: Free Press; 1997.
23. Clayton HM. Gait analysis as a predictive tool in performance horses. J Equine Vet Sci 1989; 9:335–336.
24. Back W, Schamhardt HC, Hartman W, et al. Predictive value of foal kinematics for adult locomotor performance. Res Vet Sci 1995; 59:64–69.
25. Back W, Barneveld A, Schamhardt HC, et al. Kinematic detection of superior gait quality in young trotting warmbloods. Vet Quart 1994; 16:S91–96.
26. Back W, Schamhardt HC, van Weeren PR, Barneveld A. A comparison between the trot of pony and horse foals to characterise equine locomotion at young age. Equine Vet J Suppl 1999; 30:240–244.
27. Deuel NR, Park J. The gait patterns of Olympic dressage horses. Int J Sport Biomech 1990; 6:198–226.
28. Clayton HM. Comparison of the stride kinematics of the collected, medium and extended walks in horses. Am J Vet Res 1995; 56:849–852.
29. Hodson E, Clayton HM, Lanovaz JL. Temporal analysis of walk movements in the Grand Prix dressage test at the 1996 Olympic Games. Appl Anim Behav Sci 1999; 62:89–97.
30. DeHaven RW. The Horse Protection Act – case study in industry self-regulation. Animal Welfare Forum: Equine Welfare. J Am Vet Med Assoc 2000; 216(8):1250–1253.
31. Clayton HM. Performance in equestrian sports. In: Back W, Clayton HM, eds. Equine locomotion. London: WB Saunders; 2001:193–226.
32. Clayton HM. Comparison of the stride kinematics of the collected, working, medium and extended trot in horses. Equine Vet J 1994; 26:230–234.
33. Cothran EG, MacCluer JW, Weitkamp LR, Bailey E. Genetic differentiation associated with gait within American Standardbred horses. Anim Genetics 1987; 18:285–296.
34. Wilson BD, Neal RJ, Howard A, Groenendyk S. The gait of pacers, 1: Kinematics of the racing stride. Equine Vet J 1988; 20:341–346.
35. Hildebrand M. Symmetrical gaits of horses. Science 1965; 186:1112–1113.
36. Argue CK. The kinematics of piaffe, passage and collected trot of dressage horses. PhD thesis, University of Saskatchewan, Saskatoon, 1994.
37. Rooney JR. The role of the neck on locomotion. Mod Vet Prac 1978; 59:211–213.
38. Gellman KS, Bertram JEA, Hermanson JW. Morphology, histochemistry, and function of epaxial

cervical musculature in the horse (Equus caballus). J Morphol 2002; 251(2):182–194.

39. Young IS, Alexander RMcN, Woakes AJ, et al. The synchronisation of ventilation and locomotion in horses (Equus caballus). J Exp Biol 1992; 166:19–31.

40. Kusunose R, Hatakeyama H, Kubo K, et al. [Behavioral studies on yearling horses in field environments, I: Effects of field size on the behavior of horses] [Japanese]. Bull Equine Res Inst 1985; 22:1–7.

41. Leach DH, Ormrod K. The technique of jumping a steeplechase fence by competing event-horses. Appl Anim Behav Sci 1984; 12:15–24.

42. Clayton HM, Barlow DA. The effect of fence height and width on the limb placements of show-jumping horses. J Equine Vet Sci 1989; 9:179–185.

43. Barrey E, Galloux P. Analysis of the equine jumping technique by accelerometry. Equine Vet J Suppl 1997; 23:45–49.

44. Stachurska A, Pieta M, Nesteruk E. Which obstacles are most problematic for jumping horses? Appl Anim Behav Sci 2002; 77(3):197–207.

45. Powers PNR, Harrison AJ. A study on the techniques used by untrained horses during loose jumping. J Equine Vet Sci 2000; 20:845.

46. van Weeren PR, van den Bogert AJ, Back W, et al. Kinematics of the Standardbred trotter measured at 6, 7, 8 and 9 months on a treadmill, before and after 5 months of pre-race training. Acta Anat 1993; 146:154–161.

47. Sloet van Oldruitenborgh-Oosterbaan MM, van Schamhardt HC, Barneveld A. Effects of weight and riding on workload and locomotion during treadmill exercise. Equine Exer Physiol 1995; 4:413–417.

48. Schamhardt HC, Merkens HW, van Osch GJVM. Ground reaction force analysis of horse ridden at walk and trot. Equine Exer Physiol 1991; 3:120–127.

49. Petsche VM, Derksen FJ, Berney CE, Robinson NE. Effect of head position on upper airway function in exercising horses. Equine Vet J Suppl, 1995; 18:18–22.

50. Lauk HD, Auer J, von Plocki KA. Zum Problem 'Barren' Uberblick, biomechanische Berechnungen und Verhaltungsbeobachtungen. Pferdeheilkunde 1991; 7:225–235.

51. Clayton HM. Effect of added weight on landing kinematics of jumping horses. Equine Vet J Suppl 1997; 23:50–53.

52. Deuel NR, Lawrence LM. Effects of urging by the rider on equine gallop stride limb contacts. Proc Equine Nutr Physiol 1987; 10:487–494.

53. Ueda Y, Yoshida K, Oikawa M. Analyses of race accident conditions through use of patrol video. J Equine Vet Sci 1993; 13:707–710.

54. Houpt K, Houpt TR, Johnson JL, et al. The effect of exercise deprivation on the behavior and physiology of straight-stall confined pregnant mares. Anim Welfare 2001; 10(3):257–267.

55. Mal ME, Friend TH, Lay DC, et al. Physiological responses of mares to short-term confinement and social isolation. J Equine Vet Sci 1991; 11(2):96–102.

56. Bell RA, Nielsen BD, Waite K, et al. Daily access to pasture turnout prevents loss of mineral in the third metacarpus of Arabian weanlings. J Anim Sci 2001; 79(5):1142–1150.

57. Rivera E, Benjamin S, Nielsen B, Shelle J, Zanella AJ. Behavioral and physiological responses of horses to initial training: the comparison between pastured versus stalled horses. Appl Anim Behav Sci 2002; 78(2–4):235–252.

58. Cooper JJ. Comparative learning theory and its application in the training of horses. Equine Vet J Suppl 1998; 27:39–43.

59. Lewczuk D, Pfeffer M. Investigation on the horses' stride length during endurance race competition using video image analysis. In: Conference on Equine Sports Medicine and Science. The Netherlands: Wageningen Pers; 1998:249–250.

60. Clayton HM. Classification of collected trot, passage and piaffe using stance phase temporal variables. Equine Vet J Suppl 1997; 23:54–57.

61. Clayton HM. Comparison of the collected, working, medium and extended canters. Equine Vet J Suppl 1994; 17:16–19.

8

Ingestive behavior

THE TRANSITION FROM MILK TO SOLIDS

Foals will nibble at blades of grass from their first day of life,[1–3] often targeting grass on raised ground, such as on banks, because this obviates the need (in horse foals rather than pony foals) to spread their forelegs.[4] As foals grow, they gradually increase their exploration (Fig. 8.1a) and intake of solids[5] and learn to flex their knees to access vegetation on the ground (Fig. 8.1b). The phase of playing with grass and, for that matter, drinking-water is very transient, often lasting less than a day.[6] However, a rapid increase in time spent grazing does not occur until approximately 4 months of age[5,7] (Fig. 8.2).

The consumption of a variety of non-grass substrates, including clay, bark, twigs, leaves and humus has been noted in many adult equids, with the suggestion that in moderation this response may be adaptive and provide necessary trace elements[8] or material that may facilitate gut motility. Learning about food substrates can have a profound effect on biological fitness. Indeed the availability of appropriate nutrients can have an impact not only on individual success but also on herd composition. For example in a study of a herd of horses that underwent a period of nutritional stress, male offspring had higher neonatal mortality rates in nutritionally poor years than in good years.[9]

The avoidance of poisonous plants and the selection of grass rather than other items occur concurrently between the ages of 4 and 6 weeks.[10] Foals generally feed when their mothers are feeding.[2] In a domestic setting some may acquire

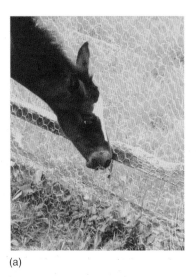 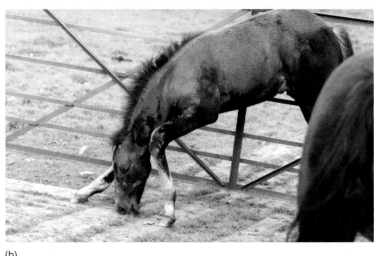

(a)   (b)

Figure 8.1 Foals (a) explore a variety of foods and (b) then develop ways of prehending them. ((a) Courtesy of Kate Ireland; (b) courtesy of Francis Burton.)

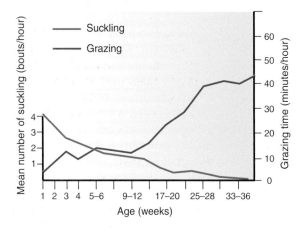

Figure 8.2 Mean time foals spend grazing and the number of bouts of nursing prior to weaning. (After Tyler.[5])

some of their dam's concentrate feed by stealth, while others are offered their own concentrate feed from birth or are given concentrate diets just prior to weaning to encourage good growth.

Although foals need a balanced diet to support adequate bone formation, the consumption of regular concentrated feed should be restricted, since it may contribute to problems of gastric acidity.[11] Furthermore, because the rate of development of stereotypic and redirected behavior is greatest

during the first 9 months of life and is related to the feeding of concentrates,[11] great care should be taken in the selection of diets for nursing mares and weanlings. Diets that most frequently cause stereotypic responses in adult crib-biters should be avoided. These include acidic diets and those that can be ingested without much chewing.

Grazing becomes more efficient as juveniles mature.[12] Juveniles also learn to avoid areas used by adults for elimination purposes.[13] Using the upper lip to isolate the selected plants, horses pass them as a bundle into the teeth and break them away using a backwards jerk of the head. Several bundles may be taken into the mouth before a bout of chewing begins.[4]

Animals seem to learn about food selection more quickly when in groups than when alone,[14] possibly reflecting an ability to learn which foods to select through social facilitation. Although several studies have failed to demonstrate observational learning per se,[15–17] at least one[18] showed that horses that observed a demonstration of an approach to feeding learned the general location of the food and therefore had a shorter latency to approach the food than control horses. Thus, stimulus enhancement may improve learning efficiency, through the transfer of information from experienced to inexperienced grazers.[19]

Observational learning studies in horses have tended to use mature subjects that are unaffiliated to one another. This represents an important possible flaw in experimental design since these may be among the least likely of all horses to be receptive to the social transmission of information. In contrast, one would predict that young foals at pasture would be more likely to use social models to learn correct food selection if their dams were effective demonstrators, because they are inexperienced foragers in a social group. Hypotheses that support this view generally assume that the greatest transfer of information occurs between a mare and her offspring. Moreover, lessons do not have to be learned by direct observation. Although yet to be demonstrated in horses, work in other species has indicated that the 'tainting' of a mother's milk as a result of her diet may provide a mechanism for such exchange.[19]

Foals between 1 and 6 weeks of age display exploration grazing which, unlike typical adult grazing, involves mouthing plants rather than ingestion. Although it is likely that a combination of mechanisms is involved in learning food selection, one of the most likely involves coprophagy (the ingestion of feces). Often seen after pawing at fecal material, coprophagy by foals peaks during the exploratory period. The dam's feces are the preferred or only fecal substrate that is explored in this way.[10,20] Old feces are rarely consumed.[8] As a feeding-exploratory behavior, coprophagy may be a method of learning about the gustatory and olfactory features of plants consumed by the dam. The significance of this activity in learning is supported by the coinciding decline in the foal's interactions with toxic plant species during this time.[10] In this way it appears that horses may circumvent the sort of observation learning typical of predatory species such as felids, by modifying their behavior in response to the transmission of information from the gastrointestinal tract to the brain.[21] Coprophagy may have additional purposes,[22] such as the acquisition of intestinal microbes and possibly deoxycholic acid, which has been found in the feces of lactating rats and is thought to play a role in the deposition of myelin.[23] For these putative reasons, hand-reared foals should be given the opportunity to perform coprophagy. It is highly unlikely to expose the foal to viable forms of endoparasite. By contrast, coprophagy is rarely seen in adults, except in those on fiber-restricted diets (see p. 201).[24]

Once valuable food sources have been located, they will be revisited after a lull that allows regrowth. Spatial memory of food patches has been demonstrated in horses,[25] and it has been suggested that this is an adaptive feature for grazers that allows them to take short-cuts through their environment.[26] The seasonal use of home ranges (see Ch. 5) supports the view that such memory may be retained from one year to the next.

FOOD SELECTION AND REJECTION

Preferences and aversions allow horses to obtain the correct nutrition for their current needs, while preventing the intake of numerous toxic plants. Post-ingestive consequences seem to influence short-term diet selection most specifically in terms of apparent energy content.[27] Because nutrients are used at different rates, they are required in different amounts in the diet. Feedback from the liver and gastrointestinal tract informs the brain of the body's current balance between nutrient supply and demand.[28] Wood-Gush[29] suggests that a 'specific hunger' for a given nutrient ensues, and the horse will then select foods that alleviate this. However, a counter argument proposes that horses eat for pleasure, and correction of specific deficiencies is improbable due to a lack of specific regulatory systems.[30]

In a study of ponies' voluntary feeding responses to different diets, meal size increased and meal frequency decreased as diets were increasingly diluted with undigestible fiber[31] (Fig. 8.3). Although ponies responded to energy dilution by increasing voluntary food intake to maintain energy intake when the diet had 25% sawdust added, increases were at a rate inadequate to maintain energy intake when the diet had 50% sawdust added.[31]

To select different foods, equids must be able to differentiate them, and this is achieved through sensory analysis. Using innate taste preferences

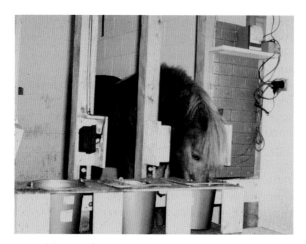

Figure 8.3 Pony being offered diets of different dilutions. Visits made to each bucket broke infrared beams and were subsequently logged to demonstrate that, to an extent, horses eat for kilojoules not volume. (Photograph courtesy of Katherine Houpt.)

or aversions alone would be undesirable since it could result in the ingestion of inappropriate material.[14,32] Therefore, prior to being prehended by horses, plants are distinguished on features of their visual appearance, including leaf shape and color, as well as their odor.[32] The importance of familiar odors in selection of food is hinted at when respiratory disorders are sufficiently profound to interfere with the horse's ability to recognize its food. Olfaction plays a particularly significant role in the way horses avoid areas contaminated with equine feces.[13,20] Although the rate of grazing is often sustained,[31,33] selectivity is hampered when the horse is grazing at night, as visual assessment of plants is impaired. This is believed to contribute to a reduction in soluble carbohydrate intake at night.[34] Once taken into the mouth, the taste and texture of plant matter provide further sensory information. More detailed differentiation between food items is facilitated by cognitive feedback that allows the visual and olfactory features of a food item to be integrated with its taste.[19]

To differentiate beneficial from detrimental feeds, horses must relate the post-ingestive consequences of ingesting a food item to the sensory stimuli that food provided before deglutition.

A learned aversion can result from ingesting a food that contains a toxin, or an excess of a nutrient, such as protein, that then acts as a toxin.[32] If toxins are present, neurons in the brainstem are stimulated, causing the animal to feel discomfort.[28] Affective feedback can then integrate information about the taste of a food to the post-ingestive consequences of that food. When this is combined with the cognitive processes that integrate taste and smell, an aversion to that food is formed and committed to memory so that the food will be rejected in future.[28]

Similarly in the horse, strong aversions to novel foods can be formed when illness *immediately* follows ingestion of a novel food. Houpt et al[35] also showed that an aversion could be formed to a novel food that caused illness, even when the novel food was given simultaneously with a familiar food. In sheep, aversions to novel foods can occur even if the post-ingestive consequences are not experienced until 12 hours after the food was tasted and ingested.[36] This is also seen in carnivores. However, in the horse, if the discomfort is delayed by as little as 30 minutes, the ability to link the discomfort to the causative food is significantly reduced.[35] A possible reason for the difference between horses and carnivores is that the latter tend to eat large sporadic meals, usually from a single source, and can therefore relate post-ingestive consequences to the last food consumed, even after a long delay.[35] In a natural situation, horses spend most of each day grazing, and consume a variety of plants. It is therefore difficult to identify the cause of discomfort after only a short delay, as more food has since been ingested.

GRAZING

Grazing is the preferred means of ingestion in adult horses, but browsing is also adopted when grass becomes particularly scarce.[37–39] Although, like horses, donkeys graze, they tend to select coarser grasses and demonstrate their greater agility as they exercise their preference for browsing. Because of their motivation to select a variety of forage, donkeys are in greater danger of ingesting poisonous plants than horses are.

Horses generally prefer legumes and grasses to shrubs and herbs[40,41] but there is apparently no correlation between gross energy of a given species of forage and the amount voluntarily consumed. Within legumes, horses are reported to prefer alfalfa pasture.[42] When grazing, horses have a preference for young growth and select leaf material rather than stems,[14,43] presumably because they are higher in carbohydrates. Studies on the preferences shown by horses for different grass species are rarely consistent and perhaps reflect variation in fiber and sugar content as the plants mature. However, timothy and white clover are often cited as preferred species.[40,44,45]

Horses spend much more time feeding on short grass than cattle.[46] Compared with cattle and sheep, horses maintain their levels of food intake even at low sward heights.[12] Having said that, dense leafy herbage is generally preferred because it provides the maximum intake per bite.[47] Apart from grasses, herbs and browse, horses will also eat bark,[48] roots,[49] soil,[50] acorns and aquatic plants.[5]

Typical domestic horse pastures have a patchy appearance not seen in free-ranging contexts.[51] Selective grazing of feeding areas and the preferential deposition of potassium-rich manure in latrine areas (see Ch. 9) combine to form well-defined lawns and roughs that are typical of horse-sick pastures.[52] Adult horses tend to avoid the long growth that characterizes latrine areas.[53,4] Once this pattern has emerged, it persists and can lead to as little as 10% of the pasture being grazed.[43] The avoidance response is attributed to the fecal content of latrine areas, urine being less repugnant.[43,54] This may be an anti-endoparasite strategy that relies on the presence of alternative grazing opportunities. Therefore, because horses kept at exceptionally high stocking rates will graze near feces in the roughs and will also defecate in the lawns, the risk of parasite infection is increased under such circumstances.[55] Indeed ponies can develop serious helminth infections within 20 days of being released onto a small pasture.[56]

Equids coexist with bovids of similar body size in many ecosystems. Although the grasses usually selected by horses have a higher fiber content than those selected by cattle, they have variable fiber content.[43] Ponies have been shown to have lower digestible organic matter intake than cattle and deer.[57] They compensate for this with a greater total dry matter intake.[58] Time spent by cattle ruminating is occupied with grazing in horses.

While grasses preferred by horses have a variable soluble carbohydrate content, they have significantly higher water contents and lower sodium concentrations than non-preferred forages.[44] Notwithstanding their tendency to develop mosaics of lawns and roughs (prized by some ecologists as a form of structural diversity), horses are recognized as economical grazers of marginal land and can be combined with goats and sheep to make the best use of pastures in poor condition.[59,60] Horses are helpful in integrated pasture management because, compared with cattle, they graze closer to the ground and use the most productive plant communities and plant species (especially graminoids) to a greater extent.

TASTE TESTS

Studies on immature horses have provided useful data on innate preferences. When given a choice between tap water and sucrose solution (at concentrations from 1.25–10 g/100 ml), foals preferred the sweet solution.[61,62] With salty (NaCl) and sour (acetic acid) flavorants, the foals rejected solutions of higher concentrations (of 0.63 g/100 ml and 0.16 ml/100 ml respectively.[61] Water made bitter by the addition of quinone hydrochloride at concentrations greater than 0.16 ml/100 ml was also rejected. Although bitterness is commonly linked to toxins,[28] some adult horses have been shown to be extremely tolerant of it, and this accounts for its variable effectiveness as a taste deterrent – for example, to prevent wood-chewing.[63] Even in foals, taste preferences can vary among individuals. For example, both Randall et al,[61] and Hawkes et al,[62] found that individual subjects rejected sucrose.

Through sampling and operant (trial-and-error) conditioning, horses can learn which foods should be ingested to meet given needs. In combination with nutritional wisdom,[64] this may account for selection and ingestion of soils that contained more iron and copper than surrounding samples.[50]

Flexibility in dietary intake is desirable since it allows horses to adapt to fluctuations in the availability of vegetation. When the availability of preferred food items is limited, horses are quick to reach a compromise between plant quality and quantity to meet their dry matter requirements.[34,60] Therefore, horses may ingest poisonous plants when they are more prevalent than safe forage or when they are dried and less detectable.[65,66] Because horses differ individually in their ability to graze selectively,[63] observing individuals as they graze a mixed sward may be worthwhile since it can help to predict their ability to avoid eating toxic plants.[67]

NATURAL INFLUENCES ON FOOD INTAKE

SOCIAL FACTORS

Among the strongest influences on a free-ranging horse's feeding behavior are the size of the group and the horse's rank within the group.[51] Leaders play a critical role in the timing of grazing,[22] and social facilitation is an important stimulant of grazing.[68] When grazing as a group, horses tend to distance themselves from conspecifics other than their preferred associates.[69] It is likely that although they are often dispersed,[4] herd members use subtle visual signals to communicate while grazing. The subtlety of such signals may account for the ability of horses to detect discrete cues in handlers.

The caution exercised by all horses when sampling novel potential foods is appropriate since horses do not regurgitate readily.[19] In some circumstances, horses can be very reluctant to eat new foods. Such neophobia is most common in horses that are currently consuming a well-balanced diet.[32] Neophobia can be overcome through social facilitation. If they are less neophobic than mature conspecifics, foals may be more able to learn preferences from experienced foragers.[10]

LACTATION AND SEASONS

Time spent grazing by mares increases with lactation, most notably in the first 3 weeks after parturition.[70] Notwithstanding the energy demands of milk production, mares have been found to have a slight tendency to forage more than stallions in all seasons.[71]

Because the duration of the photoperiod and equine appetite, as measured by voluntary food intake, are similar, a causal relationship has been suggested. Physiological responses to photoperiodic change are not immediate, sometimes occurring after a delay of up to 8 weeks.[72] Free-ranging horses take advantage of seasonal increases in the availability of foods by increasing their intake and accumulating body fat.[60] In a study of Przewalski horses under semi-natural conditions (12 mares in a 44 ha enclosure) feeding activity accounted for 40% of total activity in summer and 62% in spring.[73] The fresh weight of single stools defecated by grazing ponies peaks in the mid-summer.[74] As the quality and availability of forage declines, a peak in food searching activity occurs in autumn.[75] In winter the continued decline in availability is accompanied by a trough in the level of general activity.[73,76]

The activity of biting flies has a strong influence on the feeding behavior of horses at pasture.[77] During hot summers many activities, including feeding, are shifted to night-time.[73,78] Heavy rain also tends to inhibit grazing activity.[70]

TIME-BUDGETING

Although the only true wild horses (*E. przewalskii*) are in or from captive populations, we can use their behavior and that of feral *E. caballus* as guidelines for what could be regarded as normal equine behavioral organization. Of the major groups of behaviors, those that occupy most of a free-ranging horse's day are the search for choice grazing spots and the ingestion of forage. Equine feeding control mechanisms appear to have evolved to maintain a high gut-fill.[77]

Horses spend an average of 16–17 hours a day grazing,[79] but when forage is scarce the grazing period may exceed 19 hours[80] and horses increase their bite-frequency.[81] Horses devote much less time to chewing than ruminants, such as sheep,[82] but compensate for this by ingesting more food per unit of bodyweight per day. Peaks in foraging occur in the early morning and late afternoon[1] with bouts lasting from 30 minutes to 4 hours.[83] Both the morning and afternoon grazing bouts may be extended when forage is scarce.[84] Nocturnal ingestion naturally punctuates periods of drowsing and sleep,[85] and for this reason stable managers seeking to reduce the behavioral changes inherent to stabling should leave horses with sufficient forage for the whole night.

Time-budgets for feral horses[7] (see Fig. 1.9a–e) are similar to those of domestic horses at grass,[86] with a similar diurnal rhythm of foraging.[87] Night feeding accounted for 23% of total feeding time in pastured fillies.[88] The suggestion is that foals may learn normal feeding time-budgets from their dams,[2] and this has led to some debate about the extent to which orphan foals develop normal feeding behavior.[89,90]

While prehension may amount to 30 000 bites per day,[77] chewing rates range from 1.0 to 1.7 per second[91] with faster rates being achieved by reduced displacement of the lower jaw.[92] The type of food consumed affects the number of chews and therefore the time taken before deglutition. For example, per unit of weight, hay requires four times as many chews as oats and therefore takes four times as long to consume.[93] It has been estimated that a horse foraging exclusively on high-fiber substrates may chew 57 000 times per day, but that this can be almost halved under moderately intensive stable conditions (for example, a 500 kg horse on 5 kg of forage and 7.8 kg of concentrate).[94] This has a profound impact on salivation which, in horses, occurs only in association with mastication and not in anticipation of a meal (Table 8.1). Up to 100 liters per day has been estimated as the saliva production of a 500 kg horse on a very dry hay diet.[93] Conversely, the consequence of feeding less fiber is that there is less chewing and that the horse generates less saliva.[95] Since the buffering effects of bicarbonate are diminished under these circumstances, gastric acidity rises and the risk of gastric ulceration increases.[96]

Table 8.1 Saliva production associated with different foods

Food	Liters per kg dry matter	Liters per kg wet food	As % of swallowed bolus
Grass	4.0	0.7	11.5
Hay	4.8	4.3	17.3
Mixed feed	2.1	1.8	32

Reproduced from Harris[93], with permission.

In stabled ponies fed ad libitum, the number and frequency of feeding bouts are lowest between 1700 and 0800 hours.[86] Experimentally, satiety has been mimicked in ponies by intragastric infusions.[97] Infusions of glucose, vegetable oil and socka floc (cellulose) stimulated satiety, but in a time-dependent fashion: glucose caused immediate reduction in intake, vegetable oil took a few hours to work and the cellulose caused a reduction only in 24-hour intake.[97] The interpretation of this was that gastrointestinal cues play very little part in the immediate control of intake, but that metabolic cues related to caloric availability controlled intake by regulating the size and/or frequency of meals. Interestingly a sodium chloride infusion reduced intake, not by stimulating satiety but by causing malaise. The ponies developed a learned aversion to the nasogastric tube after receiving the sodium chloride, whereas after the other infusions they actually seemed to welcome the tubing process (Sarah Ralston, personal communication 2002).

HUMAN INFLUENCES ON FOOD INTAKE

TIMING AND CONTENT

In the domestic situation, food is concentrated to give performance horses readily digested energy resources that can therefore be consumed more rapidly than less energy-dense (more natural) forages. In a bid to reduce the chances of colic, it is usual to restrict access to concentrated food immediately before and after strenuous exercise. It is not clear whether this traditional practice is effective. The effect of exercise itself is interesting since, compared with non-exercised animals, exercised horses modify their grazing behavior by taking fewer, but larger, bites.[98]

The provision of long fiber such as hay in nets and raised feeders to prevent wastage by soiling in the bedding confounds the horse's natural grazing posture. It has been suggested that some horses demonstrate their motivation to graze when they displace forage from these devices onto the stable floor.[99] Having said that, the most profound imposed impediment to natural behaviors is the increase in concentrated parts of the diet relative to feral menus and the accompanying reduction in fibrous components.

Bulky foods that make a considerable contribution to gut-fill and thermal load are avoided in racehorses because they are thought to compromise lung-volume and racing performance. Furthermore, fiber and the saliva that must be swallowed with it add to the non-functional weight that the horse must carry. Hay has also fallen out of favor with some horse-keepers because of its role in the etiology of chronic obstructive pulmonary disease[94] and the suggestion that attempts to reduce its allergen content by soaking may decrease its nutritive value.[100,101] All of these factors mean that horses are often denied the opportunity to fulfill their behavioral needs to forage to maintain gut-fill, even though their nutritional needs may be met. Because horses evolved to be trickle feeders, the stomach of an adult horse is relatively small (9–15 liters) and inelastic.[93] It empties within about 20 minutes, and its rate of emptying is a function of the physical qualities of the current meal. Restrictions on feeding behavior, and especially the provision of discrete meals, lead to digestive anomalies and behavioral frustration.

The physical form of food is known to influence the rate of chewing[102] and the energy[103] required for ingestion. The addition of chaff, a traditional means of increasing the time taken to consume concentrated feeds, works simply by increasing the total forage content of the ration. High-energy hay replacers, such as haylage, have been associated with the development of wood-chewing in foals.[11] Haylage is often fed in restricted

quantities and may result in the redirection of oral behavior due to increased motivation to forage because of decreased gut-fill[104] or other feedback mechanisms.[105]

Food presented as highly compounded pellets may be less attractive to horses than softer substrates.[106] While foodstuffs are dried to make them easier to store and handle, this may also make their flavors less accessible and reduce their palatability. In the case of hay, some horses learn to remedy this dryness by dunking mouthfuls in water, either because moisture makes it more pleasing to the palate, or makes it easier to swallow,[4,24] or less painful to swallow if there is concurrent dental pain (Caroline Hahn, personal communication 2002).

In the free-ranging state, the primary function of movement within a home range is the selection of habitat that allows horses to maximize their intake of high-quality food.[107,108] Similarly, the tremendous variability in the shape and quality of pastures offered to horses in domestic contexts influences the amount of locomotion required to forage on them optimally (although it has been estimated that horses take 10 000 steps per day) when grazing (Katherine Houpt, personal communication 2002). Pasture shapes of equal length and breadth evoke more even grazing than do rectangular paddocks.[109] When exposed to a new pasture, horses rapidly detect patches of their preferred grasses and concentrate foraging activities within them.[91] The use of fertilizers increases the intake per bite by encouraging leaf rather than stem growth.[110]

Free-ranging horses regularly consume soil,[76] but it is not clear what elements they are seeking when they do so. It has been suggested that sodium, iron and copper supplementation are among the benefits of this activity.[50,111] Voluntary salt intake is noted to increase in stabled horses when they are not exercised.[112] This is surprising because generally exercise increases the voluntary food intake of horses offered food ad libitum[113] and salt consumption could be expected to rise to reflect salt losses through sweating. However, the oral occupation that salt-licking offers to stabled horses with unmet oral needs should not be overlooked here. Ponies fed an all-concentrate diet spend more time licking salt than those on a hay diet.[114] Occasionally, the use of saltlicks may become excessive and result in polydipsia (see subsection on drinking, p. 206).[115]

VARIETY

Although strong seasonal variation may occur in diet quality, the grass content of diets rarely falls below 80% in open-range situations.[76] When offered a choice of edible plants, horses tend to select grasses to meet their immediate energy needs and then seem to select more forbs in a form of supplementation.[116] Schafer[117] suggests that Icelandic ponies have been observed selecting medicinal plants with the surrounding grasses. He proposes that this is helpful in a bid to 'avoid worm infections' and he offers the consumption of chestnut leaves as another example of pharmacognosy, suggesting that this causes a demonstrable improvement in vigor.[117]

Most stabled horses are provided with a single forage.[118] They therefore have no opportunity to blend substrates to suit their individual needs. The effects of such monotony are as yet unclear, but it seems plausible that providing multiple forages may improve the welfare of stabled horses by enriching their environments and allowing them to perform highly motivated foraging behavior patterns.[119] Further, it is proposed that this approach may reduce the chances of

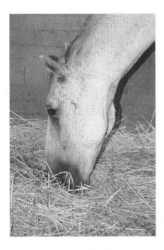

Figure 8.4 Horse eating straw bedding.

intestinal obstruction by decreasing the amount of straw that stabled horses consume (Fig. 8.4).[119] Having said that, in the absence of any better forage source, horses in developing countries are commonly fed large quantities of straw with no apparent ill-effects on gut motility (Caroline Hahn, personal communication 2002).

BEHAVIOR ASSOCIATED WITH INGESTION

Locomotion is an integral part of grazing behavior, and horses cover large areas because they seldom take more than two mouthfuls in one spot before moving on to the next.[20,30,40,45] Because stabled horses are generally offered forage in one site, they are not driven to move between food sources. Although the extent to which they can move in a stable is limited, it would be useful to increase locomotion if we are seeking to mimic free-ranging feeding strategies. As horses travel between food items in a pasture, they accelerate to a maximum foraging velocity by increasing both the length and frequency of strides.[120] On sloping pasture the dedicated use of certain routes becomes apparent with the formation of tracks that facilitate grazing. The spacing of the tracks depends on the incline.[121]

Submersion of the muzzle may be required when horses feed on aquatic vegetation.[4] Meanwhile, pawing may occur as horses forage for roots under soil[49] or grass under snow that is too deep to be pushed aside with their muzzles.[76] Pawing is also reported in horses as a means of breaking ice over watering holes.[117]

While vocalization and walking occur more often before than after feeding,[33] presumably as a result of anticipation, a significant elevation in heart rate occurs in ponies both before and during feeding.[122] Meanwhile, in horses fed large meals episodically, there is a transient post-prandial hypovolemia[123] and an increase in blood flow to the feet.[124] Although their function is obscure, these changes are thought to be of clinical significance in the etiology of laminitis and may relate to the persistent increase in hoof wall temperature for 16–40 hours after vasodilation.[125] As an aside, it may be that lack of locomotion between mouthfuls of food is a contributory factor in the emergence of laminitis.

Although increased surveillance is a benefit of social living for prey animals, such as the horse, vigilance by individuals within a group always persists. The rate of looking-up during grazing and drinking[22] and social spacing are important anti-predator strategies that are mathematically related to herd size. For example, when the number of Thoroughbred yearlings in experimental groups at pasture was increased from 2 to 12, the mean distance between them increased from 5 meters to as much as 50 meters.[126]

Social facilitation strongly influences behaviors associated with grazing in the horse.[68] This is illustrated by the finding that locomotion as an adjunct to grazing is significantly greater for a lone horse than for those in a group.[126] Meanwhile, the duration of grazing bouts increases linearly as the group size increases up to four.[126] This could reflect competition between grazing horses or possibly decreased anxiety as a result of increased predator vigilance.

A study of stabled Shetland ponies, showed that social facilitation was crucial for the stability of time budgets and that visual, more than olfactory or auditory, contact with conspecifics facilitated feeding behavior.[127] However, the presence of conspecifics is not equally helpful for all members of a group, since when feeding from a shared trough, in the presence of high-ranking pen-mates, subordinate horses are less likely to be disturbed if solid partitions between feeding bays are used. The use of computer-controlled feeding stations may help to reduce disturbance of lower-ranked members of a group, although attention must be paid to the design of feeding bays so that entering and leaving are facilitated.[128,129] Stable designs that give horses the choice of visual contact or privacy (Fig. 8.5) are an appropriate response to these findings.

Strangely, fluctuations in the R–R intervals that are common features of equine heart function and possibly represent respiratory sinus arrhythmia are absent during feeding periods.[130] Perhaps there is an increase in vagal tone associated with

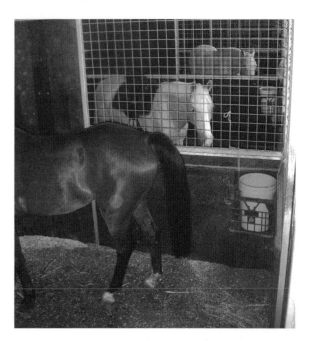

Figure 8.5 Partial barriers between stalls allow horses to choose between visual contact with neighbors or privacy. This simple form of environmental enrichment can help to reduce distress in stabled animals. (Photograph courtesy of Centennial Parklands Equestrian Complex, Sydney, NSW, Australia.)

gastrointestinal activity that means that feeding has an effect on autonomic activity in the same way that crib-biting bouts are associated with reductions in heart rate.[131]

THE RELATIONSHIP BETWEEN NUTRITION AND BEHAVIOR

The relationship between diet and behavior is fascinating. For example, there is a report that a group of horses in New Zealand with deteriorating 'behavior and manners' responded to parenteral administration of vitamin E-selenium.[132] Horses on pasture, however, have higher plasma serotonin and tryptophan levels than those in stalls fed grain (unpublished data from Sarah Ralston, personal communication 2002). Many equestrians report that horses and especially ponies become 'hot', 'fizzy' or 'corned-up' – in other words, more reactive and less tractable – when fed more oats and less hay. This may reflect a shift in the glycemic peak that merits further scientific study. There is evidence that replacing starch and sugars with fat and fiber may diminish spontaneous locomotion and reactivity to a variety of novel stimuli.[133,134] Those who report 'not resting properly' (restlessness) as one of the more common undesirable behavior patterns in sport horses[135] should consider the role of over-nutrition in the emergence of the problem.

Paradoxically, changing the diet of ponies from hay to oats has been reported to cause a transient augmentation of total sleep time with increases in both slow-wave sleep and REM sleep.[136] After 4 days, however, sleep patterns in these animals had returned to normal. It may be that the post-prandial changes in the lower limbs of these animals as a result of the dietary imposition, resulted in spending more time in recumbency, and that sleep was the consequence of the physiological stimulation that also resulted from the novel carbohydrate load. Fasting is associated with similar transient increases in both slow-wave sleep and REM sleep.[85]

It is possible that some diets may better equip horses to cope with stressors associated with competition and fatigue.[134] A crossover study demonstrated that foals coped better during weaning if they were allowed access to a supplement in which starch and sugar were replaced by fat and fiber, before separation from the dams. Similar amelioration of stress-related behaviors, such as vocalization, has been noted in foals supplemented with zinc.[134]

DYSPHAGIA

Reasons for dysphagia can include trigeminal nerve injuries which may cause the mouth to gape.[4] Difficulty in swallowing is also noted in white muscle disease, botulism and some cases of poisoning. Dental problems may cause refusal of hard dry foods, irregular chewing and the tilting of the head while chewing. Dropping of food may also be associated with dysfunction of the facial nerve. Horses with esophagitis may lower the neck and extend the head, while those with stomatitis may loll out their tongues and those

with choke often show repeated arching of the neck. While involuntary chewing and tongue flicking have been described as symptoms of Yellow-star thistle poisoning,[4] bruxism (tooth grinding) is generally regarded as a sign of generalized low-grade discomfort for example as a result of gastric ulcers.[137]

ANOREXIA AND HYPOPHAGIA

In normal horses the reasons for failing to meet nutritional requirements are often related to social consequences or distracting arousal. Subordinate members of a group may be bullied away from a limited supply of food, especially if it is not dispersed appropriately. In addition, horses that eat slowly may miss out if peers can consume more than their share of the ration. Horses may also fail to feed when distressed by the move to a new environment, or the departure of a favored affiliate, or by the arousal resulting from activities on the yard, such as the arrival of conspecifics.[83]

When horses are given an equal opportunity to feed, disease is the primary cause of a reduced food intake. For example, febrile states are a common finding for practitioners called to acutely inappetant horses. Pain may not only reduce appetite but also affect behaviors associated with eating. For example, an individual may be less likely to approach to food and defend its rations. In donkeys such changes in behavior can mark the onset of estrus but nevertheless should be taken very seriously because they may be the only indication of illness that may be grave but masked by the species' apparent tolerance of discomfort.[138] Feeding responses to disease in the donkey are important, since anorexia, a frequent consequence of pain, can lead to hyperlipemia and death.[139]

While dental erosion can lead to inadequate mastication, dysphagia and food being lost from the mouth during mastication (so-called 'quidding'[140]), buccal pain can even cause reluctance to approach food. With horses that present with weight-loss, time spent observing them as they interact with a variety of foods can be extremely helpful in diagnosing the problem. For example, this may help to determine the extent of quidding versus inappetance or the preference a horse may have developed for soft or moistened food. Intriguingly, patterns of feeding behavior are altered markedly as a legacy of dysautonomia.[141]

Among the best approaches to improving food consumption in a sick horse, one should consider:

- warming the food to release volatile flavorants – this works best if the horse has encountered that sort of warmed food when healthy
- dampening the food to reduce the effort involved in chewing (this is especially helpful if the horse is experiencing oral pain), or adding dissolved attractive components to lubricate the passage of food and facilitate deglutition
- feeding small amounts at a time in a bid to mimic the trickle effect, and avoid the horse being overwhelmed with food to sustain a healthy interest in the food
- feeding within sight (but not physical contact) of an affiliate that is eating.

HYPERPHAGIA

The prodigious appetite of horses is well recognized, and it is suggested that the ability of oropharyngeal stimuli to override metabolic or gastrointestinal feedback within a single feeding session contributes to the horse's susceptibility to colic and metabolic disorders.[142] The rate of eating and size of meal in ponies is negatively correlated with pre-prandial plasma glucose concentrations.[86] Gorging and bolting of food may therefore occur after a period of food restriction and can lead to esophageal obstruction.[137] Because they precipitate excess acidity, periods without food can rapidly lead to severe gastric ulceration.[143] Clearly, therefore, management regimens that facilitate trickle rather than episodic feeding are desirable.

A rapacious appetite is sometimes accompanied by inadequate mastication that may compromise the horse's ability to buffer gastric acidity and digest its food. Veterinarians are rarely consulted about horses that are eating too rapidly, since it is rarely a sign of ill-health. However, there are clear behavioral reasons for this to occur, and owners should consider the role of current or even previous competition from other horses as among the most likely. Feeding more fiber to increase the sense of gut-fill prior to the presentation of discrete concentrated meals is the best approach to these cases. Furthermore, increasing the fiber content of concentrated meals themselves by introducing chaff is more effective than attempts to thwart ingestion by the use of physical obstacles such as bricks within the feeding device.

Practitioners should be aware that over-feeding of laminitic ponies (that through no fault of their own are depreciating rapidly in market value with age) may sometimes continue contrary to veterinary advice to ensure that euthanasia ensues and the insured value can be realized.

WOOD-CHEWING AND BED-EATING

Food restriction is a common feature of stable management because of the appeal of concentrated foods that can be consumed rapidly, often in less than 3 hours. Although when offered food constantly, ponies consumed 80% of their daily intake in an average of 10 separate meals,[86] most owners provide feed at frequencies and times that suit them rather than their horses' gastrointestinal function. This often leads to the imposition of fasting at night.[144] Food and fiber restriction may prompt horses to consume straw provided as bedding, and this has been linked to impaction colic.[145]

Bark chewing is a common feature of horses on irrigated pastures that have less fiber content than natural pastures (Fig. 8.6).[48] Sometimes referred to as a normal vestige of browsing behavior, wood-chewing is of importance because, although it is not sufficiently invariant to be classed as a stereotypy, it may be associated with or precede the development of crib-biting.[146] The tendency to chew wood can be reduced by increasing the fiber content of the ration. While helping to normalize gut function, this intervention can also save stables from rapidly being destroyed by their occupants. Horses can ingest approximately 1.5 kg of timber per day.[147]

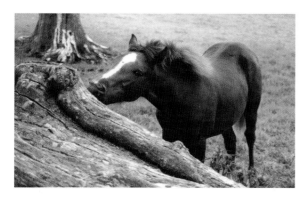

Figure 8.6 Although wood-chewing is regarded by some as unwelcome, many ethologists consider it a normal analogue of bark-chewing, a normal feature of the repertoire of free-ranging horses. (Photograph courtesy of Francis Burton.)

It is accepted that horses fed low-forage diets spend significantly more time chewing wood than horses fed hay.[105,148] Further, Krzak et al[112] reported that wood-chewing increased when the stomachs of horses were at their emptiest. Lignophagia is unwelcome because it can cause intestinal obstruction.[149] It is suggested that fiber restriction reduces hindgut pH and that this leaves horses fundamentally unsated, but it also has the effect of eliciting abnormal oral behaviors.[105] While my own studies have shown an increase in intraspecific aggression in horses on so-called 'complete' diets, others have noted an increased nervousness as well as wood-chewing in ponies deprived of hay.[150] When forage is in short supply, many owners report increased aggression among horses at pasture. Along with biting of the stable, wood-chewing was the main oral behavior that was reduced by giving stabled horses non-therapeutic oral doses of virginiamycin.[105] A suggested mechanism for this phenomenon involves the reduction of fermentative acidosis in the hindgut by changing the population of hindgut flora. The remedial elevation of a horse's hindgut pH with antimicrobials may be an expensive alternative to increasing its fiber intake.

Fiber restriction has been associated with the ingestion of a variety of unusual substrates (so-called pica), including shavings and sawdust (in bedding), hair[151] (from the manes and tails of other horses) and feces.[83] Having said that,

foals mouth and chew many of these items as a normal part of object play.[6]

COPROPHAGY

In all foals coprophagia is a normal behavior with a variety of suggested functions (see above). In free-ranging horses, there are rare reports of foals and their dams consuming old fecal material as a consequence of food shortage.[50] Fiber-restricted rations,[8,152] frustration (which probably results from the same deficit), and underfeeding in general[83] can lead to an adult horse consuming its own feces or those of a conspecific. The digestible energy content of equine fecal material is sufficient to suggest that this substrate may help to nourish a horse.[83]

There are anecdotal reports of horses consuming the blood and even the flesh of freshly dead rabbits, some of which are said to have been killed by the horses themselves.[153] It is interesting to contemplate the sort of nutritional deficit that could generate the motivation to perform this behavior. Generally speaking practitioners should investigate the possibility of a dietary deficiency and screen blood biochemistry before labeling an unusual craving 'depraved'.

GEOPHAGIA

Occasionally, horses lick and chew at soil but it is not yet clear whether they do so to resolve nutritional deficiencies or because they simply enjoy the activity.[50] Involuntary soil ingestion occurs mainly during grazing, because soil adheres to vegetation.[154] Incisor erosion may sometimes result and may even mimic damage caused by crib-biting. Sand colic is associated with the ingestion of some soil types either during eating or drinking.[82]

ORAL STEREOTYPIES
Licking and crib-whetting

Although rarely reported as problems by owners, licking and crib-whetting are sometimes seen as appetitive behaviors before crib-biting or may become stereotypic in their own right. The approach to their management follows that of other redirected and stereotypyic oral activities.

Crib-biting and wind-sucking

A crib-biting horse repeatedly seizes fixed objects with its incisor teeth and pulls back while making a characteristic grunting noise that signifies the passage of air into the esophagus. A wind-sucker achieves the same characteristic neck posture and grunt without holding onto any fixed object. It is believed that crib-biters may become wind-suckers – for example, if no substrate is available or if this component of the behavior is punished.[155] Horses that merely hold onto a fixed object without grunting are said to show grasping.[156] These behavior patterns have been linked to various forms of ill-health, including tooth wear, colic and a failure to maintain bodyweight. Radiography of horses as they were crib-biting challenged the traditional view that crib-biters actively ingest air, because there was no movement of the tongue as one would expect in true swallowing.[157] Instead, each horse showed an explosive distension of the proximal esophagus (Fig. 8.7) that prompted no

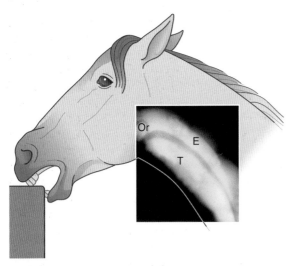

Figure 8.7 Composite image from three stills captured during fluoroscopy of the cranial half of a horse's neck during a bout of crib-biting. Air is visible in the esophagus (E), trachea (T) and oropharynx (Or). (Reproduced by permission of the University of Bristol, Dept of Clinical Veterinary Science.)

peristalsis. Much of the air exited the proximal esophagus between crib-bites by returning through the cranial esophageal sphincter into the pharynx. This may explain why tympanitic colic (abdominal pain associated with wind or flatulence) is not seen in all crib-biting horses.

Risk factors

Epidemiological studies have identified husbandry factors that are associated with peaks in the prevalence of abnormal behavior in racehorses.[118,148] These management factors include small amounts of daily forage (less than 6.8 kg) and stable designs that limit the amount of communication possible between neighboring horses. This association is somewhat predictable because one would expect horses to behave normally if they have plenty of food and company. However, when interpreting the results of surveys, it is important not to arrive at cause-and-effect conclusions. Although cross-sectional studies have revealed and quantified the association between certain management practices and stereotypic behavior, it must be remembered that all such studies are essentially retrospective.

Further light has been shed on the causal factors influencing the development of stereotypic behaviors by a 4-year prospective study of a population of 225 young Thoroughbred and part-Thoroughbred horses.[11] Dynamic cohorts were followed for between 1 and 4 years, with each foal being observed directly during the pre-weaning period, at weaning and at regular intervals post-weaning. The study found that crib-biting was initiated by 10.5% of this population at a median age of just 20 weeks (Fig. 8.8).

After weaning, youngsters given concentrate feed have a significantly greater risk of developing crib-biting than those not given concentrate, while those fed on hay replacers (such as silage or haylage) rather than hay have a significantly greater risk of developing wood-chewing.[11]

The strong effect of weaning is of considerable importance. Weaning is a stressful time for the juvenile, and abrupt weaning has been implicated as a source of emotional anxiety, because of

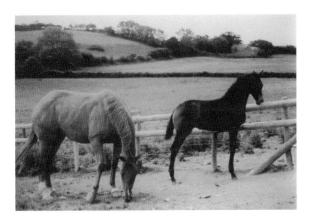

Figure 8.8 Crib-biting foal. (Photograph courtesy of Caroline Bower.)

numerous management changes at weaning time.[158–160] These include:

- withdrawal of opportunities to suckle
- breaking of the mare–foal bond
- altered feeding practices
- introduction to drinking water (in one study of 15 foals, only 7 were observed to drink before weaning[2])
- novel housing
- new social groupings
- the amount of human contact often being increased.

Although the use of creep feeds may benefit the foal nutritionally, they may compromise the health of the gastric mucosa[161] and do little to meet the behavioral needs of non-nutritive suckling. After traditional total and abrupt weaning, which involves permanent, sudden separation from the mare, foals frequently attempt to redirect suckling behavior toward the genital regions of conspecifics. It is believed that the thwarted motivation to suckle at this time may contribute to the emergence of crib-biting and wood-chewing in some individuals.

Crib-biting may also originate from specific dietary problems in young horses. For example, foals that received concentrates after weaning were four times more likely to develop crib-biting than those that did not.[11] It has been suggested that normal gut motility and transit times in crib-biting horses may depend on physical flushing by saliva associated with their crib-biting behavior.[162,163] Furthermore, crib-biting may increase the flow of alkaline saliva and reduce gastric acidity[145] associated with feeding concentrates.[164] Compared with the company of other distressed freshly weaned peers, the presence of calm, grazing horses may help to reduce the distress of weaning for paddock-weaned foals, even if they have been abruptly separated from their dams.[11] Because links between distress and gastric ulcers have been proposed in foals[165,166] and established in other species,[167,168] strategies that help to reduce the emotional impact of weaning are likely to be of benefit at an organic level.

The relationship between oral stereotypies and gastrointestinal health

The significance of gastric ulceration in intensively managed (food-restricted) horses is now widely recognized, with 82% of racehorses[169] and 51% of Thoroughbred foals under the age of 3 months[170] showing lesions.

Epidemiological risk factors for oral stereotypies that relate to diet (such as small amounts of daily forage) could have the effect of increasing gastric acidity.[151,117] Saliva is the natural buffer to excess gastric acidity; however, in horses, its production depends on pressure being exerted on the parotid salivary gland, primarily as an adjunct to chewing. If insufficient time is spent grazing or eating forage, horses may produce saliva of insufficient volume and quality to buffer their stomach contents. It has therefore been proposed that cribbiting may originate in an *attempt* by the horse to produce additional saliva.[145] This is supported by there being a trend towards increased water consumption by crib-biters compared with normal horses.[171] The fact that the attempt may not always be successful may be one reason why the biting behavior develops stereotypic characteristics.

The putative links between weaning and crib-biting have been explored because of the causative role of concentrate feeding in the emergence of gastric ulcers.[161] Furthermore, because the original eliciting causes of the stereotypy are more apparent in youngsters, which have been exposed to fewer variables than older animals, a cohort of young horses was recruited to explore this hypothesis.[161] After an initial assessment of behavior, and endoscopic examination of the gastric lining, horses were randomly allocated to antacid or control diets. Initially, the stomachs of crib-biting foals were significantly more ulcerated, eroded and inflamed than the stomachs of normal foals. However, the use of antacid diets resulted in a significant improvement in the condition of their stomachs. Crib-biting behavior declined in all foals (a finding that challenges the concept of emancipation) but the decline was especially marked in those maintained on the antacid diet.[161] These results are of great interest, because they indicate humane approaches to the prevention and treatment of oral stereotypies in young horses. Having said that, we should be careful not to oversimplify the etiology of crib-biting. The role of the hindgut pH in the motivation to crib-bite is becoming clearer, with virginiamycin reducing the frequency of crib-biting after being added to meals for 2 weeks, despite its decreasing the pH of food (Clegg & McGreevy, unpublished data).

Physiological associations with crib-biting

Plasma cortisol levels in crib-biters are higher than in normal horses under a variety of treatments,[172] which suggests that they are particularly susceptible to stress. Crib-biters are often regarded as being less able than normal horses to maintain bodyweight. Although this is sometimes blamed on incisor erosion (Fig. 8.9), it more commonly arises because they are occupied with performing their stereotypy and therefore they rest less than normal horses.[173] This may be an important cost for crib-biting horses as they expend energy that would otherwise have been conserved at rest. The tendency for crib-biters to spend less time eating is also likely to contribute to a relative energy deficit and consequent unthriftiness when on a critical plane of nutrition.

A significant reduction in oro-cecal motility has been reported in crib-biters prevented from eating and crib-biting.[163] This suggests that normal gut function in these animals is affected

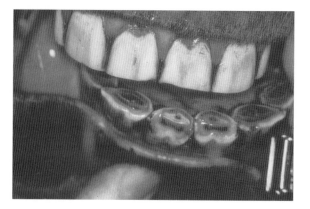

Figure 8.9 Erosion on the tables of the mandibular incisors of a crib-biter. (Reproduced by permission of the University of Bristol, Dept of Clinical Veterinary Science.)

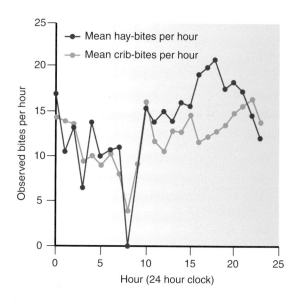

Figure 8.10 Diurnal rhythm in the bite rates for crib-biting and eating hay (from 64 days of observation). Horses were stabled with ad libitum hay. Between 0830 hours and 0930 hours they were turned out in paddocks.

by oral activity. However, horses on 'nutritionally complete' diets, with no forage component, showed an association between crib-biting and increased total gut-transit time.[173] These data suggest that eating and crib-biting may be partial substitutes for each other and that there is a triangular relationship between diet, gut activity and crib-biting. Certainly, in terms of their diurnal distribution, eating and crib-biting tend to occur together (Fig. 8.10). Studies of gut mobility are important because increased total gut transit times may predispose horses to simple colonic obstruction and distension colic.[174]

The consequences of preventing crib-biting are of interest because they help to clarify the possible function of oral stereotypies. Studies using purpose-built projection-free looseboxes have compared short-term deprivation of crib-biting with the temporary withdrawal of forage. Intriguingly, neither deprivation of food nor of opportunities for crib-biting alone was associated with a plasma stress response.[162,175] However, when the horses were deprived of both food and the opportunity to crib-bite, they showed a significant rise in the plasma stress response. This exposes the link between foraging and crib-biting and explains why restricted feeding is a management factor associated with an increase in abnormal behavior. There was also a significant reduction in oro-cecal motility recorded in crib-biters deprived of food and opportunities for crib-biting, which implies that normal gut function in these animals depends on their being given ad libitum access to food and to suitable crib-biting substrates. Crib-biters deprived of the opportunity to stereotype ate more than normal horses, suggesting that they had greater oral needs.

The suggestion that crib-biters underwent relative gut stasis when deprived of food and the opportunity to crib-bite, should be borne in mind when owners elect to stable their horses overnight with a haynet that will be emptied by morning. Methods of making horses work harder to gather their forage ration, e.g. by using haynets with especially small holes (so-called restrictor nets), can protract feeding times and may therefore have a beneficial effect on gut function as well as time-budgeting in general. However, this may not be beneficial for all individuals since, for some, the frustration associated with working for forage may represent an additional stressor.

Beyond proximate gastrointestinal effects, crib-biting may bring more subtle rewards that could account for its persistence in the absence of gastric insults. Dopamine may activate basal ganglia motor systems to reinforcing crib-biting via a reward mechanism. It has been suggested that stress stimulates the release of endorphins, triggering excessive dopaminergic activity within the striatum.[176] In rats, the release of dopamine by endorphins has been shown to depend on activation of NMDA receptors.[177] When nine crib-biting horses were treated with the NMDA receptor antagonist dextromethorphan (1 mg/kg, i.v.) – the active ingredient in most cough mixtures – eight showed a reduced cribbing rate compared with baseline.[178] This pathway certainly merits further investigation so that we can better understand the way in which crib-biting may be self-reinforcing and therefore prone to emancipation.

Treatment of oral stereotypies

At some stage, most owners resort to physical restriction in an attempt to prevent the performance of abnormal oral behaviors.[162] One of the most common methods involves the use of a tight collar (Fig. 8.11) designed to make crib-biting so uncomfortable or painful to perform that the horse stops. The effect of these collars was studied in a group of 12 horses fitted with the collars for 24 hours.[175] After the removal of the collars, the horses performed crib-biting at a higher rate than before the collars were fitted. This post-inhibitory rebound demonstrates that the motivation to crib-bite increases during periods of physical prevention.

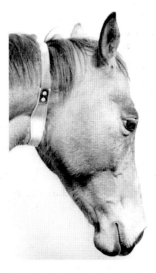

Figure 8.11 Collar used to make crib-biting uncomfortable or less gratifying. (Reproduced by permission of the University of Bristol, Dept of Clinical Veterinary Science.)

Despite welfare concerns, surgical responses to crib-biting continue to be developed. For example, laser-assisted removal of 10 cm of the ventral branch of the spinal accessory nerve and 34 cm sections of the paired omohyoideus and sternothyrohyoideus muscles is reported to result in elimination of the behavior in 10 horses that were followed up for a minimum of 7 months.[179] This intervention presumably makes the distension of the proximal esophagus difficult and therefore makes the behavior less gratifying.

From rebound work it is argued that the reason collars, electric shock 'treatments' and surgical removal of neck muscles or nerves, often prove unsuccessful is because the motivation to crib-bite in horses is sustained.

The relationship between gut acidity and the incidence of oral activities such as crib-biting, grasping and wind-sucking[104,161,180] is becoming clear and has prompted the development of novel feeding practices, especially regimens that are likely to be particularly useful at weaning. Similarly, the addition of dietary antacids reduces the intensity and frequency of the response in emancipated crib-biters, especially post-feeding.[180] Unfortunately we have no direct evidence to date that shows that resolution of gastric ulceration reduces the frequency of crib-biting, but nevertheless it is prudent to check crib-biters for gastric ulcers. The extent to which an individual horse should be allowed to crib-bite (e.g. on tailor-made surfaces that are cushioned to reduce incisor wear) depends on its colic history. High-risk animals should be managed in ways that minimize the primary need to crib-bite. Moreover, owners of all crib-biters should maximize periods at pasture and, where it is necessary to supplement feed, the fiber component of the total diet. By maintaining a high meal frequency they can give their horses the chance to emulate trickle feeding and thus reduce gastric acidity.

DRINKING

Nursing foals rarely drink water, since they rely on milk for their supply of fluids.[2,51] The youngest age at which foals have been observed to drink water is 3 weeks.[2] Drinking in weaned animals is related to ambient temperature, water availability and lactational status.[2]

Movement to water is usually, although not exclusively, made by the entire herd.[2] In pastured horses, trips to water most commonly occur in the afternoon.[2] Horses submerge their lips below the surface of the water to drink (Fig. 8.12) and generate a pressure gradient by movement of the tongue in combination with swallowing at the rate of once per second.[4] The importance of the pressure gradient was hinted at by reports of the postoperative behavior of horses that underwent the outdated buccostomy approach to crib-biting and wind-sucking. Such horses were often said to take 2 or 3 days to learn to drink with fistulae in their cheeks. Although it was assumed that these horses were struggling to create a pressure gradient within their altered mouths, we should not discount the contemporaneous buccal pain as a likely postoperative side-effect that would have made drinking uncomfortable.

Hydration levels depend on voluntary fluid intake and are affected by exertion, ambient temperature, humidity, gut-fill, the speed of water conservation responses, such as antidiuretic hormone release, and the accessibility of transcellular reserves, such as those in the gastrointestinal tract.

Although horses in the exceptionally hostile heat of the Namib Desert have been noted to

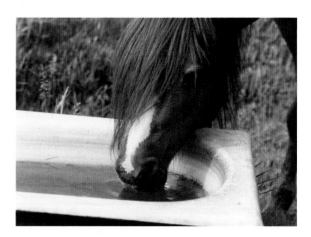

Figure 8.12 Horses drink by immersing their lips. (Photograph courtesy of Francis Burton.)

consume an average of 30 liters per day,[181] those in a cool environments may drink much less.[182] The water intake of stabled horses is in the range 2–4 liters per kilogram of dry-matter food consumed,[183] the variation being a reflection of the variable amount of chewing, and therefore salivation, required for dry hay versus, for example, cereals.[93] While water intake for working horses is also related to exercise and can send daily requirements up to 90 liters,[184] for free-ranging horses, trips to water may vary in their frequency according to the location of forage sources and the environmental temperature.[2] Horses usually visit their water source at least once per day, whereas those foraging farther from their water source may schedule visits up to 72 hours apart.[185] Some Namib horses can survive for 100 hours without water.[181]

Drinking is a social activity undertaken by the group as a whole and it is usually completed within 30 minutes.[49] Competition for fresher, unmuddied water means that the higher-ranking members of a band drink first, as do the more dominant bands.[4] Most commonly undertaken in daylight, especially toward dusk, visits to water involve increased exposure to predation and the chance of encountering other bands. Swift departures from watering holes, which reduce the opportunity for unwelcome interactions, have been remarked upon.[186]

For the owners of performance horses, voluntary fluid intake can prove pivotal to success. Although intake is known to vary with the supply of water, its individual characteristics (such as flavor) and the behavior of conspecifics, the pattern of drinking is generally tailored to meet homeostatic demands. In winter, very cold water can be aversive and decrease voluntary water intake to the extent of dehydration and even colic, whereas offering horses a choice of chilled water and ambient warm water in hot weather produces no preferences or qualitative differences in drinking behavior.[187]

Despite fears articulated in lay texts of inappropriate flushing of undigested food particles into the small intestine, most equine scientists seem to agree that, as long as water has not been withheld for an extended period, a horse can safely drink before, during and after feeding.[184] Thirst tends to increase after feeding,[184] and large meals tend to cause a rapid and short-lived decrease in plasma volume.[188] So, rather than hampering digestion, drinking may actually facilitate it. When food and water are freely available 89% of drinking occurs within a period from 10 minutes before to 30 minutes after feeding.[189] The flushing effect is of negligible consequence because, when the stomach is full, water tends to pass along the lesser curvature, leaving the food largely undisturbed[190,191] and, in any case, almost all digestion in the horse is post-gastric.[93] By the same token we should accept that the provision of dry foods is unnatural, and for this reason the habit of some horses to dunk their hay should be regarded as a behavioral need and certainly not something to be prevented or even discouraged.

As long as it has no harmful effects on gut motility,[192] intermittent water delivery is not thought to have a negative impact on psychological well-being of stabled horses.[193] The method by which water is supplied can affect both drinking behavior and fluid balance in the horse. For example, a preference for buckets over pressure valve bowls and a failure to maintain fluid balance in some horses using the latter system have been demonstrated.[194] This may have harmful effects on horses that have an increased requirement for water. Therefore if a horse is normally watered using an automatic system, supplementation with water from a bucket may help to ensure rehydration after exertion.

Hygiene is of concern, since automatic water bowls and buckets may become contaminated with food or fecal material.[195] Regardless of the receptacle from which horses drink, stable managers sometimes report reduced water intake after the use of potent agents to clean water containers. This is because, even after thorough rinsing, some of the stronger detergents, disinfectants and soaps can leave traces of unpleasant smells and tastes.

Changes in routine, such as prevail in international travel and many competitive contexts, can disturb the natural tendency of horses to drink at around feeding time. Until compensation is effected, which can take up to 7 days, the welfare and performance of horses disturbed in this way can be compromised.[196]

Reluctance to drink can be a neophobic response in that many horses and most donkeys[138] are suspicious of novel odors and flavors in their drinking water. Having evolved to occupy a home range, horses are unlikely to have to encounter new water sources in nature and are innately wary of contaminants. Many equestrian competitors counter this neophobia by using flavorants, such as molasses or peppermint cordial, in the drinking water at home so that the same ingredient can be added to water offered at competitions.[197] Equine hospitals should consider the same approach in anticipation of elective surgery. It seems that simply offering a variety of familiar flavors may enhance overall consumption, perhaps as a product of exploratory behavior.[197] Meanwhile, horses that consistently prefer drinking muddy to clean water may be attempting to remedy a mineral deficiency.[24]

Inadequate water intake has been identified as a cause of impaction colic[198] and should certainly be avoided when horses are required to make the transition between pasture and stabling.[94] Horses affected by tetanus are sometimes seen to immerse their muzzle into water without being able to consummate the behavior by drinking. Meanwhile some normal donkeys are said to refuse to drink from troughs if the water level is so low that they have to put their head so far into the trough that they can no longer see around them.[138] Notwithstanding the normal reluctance on the part of horses to drink water from novel sources or via novel receptacles, any suspicion of adipsia should prompt immediate action, including monitoring of water intake and drinking behavior as well as inspection of the water source to eliminate possible contaminants.[83]

Because horses drink in response to falls in plasma volume and increases in plasma osmolality (experimental increases in plasma osmolality over a threshold of 3% prompt drinking[189]), any factor that alters these parameters can cause thirst.[183] Where furosemide (frusemide) has been administered – for example, to prevent exercise-induced pulmonary hemorrhage – horses can be expected to show increased thirst and to crave salt.[199]

Pathologies that lead to polydipsia and polyuria are dealt with thoroughly in other texts. Before a behavioral cause is proposed, polydipsic horses should be assessed for evidence of various pathologies that increase demand for water including diarrhea, diabetes and Cushing's disease. Stereotypic interaction with water may not necessarily involve increased water consumption, because water may be splashed and dribbled rather than simply drunk. It has been associated with frustrating environments but, paradoxically, in tie-stalled mares it has been reported only in those given continuous access to water.[193,195] Oral stereotypies are associated with increases in both water intake and frequency of visits to water buckets (Clegg & McGreevy, unpublished data). Excessive water intake in the absence of medication or disease has been noted as a consequence of stereotypic salt-licking[114] but primary psychogenic polydipsia is more common.[183] When seen in association with feeding in stabled horses, polydipsia should not be confused with a salivation deficit or a product of thwarted oral motivation, as reported in horses fed scheduled feeds from automated devices.[183]

SUMMARY OF KEY POINTS

- Food selection allows horses to adjust their intake of nutrients to suit their current situation, while avoiding poisonous alternatives.
- A horse is born with innate dietary preferences which generally include:
  - sweet-tasting foods
  - grasses high in fiber and carbohydrate
  - short, young growth.
- There is individual variation in preferences and aversions.
- Horses may learn from conspecifics and personal experience which foods to select.
- Concentrated feeds are associated with reduced saliva production and increased gastric acidity.
- Periods without food are associated with increased gastric acidity and risk of gastric ulceration.
- Lack of forage is the most important management factor linked with the development of stereotypic behaviors in cross-sectional epidemiological studies.
- Lack of forage and the provision of concentrate feed are important causal factors that precede the development of oral stereotypies in young horses in prospective epidemiological studies.

- It does not appear easy for horses to copy novel behavior patterns, which suggests that imitation of stereotypies is unlikely.
- Crib-biting is associated with disorders of the digestive system. There is a significant association between stomach ulceration and crib-biting in foals.
- Dietary treatments that reduce the incidence and severity of oral stereotypies offer humane avenues of treatment and prevention.
- The way in which water is supplied to horses can affect both drinking behavior and fluid balance.

CASE STUDY

A 4-month-old Warmblood colt was spotted repeatedly grasping at the top of a gatepost and occasionally licking it while the rest of the group, including its dam, idled in the same corner of the paddock. On closer scrutiny the owners found no evidence of wood-chewing and did not detect a grunting sound coincident with the behavior. The foal was not receiving creep feed but the mare, the highest-ranking adult in the group, was receiving concentrated feed every evening. None of the four adult horses in the paddock showed similar behaviors.

Video surveillance was used for this case. Because of its repetitive nature, the invariantly arched neck posture and the appetitive licking associated with it, the behavior was diagnosed as an early form of stereotypic crib-biting.

The grasping behavior was regarded with concern because of the likelihood of its becoming stylized into crib-biting and the probability of its becoming emancipated after weaning, so measures were taken to reduce management factors associated with its appearance. All gateposts in the paddock were coated very generously with a proprietary taste deterrent. The fence-line was protected with a single line of electrified wire. The sward in the paddock was low, so hay was fed to the group on a daily basis. It was delivered to the centre of the enclosure rather than being placed near the gateway where concentrates had previously been offered. This was intended to break down any association between eating and reaching for the gatepost. The hay was placed on the ground in the short term to avoid there being any uprights in close proximity to the feeding horses and to normalize their posture.

Hay from three farms was sourced, and samples of each were offered in seven separate piles, which allowed the five horses a pile each and two forage sources to choose from if displaced. Alternating the source of the hay in adjacent piles meant that the mare and foal had a choice of forages. When the pair were brought in for supervised supplementary feeding of the dam, it became clear that she was dropping a considerable amount of grain while chewing. Great care was taken to ensure that no dropped grain was left lying around for the foal to consume. Meanwhile, the mare received dental treatment that resolved the quidding.

Before weaning was attempted, a mare-and-filly-foal dyad was located by means of an advertisement in a local newspaper and brought to the paddock. The foals bonded extremely well and one month later the visiting mare was removed. Two weeks later the resident mare was removed and the colt was observed carefully for signs of the grasping response. None was seen. The pair of weanlings were kept at pasture throughout the winter. Ad libitum hay feeding was maintained and small amounts of concentrated food with a dietary antacid supplement were introduced very gradually. Although the amount fed to the youngsters was small it was nonetheless divided into three feeds to reduce its effect on gastric pH. Four years later the colt's behavior remains normal. The owners have not challenged him with traditional feeding regimens and intend to keep the time he spends in the stable to a minimum. None of the dam's subsequent foals have shown signs of similar behaviors.

REFERENCES

1. Tyler SJ. The behaviour and social organisation of the New Forest ponies. Anim Behav Monogr 1972; 5: 85–196.
2. Crowell-Davis SL, Houpt KA, Carnevale J. Feeding drinking behaviour of mares and foals with free access to pasture and water. J Anim Sci 1985; 60(4):883–889.
3. Weaver LT. Milk and neonatal gut: comparative lessons to be learnt. Equine Vet J 1996; 18(6):427–429.
4. Waring GH. Horse behavior. Park Ridge, NJ: Noyes; 1983.

5. Tyler SJ. The behaviour and social organisation of the New Forest ponies. Dissertation, University of Cambridge, UK, 1969.

6. McDonnell SM, Poulin A. Equid play ethogram. Appl Anim Behav Sci 2001; 78(2–4):263–295.

7. Boy V, Duncan P. Time-budgets of Camargue horses, I: Developmental changes in the time-budgets of foals. Behaviour 1979; 71:187–202.

8. Crowell-Davis SL. Developmental behavior. Vet Clin North Am Equine Pract: Behav 1986; 2(3):573–590.

9. Monard AM, Duncan P, Fritz H, Feh C. Variations in the birth sex ratio and neonatal mortality in a natural herd of horses. Behav Ecol Sociobiol 1997; 41(4):243–249.

10. Marinier SL, Alexander AJ. Coprophagy as an avenue for foals of the domestic horse to learn food preferences from their dams. J Theor Biol 1995; 173:121–124.

11. Waters AJ, Nicol CJ, French NP. Factors influencing the development of stereotypic and redirected behaviours in young horses: findings of a four year prospective epidemiological study. Equine Vet J 2002; 34(6):572–579.

12. Mesochina P, Peyraud JL, Duncan P, et al. [Grass intake by growing horses at pasture: a test of the effects of the horses' age and sward biomass] [French]. Ann Zootech 2000; 49(6):505–515.

13. Ödberg FO, Francis-Smith K. A study of eliminative and grazing behaviour—the use of the field by captive horses. Equine Vet J 1976; 8(4):147–149.

14. Forbes JM. Voluntary food intake and diet selection in farm animals. Wallingford, Oxon: CAB International; 1995.

15. Baer KL, Potter GD, Friend TH, Beaver BV. Observation effects on learning in horses. Appl Anim Ethol 1983; 11:123–129.

16. Baker AEM, Crawford BH. Observational learning in horses. Appl Anim Behav Sci 1986; 15:7–13.

17. Lindberg AC, Kelland A, Nicol CJ. Effects of observational learning on acquisition of an operant response in horses. Appl Anim Behav Sci 1999; 61(3):187–199.

18. Clarke JV, Nicol CJ, Jones R, McGreevy PD. Effects of observational learning on food selection in horses. Appl Anim Behav Sci 1996; 50:177–184.

19. Provenza FD, Cincotta RP. Foraging as a self-organisational learning process; accepting adaptability at the expense of predictability. In: Hughes RN, ed. Diet selection. Oxford: Blackwell Scientific; 1993.

20. Francis-Smith K, Wood-Gush DGM. Coprophagia as seen in Thoroughbred foals. Equine Vet J 1977; 9:155–157.

21. McLean AN. Cognitive abilities — the result of selective pressures on food acquisition? Appl Anim Behav Sci 2001; 71:241–258.

22. Crowell-Davis SL, Houpt KA. Coprophagy by foals: effect of age and possible functions. Equine Vet J 1985; 17(1):17–19.

23. Moltz H, Lee TM. The maternal pheromone of the rat: identity and functional significance. Physiol Behav 1981; 26:301–306.

24. McGreevy PD. Why does my horse ...? London: Souvenir Press; 1996.

25. McCall CA, Potter GD, Friend TH, Ingram RS. Learning abilities in yearling horses using the Hebb-Williams closed field maze. J Anim Sci 1981; 53(4):928–933.

26. Nicol CJ. Farm animal cognition. J Anim Sci 1996; 62(3):375–391.

27. Cairns MC, Cooper JJ, Davidson HPB, Mills DS. Ability of horses to associate orosensory characteristics of foods to their post-ingestive consequences in a choice test. Havemeyer Workshop on Horse Behaviour and Welfare, Holar, Iceland, 2002: 5–9.

28. Forbes JM. Dietary Awareness. Appl Anim Behav Sci 1998; 57:287–297.

29. Wood-Gush DGM. Elements of ethology. New York: Chapman & Hall; 1983.

30. Fraser AF. The behaviour of the horse. Wallingford, Oxon: CAB International; 1992.

31. Laut JE, Houpt KA, Hintz HF, Houpt TR. The effects of caloric dilution on meal patterns and food intake of ponies. Physiol Behav 1985; 35(4):549–554.

32. Forbes JM. Natural feeding behaviour and feed selection. In: van der Heide D, Huismam EA, Karis E, Osse JWM, Verstegen MWA, eds. Regulation of feed intake. Wallingford, Oxon: CAB International; 1999.

33. Houpt KA, O'Connell MF, Houpt TA, Carbonaro DA. Nighttime behaviour of stabled and peri-parturient ponies. Appl Anim Behav Sci 1986; 15:103–111.

34. Duncan P. Horses and grasses—the nutritional ecology of equids and their impact on the Camargue. New York: Springer; 1992.

35. Houpt KA, Zahorik DM, Swartzman-Andert JA. Taste aversion learning in horses. J Anim Sci 1990; 68:2340–2344.

36. Burritt EA. Provenza FD. Ability of lambs to learn with a delay between food ingestion and consequences given meals containing novel and familiar foods. Appl Anim Behav Sci 1991; 32:179–189.

37. Fraser AF, Brownlee A. Veterinary ethology and grass sickness in horses. Vet Rec 1974; 95(9):448.

38. Hansen RM. Foods of free-roaming horses in Southern New Mexico. J Range Manag 1976; 29(4):437.

39. Putman RJ, Pratt RM, Ekins JR, Edwards PJ. Food and feeding behaviour of cattle and horses in the New Forest Hampshire. J Appl Ecol 1987; 24:369–380.

40. Archer M. Preliminary studies on the palatability of grasses, legumes and herbs to horses. Vet Rec 1971; 89:236.

41. Collery L. Observations of equine animals under farm and feral conditions. Equine Vet J 1974; 6:170.

42. Merritt TL, Washko JB, Swain RH. Pasture preferences of horses. Mimeo: Pennsylvania State University; 1969. H-69–1.

43. Archer M. Grazing patterns of horses. Br Vet J 1977; 133:98.

44. Archer M. The species preferences of grazing horses. J Br Grassland Soc 1973; 28:123.

45. Houpt KA, Wolski TR. Domestic animal behavior for veterinarians and animal scientists. Ames: Iowa State University Press; 1982.

46. Menard C, Duncan P, Fleurance G, et al. Comparative foraging and nutrition of horses and cattle in European wetlands. J Appl Ecol 2002; 39(1):120–133.

47. Stobbs TH. The effect of plant structure on the intake of tropical pastures, II: Differences in sward structure,

nutritive value and bite size of animals grazing Setaraia anceps and Chloris gayana at various stages of growth. Aust J Agric Res 1973; 24:821–829.

48. Keenan DM. Bark chewing by horses grazed on irrigated pasture. Aust Vet J 1986; 63(7):234–235.

49. Feist JD, McCullough DR. Behaviour patterns and communication in feral horses. Z Tierpsychol 1976; 41:337–371.

50. McGreevy PD, Hawson LA, Habermann TC, Cattle SR. Geophagia in horses: a short note on 13 cases. Appl Anim Behav Sci 2001; 71:119–215.

51. Carson K, Wood-Gush DGM. Equine Behaviour, II: A review of the literature on feeding, eliminative and resting behaviour. Appl Anim Ethol 1983; 10:179–190.

52. DiPietro JA, Ewert KE, Todd KS Jr. Ivermectin treatment of horses: effect on the distribution of lawns and roughs in horse pastures. Vet Parasitol 1993; 48(1/4):241–246.

53. Edwards PJ, Hollis S. The distribution of excreta on New Forest grassland used by cattle ponies and deer. J Appl Ecol 1982; 19(3):953–964.

54. Archer M. Studies on producing and maintaining balanced pastures for studs. Equine Vet J 1978; 10(1):54–59.

55. Medica DL, Hanaway MJ, Ralston SL, Sukhdeo MVK. Grazing behaviour of horses on pasture: predisposition to strongylid infection. J Equine Vet Sci 1996; 16(10):421–427.

56. Round MC. Some aspects of naturally acquired helminthiasis of horses. Equine Vet J 1971; 3:31–37.

57. van Wieren SE. Do large herbivores select a diet that maximizes short-term energy intake rate? Forest Ecol Manage 1996; 88(1/2):149–156.

58. Dulphy JP, Jouany JP, Theriez M. [Comparison of the ability of different species of domestic herbivores to ingest and digest forages distributed in feeding troughs] Aptitudes comparées de differentes especes d'herbivores domestiques a ingerer et digerer des fourrages distribues a l'auge. Ann Zootech 1994; 43(1):11–32.

59. Somlo R, Bonvissuto G, Shriller A, et al. [Effect of range condition on the seasonal diets of herbivores and on multiple grazing in the western mountains and plateaus of Patagonia] La influencia de la condicion del pastizal sobre la dieta estacional de los herbivoros y e pastoreo multiple en sierras y mesetas occidentales de Patagonia. Revista Argentina de Produccion Animal 1994; 3/4:187–207.

60. Gudmundson O, Dyrmundsson OR. Horse grazing under cold and wet conditions; a review. Livestock Prod Sci 1994; 40(1):57–63.

61. Randall RP, Schurg WA, Church DC. Response of horses to sweet, salty, sour and bitter solutions. J Anim Sci 1978; 47:51–55.

62. Hawkes J, Hedges M, Daniluk P, et al. Feed preferences of ponies. Equine Vet J 1985; 17:20–22.

63. Marinier SL, Alexander AJ. Selective grazing behavior in horses: development of methodology and preliminary use of tests to measure individual grazing ability. Appl Anim Behav Sci 1991; 30(3–4):203–221.

64. Kiley-Worthington M. The behaviour of horses—in relation to management and training. London: JA Allen; 1987.

65. Colon JL, Jackson CA, del Piero F. Hepatic dysfunction and photodermatitis secondary to alsike clover poisoning. Compend Contin Educ Practicing Vet 1996; 18(9):1022–1026.

66. McBarron EJ. Poisonous plants—handbook for farmers and graziers. Department of Agriculture, NSW: Inkata Press; 1983.

67. Marinier SL, Alexander AJ. Use of field observations to measure individual grazing ability in horses. Appl Anim Behav Sci 1992; 33(1):1–10.

68. Rifa H. Social facilitation in the horse (Equus caballus). Appl Anim Behav Sci 1990; 25:167–176.

69. Hansen DK, Rouquette FM Jr, Florence MJ, et al. Grazing behavior of yearling horses, I: Time spent grazing different forages. Forage Research in Texas, Texas A & M University 1987; 17–21.

70. Martin-Rosset W, Doreau M, Cloix J. [Activities of a herd of draught brood mares and their foals on pasture] Etudes des activities d'un troupeau de poulinières de trait et de leurs poulains au paturage. Ann Zootech 1978; 27(1):33–45.

71. Duncan P. Time-budgets of Camargue horses, II: Time-budgets of adult horses and weaned sub-adults. Behaviour 1980; 72:26–49.

72. Fuller Z, Cox JE, Argo CM. Photoperiodic entrainment of seasonal changes in the appetite, feeding behaviour, growth rate and pelage of pony colts. Anim Sci 2001; 72(1):65–74.

73. Berger A, Scheibe KM, Eichhorn K, et al. Diurnal and ultradian rhythms of behaviour in a mare group of Przewalski horse (Equus ferus przewalskii), measured through one year under semi-reserve conditions. Appl Anim Behav Sci 1999; 64(1):1–17.

74. Choung CC, Kang MS, Ha SC. Grazing behaviour of Cheju native ponies. [Korean] Korean J Anim Sci 1994; 36(4):428–433.

75. Gill J. Circadian pattern of motor activity in horses in dependence of age and season [Polish]. Medycyna Weterynaryjna 1992; 48(4):183–185.

76. Salter RE, Hudson RJ. Feeding ecology of feral horses in Western Alberta. J Range Management 1979; 32(3):221–225.

77. Mayes E, Duncan P. Temporal patterns of feeding behaviour in free-ranging horses. Behaviour 1986; 96(1/2):105–129.

78. Kaseda Y. Characteristics of the horse tracks on the slopes of Misaki pasture in Toi Cape [Japanese]. Jpn J Zootech Sci 1983; 51(9):642–648.

79. Gallagher JR, McMeniman NP. Grazing behaviour of horses in S.E. Queensland pastures. Recent advances in animal nutrition in Australia 1989, Department of Biochemistry, Microbiology and Nutrition, University of New England, Armidale, Australia; 1989. 11A.

80. Rubenstein DI. Behavioural ecology in island feral horses. Equine Vet J 1981; 13:27–34.

81. Rogalski M. Behaviour of the horse at pasture [Polish]. Kon Polski 1970; 5:26–27.

82. Dulphy JP, Martin-Rosset W, Dubroeucq H, et al. Compared feeding patterns in ad libitum intake of dry forages by horses and sheep. Livestock Prod Sci 1997; 52(1):49–56.

83. Ralston SL. Feeding behavior. Vet Clin North Am Equine Pract 1986; 2(3):609–621.

84. Arnold GW. Comparison of the time budgets and circadian patterns of maintenance activities in sheep, cattle and horses grouped together. Appl Anim Behav Sci 1984; 13(1–2):19–30.

85. Dallaire A. Rest behavior. Vet Clin North Am Equine Pract: Behav 1986; 591–607.

86. Ralston SL, van den Broek G, Baile CA. Feed intake and associated blood glucose, free fatty acid and insulin changes in ponies. J Anim Sci 1979; 49(3):838–845.

87. Kern D, Bond J. Eating patterns of ponies fed ad libitum. J Anim Sci 1972; 35:285.

88. Doreau M, Martin-Rosset W, Petit D. [Nocturnal feeding activities of horses at pasture] Activities alimentaires nocturnes du cheval au paturage. Ann Zootech 1980; 29(3):299–304.

89. Glendinning SA. A system of rearing foals on an automatic calf-feeding machine. Equine Vet J 1974; 6:12–16.

90. Houpt KA, Hintz HF. Some effects of maternal deprivation on maintenance behaviour, spatial relationships and responses to environmental novelty in foals. Appl Anim Ethol 1983; 9:221–230.

91. Okuda Y, Ngata Y, Kubo K, et al. Grazing behaviour and heart rate of young Thoroughbreds on pasture. Bull Equine Res Inst Jpn 1980; 17:8–20.

92. Ruckebusch Y, Vigroux P, Candau M. Analyse du comportement alimentaire chez les equides. CR Journée d'Etude CEREOPA, Paris, 1976; 69–72.

93. Harris PA. How understanding the digestive process can help minimise digestive disturbances due to diet and feeding practices. In: Harris PA, Gomarsall G, Davidson HPB, Green R, eds. Proceedings of the BEVA Specialist days on Behaviour and Nutrition. Equine Vet J 1999; 45–49.

94. Cuddeford D. Why feed fibre to the performance horse today? In: Proceedings of the BEVA Specialist days on Behaviour and Nutrition. Harris PA, Gomarsall G, Davidson HPB, Green R, eds. Equine Vet J 1999; 50–54.

95. Meyer H, Coenen M, Gurer C. Investigations of saliva production and chewing in horses fed various feeds. In: Proceedings of the 9th Equine Nutrition and Physiology Symposium, East Lansing, Michigan, 1985:38–41.

96. Pagan JD. Gastric ulcers in horses: a widespread but manageable disease. World Equine Vet Rev 1997; 2:28–30.

97. Ralston SL, Baile CA. Effects of intragastric loads of xylose, sodium chloride and corn oil on feeding behaviour of ponies. J Anim Sci 1983; 56(2):302–308.

98. Duren SE, Dougherty CT, Jackson SG, Baker JP. Modification of ingestive behaviour due to exercise in yearling horses grazing orchardgrass. Appl Anim Behav Sci 1989; 22(3–4):335–345.

99. Heleski CR, Shelle AC, Nielsen BD, Zanella AJ. Influence of housing on weanling horse behaviour and subsequent welfare. Appl Anim Behav Sci 2002; 78(2–4):297–308.

100. Warr EM, Petch JL. Effects of soaking hay on its nutritional quality. Equine Vet Educ 1992; 5:169–171.

101. Blackman M, Moore-Colyer MJS. Hay for horses: the effect of three different wetting treatments on dust and nutrient contents. Anim Sci 1998; 66:745–750.

102. Bergero D, Nardi S. [Eating time of some feeds for saddle horses reared in Italy] Tempi di consumo di alcuni alimenti in cavalli da sella allevati in Italia. Obiettivi e Documenti Veterinaria 1996; 17(1):63–67.

103. Vernet J, Vermorel M, Martin-Rosset W. Energy cost of eating long hay, straw and pelleted food in sport horses. Anim Sci 1995; 61(3):581–588.

104. Nicol CJ. Stereotypies and their relationship to management. In: Harris PA, Gomarsall G, Davidson HPB, Green R, eds. Proceedings of the BEVA Specialist days on Behaviour and Nutrition. Equine Vet J 1999; 11–14.

105. Johnson KG, Tyrell J, Rowe JB, Pethick DW. Behavioural changes in stabled horses given nontherapeutic levels of virginiamycin. Equine Vet J 1998; 30(2):139–143.

106. Hintz HF, Loy RC. Effects of pelleting on the nutritive value of horse rations. J Anim Sci 1966; 25:1059.

107. Duncan P. Determinants of the use of habitat by horses in a Mediterranean wetland. J Anim Ecol 1983; 52(1):93–109.

108. Crane KK, Smith MA, Reynolds D. Habitat selection patterns of feral horses in south-central Wyoming. J Range Manage 1997; 50(4):374–380.

109. Kusunose R, Hatakeyama H, Ichikawa F, et al. Behavioural studies on yearling horses in the field environment, 3: Effects of the pasture shape on the behaviour of horses. Bull Jpn Equine Res Inst 1987; 24:1–5.

110. Stobbs TH. The effect of plant structure on the intake of tropical pastures, I: Variation in the bite size of grazing cattle. Aust J Agric Res 1973; 24: 809–819.

111. Salter RE, Pluth DJ. Determinants of mineral lick utilization by feral horses. Northwest Sci 1980; 54:109–118.

112. Krzak WE, Gonyou HW, Lawrence LM. Wood chewing by stabled horses: diurnal pattern and effects of exercise. J Anim Sci 1991; 69:1053–1058.

113. Sasimowski E, Budzynski M, Jelen B, et al. [Observations on the behaviour of horses in an open stable and the fodder consumption when offered ad libitum] Obserwacje nad zachowaniem sie koni w warunkach wolnowybiegowej stajni I pobieraniem przez nie paszy zadawanej ad libitum. Prace I Materialy Zootechniczne 1979; 20:69–86.

114. Willard JG, Willard JC, Baker JP. Dietary influences on feeding behaviour in ponies. J Anim Sci 1973; 37:227.

115. Buntain BJ, Coffmann JR. Polyuria and polydipsia in a horse induced by psychogenic salt consumption. Equine Vet J 1981; 13:266–268.

116. Olson-Rutz KM, Marlow CB, Hansen K, et al. Packhorse grazing behaviour and immediate impact on timberline meadow. J Range Manage 1996; 49(6):546–550.

117. Schafer M. The Language of the horse. London: Kaye & Ward; 1975.

118. McGreevy PD, Cripps PJ, French NP, et al. Management factors associated with stereotypic and redirected behaviour in the Thoroughbred horse. Equine Vet J 1995; 27:86–91.

119. Goodwin D, Davidson HPB, Harris P. Foraging enrichment for stabled horses: effects on behaviour and selection. Equine Vet J 2002; 34(7):686–691.

120. Shipley LA, Spalinger DE, Gross JE, et al. The dynamics and scaling of foraging velocity and encounter rate in mammalian herbivores. Funct Ecol 1996; 10(2):234–244.

121. Kaseda Y. Seasonal changes in time spent grazing and resting of Misaki horses [Japanese]. Jpn J Zootech Sci 1980; 54(7):464–469.

122. Youket RJ, Carnevale JM, Houpt KA, Houpt TR. Humoral, hormonal, and behavioural correlates of feeding in ponies: the effects of meal frequency. J Anim Sci 1985; 61:1103–1110.

123. Clarke LL, Ganjam VK, Fitchenbaum B, et al. Effect of feeding on renin angiotensin-aldosterone system in the horse. Am J Physiol 1988; 254:5R24–R530.

124. Hoffman KL, Wood AKW, Griffiths KA, et al. Postprandial arterial vasodilation in the equine distal thoracic limb. Equine Vet J 2001; 33(3):269–273.

125. Pollitt CC, Davies CT. Equine laminitis: its development coincides with increased sublamellar blood flow. Equine Vet J Suppl 1998; 26:125–132.

126. Kusunose R, Hatakeyama H, Ichikawa F, et al. Behavioural studies on yearling horses in field environments, 2: Effects of group size on the behaviour of horses. Bull Jpn Equine Res Inst 1986; 23:1–6.

127. Sweeting MP, Houpt CE, Houpt KA. Social facilitation of feeding and time budgets in stabled ponies. J Anim Sci 1985; 60(2):369–374.

128. Pirkelmann H. [Behaviour of horses at electronic controlled concentrate feeding stations] Verhalten von Pferden an rechnergesteuerten Futterautomaten. Ktbl-Schrift 1991; 344:116–127.

129. Fleege G. [Behaviour of horses held in groups with individual feeding] Verhalten von Pfereden bei individueller Fressplatzzuweisung in Grupenhaltung. Ktbl-Schrift 1991; 344:128–139.

130. Matsui K, Sugano S, Sawasaki T. Relationship between diurnal variation in R–R interval and feeding behaviour in the horse. J Equine Sci 1994; 5(4):131–135.

131. Minero M, Canali E, Ferrante V, et al. Heart rate and behavioural responses of crib-biting horses to two acute stressors. Vet Rec 1999; 145(15):430–433.

132. Dewers HF. A possible vitamin E-responsive condition in adult horses. NZ Vet J 1981; 29(5):83–84.

133. Holland JL, Kronfield DS, Meacham TN. Behaviour of horses is affected by soy lecithin and corn oil in the diet. J Anim Sci 1996; 74(6):1252–1255.

134. Kronfeld D, Holland J, Hoffman R, Harris P. Dietary influences on behaviour and stress. The role of the horse in Europe. Equine Vet J Suppl 1999; 28:64.

135. Lopez Olivia M, Gonzalez G, Corbeira P, et al. [Undesirable behaviours in sport horses subject to the rigors of management, training and competition] Manifestaciones conductuales indeseables en los equinos deportivos sometidos a exigencias de manejo, entrenamiento y competicion. Revistas de Medicina Veterianria 1999; 80(2):125–128.

136. Dallaire A, Ruckebusch Y. Sleep patterns in the housed pony under different dietary conditions. Can J Comp Med 1974; 38:65–71.

137. Eades SC, Booth AJ, Hansen TO, et al. The gastrointestinal and digestive system. In: Higgins AJ,

Wright IM, eds. The equine manual. London: WB Saunders; 1995:453–539.

138. Taylor TS, Matthews NS. Mammoth asses – selected behavioural considerations for the veterinarian. Appl Anim Behav Sci 1998; 60(2–3):283–289.

139. Harris PA, Frape DL, Jeffcott LB, et al. Equine nutrition and metabolic diseases. In: Higgins AJ, Wright IM, eds. The equine manual. London: WB Saunders; 1995:123–186.

140. Naylor JM, Freeman DE, Kronfield DS. Alimentation of hypophagic horses. Compend Cont Ed Pract Vet 1984; S93-S99.

141. Doxey DL, Tothill S, Milne EM, Davis Z. Patterns of feeding and behaviour in horses recovering from dysautonomia (grass sickness). Vet Rec 1995; 137(8):181–183.

142. Ralston SL. Regulation of feed intake in the horse in relation to gastrointestinal disease. Pferdeheilkunde Sonderausgabe 1992; 15–18.

143. Murray MJ, Eichorn ES. Effects of intermittent feed deprivation, intermittent feed deprivation with ranitidine administration and stall confinement with ad libitum access to hay on gastric ulceration in horses. Am J Vet Res 1996; 57(11):1599–1603.

144. Doreau M. [Feeding behaviour of horses in stables] Comportement alimentaire du cheval a l'écurie. Ann Zootech 1978; 27(3):291–302.

145. Greet TRC, Rossdale PD. The digestive system. In: Hayes MH, Rossdale PD, eds.Veterinary notes for horse owners. London: Stanley Paul; 1987:5–24.

146. Nicol CJ. Understanding equine stereotypies. The role of the horse in Europe. Equine Vet J Suppl 1999; 56–57.

147. Houpt KA. Oral vices of horses. Equine Pract 1982; 4(4):16–25.

148. Redbo I, Redbo-Torstensson P, Ödberg FO, et al. Factors affecting behavioural disturbances in race-horses. Anim Sci 1998; 66:475–481.

149. Green P, Tong JMJ. Small intestinal obstruction associated with wood chewing in two horses. Vet Rec 1988; 123:196–198.

150. Haenlein GFW, Holdren RD, Yoon YM. Comparative responses of horses and sheep to different physical forms of alfalfa hay. J Anim Sci 1966; 25:740–743.

151. Willard JG, Willard JC, Wolfram SA, Baker JP. Effect of diet on cecal pH and feeding behaviour of horses. J Anim Sci 1977; 45:87–93.

152. Nagata Y. Effects of various degrees of size and hardness of complete pelletized feed on feeding behaviour of horses. Exp Reprod Equine Health Lab (Japan) 1971; 8:72.

153. McDonnell S. Carnivorous horses. The Horse October 2002, article 3832.

154. Herlin AH, Andersson J. Soil ingestion in farm animals: a review. Report—Department of Agricultural Biosystems and Technology, Swedish University of Agricultural Sciences 1996; 105:35.

155. Sambraus HH, Rappold D. Crib-biting and wind-sucking in horses. Pferdeheilkunde 1991; 7:211–216.

156. Owen RR. Crib-biting and wind-sucking—that equine enigma. In: Hill CSG, Grunsell FWG, eds. The veterinary annual 1982; Bristol: Wright Scientific Publications; 1982:156–168.

157. McGreevy PD, Richardson JD, Nicol CJ, Lane JG. A radiographic and endoscopic study of horses

performing an oral stereotypy. Equine Vet J 1995; 27:92–95.

158. McCall CA, Potter GD, Kreider JL. Locomotor, vocal and other behavioural responses to varying methods of weaning foals. Appl Anim Behav Sci 1985; 14(1):27–35.

159. McCall CA, Potter GD, Kreider JL, Jenkins WL. Physiological responses in foals weaned by abrupt or gradual methods. J Equine Vet Sci 1987; 7(6):368–374.

160. Apter RC, Householder DD. Weaning and weaning management of foals: a review and some recommendations. J Equine Vet Sci 1996; 16(10):428–435.

161. Nicol CJ, Davidson HPD, Harris PA, et al. Study of crib-biting and gastric inflammation and ulceration in young horses. Vet Rec 2002: 151(22):658–662.

162. McGreevy PD, Nicol CJ. Prevention of crib-biting: a review. Equine Vet J Suppl 1998; 27:35–38.

163. McGreevy PD, Nicol CJ. Physiological and behavioural consequences associated with short-term prevention of crib-biting in horses. Physiol Behav 1998; 65:15–23.

164. Nadeau JA, Andrews FM, Mathew AG, et al. Evaluation of diet as a cause of gastric ulcers in horses. Am J Vet Res 2000; 61:784–790.

165. Borrow HA. Duodenal perforations and gastric ulcers in foals. Vet Rec 1993; 132:12,297–299.

166. Furr MO, Murray MJ, Ferguson DC. The effects of stress on gastric ulceration, T3, T4, reverse T3 and cortisol in neonatal foals. Equine Vet J 1992; 24:1,37–40.

167. Tarara EB, Tarara RP, Suleman MA. Stress-induced gastric ulcers in vervet monkeys (Cercopithecus aethiops): the influence of life history factors, Part II. J Zoo Wildlife Med 1995; 26:1,72–75.

168. Henrotte JG, Aymard N, Allix M, Boulu RG. Effect of pyridoxine and magnesium on stress-induced gastric ulcers in mice selected for low or high blood magnesium levels. Ann Nutr Metabol 1995; 39:5,285–290.

169. Vatistas NJ, Snyder JR, Carlson G, et al. Cross-sectional study of gastric ulcers of the squamous mucosa in Thoroughbred racehorses. Equine Vet J 1999; 29:34–39.

170. Murray MJ, Schusser GF, Pipers FS, Gross SJ. Factors associated with gastric lesions in Thoroughbred horses. Equine Vet J 1998; 28(5):368–374.

171. McGreevy PD. The functional significance of stereotypies in the stabled horse. PhD thesis, University of Bristol, 1995.

172. Pell S, McGreevy PD. The prevalence of abnormal and stereotypic behaviour in Thoroughbreds in Australia. Aust Vet J 1999; 77(10):678–679.

173. McGreevy PD, Webster AJF, Nicol CJ. A study of the digestive efficiency, behaviour and gut transit times of crib-biting horses. Vet Rec 2001; 148:592–596.

174. Hillyer MH, Taylor FGR, Proudman CJ, et al. Case control study to identify risk factors for simple colonic obstruction and distension colic in horses. Equine Vet J 2002; 34(5):455–463.

175. McGreevy PD, Nicol CJ. The effect of short term prevention on the subsequent rate of crib-biting in

Thoroughbred horses. Equine Vet J Suppl 1998; 27:30–34.

176. Dodman NH, Shuster L, Court MH, Dixon R. Investigation into the use of narcotic antagonist in the treatment of a stereotypic behavior pattern (crib-biting) in the horse. Am J Vet Res 1997; 48:311–319.

177. Dourmap N, Costentin J. Involvement of the glutamate receptors in the striatal enkephalin-induced dopamine release. Eur J Pharmacol 1994; 253:R9–R11.

178. Rendon RA, Shuster L, Dodman NH. The effect of the NMDA receptor blocker, dextromethorphan, on cribbing in horses. Pharmacol Biochem Behav 2001; 68(1):49–51.

179. Delacalle J, Burba DJ, Tetens J, Moore RM. YAG laser-assisted modified Forssell's procedure for treatment of cribbing (crib-biting) in horses. Vet Surg 2002; 31(2):111–116.

180. Mills DS, MacLeod CA. The response of crib-biting and windsucking in horses to dietary supplementation with an antacid mixture. Ippologia 2002; 13(2):1–9.

181. Goergen R. Life on the edge. New Scientist 2001; 2305:30–33.

182. Tasker JB. Fluid and electrolyte studies in the horse, III: Intake and output of water, sodium and potassium in normal horses. Cornell Vet 1967; 57:649–657.

183. Houpt KA. Thirst of horses: the physiological and psychological causes. Equine Pract 1987; 9:28–30.

184. Hinton H. On the watering of horses—a review. Equine Vet J 1978; 10:27–31.

185. Bannikov AG. Special natural conditions of the biotope of the Przewalski wild horse and some biological features of this species. [Russian] Equus 1961; I:13–21.

186. Ganskopp D, Vavra M. Habitat use by feral horses in the northern sagebrush. J Range Manage 1986; 39(3):207–212.

187. McDonnell SM, Kristula MA. No effect of drinking water temperature (ambient vs. chilled) on consumption of water during hot summer weather in ponies. Appl Anim Behav Sci 1996; 49(2):159–163.

188. Houpt KA, Perry PJ, Hintz HF, Houpt TR. Effect of meal frequency on fluid balance and behaviour in ponies. Physiol Behav 1988; 42(5):401–407.

189. Sufit E, Houpt KA, Sweeting M. Physiological stimuli of thirst and drinking patterns in ponies. Equine Vet J 1985; 17(1):12–16.

190. Richardson C. Cassell's new book of the horse, vol 4. London: Waverley; 1911.

191. Linton RG. Animal nutrition and dietetics. Edinburgh: Green; 1927.

192. Mansmann RA, Woodie B. Equine transportation problems and some preventives: a review. J Equine Vet Sci 1995; 15:141–144.

193. McDonnell SM, Freeman DA, Cymbaluk NF, et al. Behavior of stabled horses provided continuous or intermittent access to drinking water. Am J Vet Res 1999; 60(11):1451–1456.

194. Nyman S, Dahlborn K. Effect of water supply method and flow rate on drinking behavior and fluid balance in horses. Physiol Behav 2001; 73(1–2):1–8.

195. Freeman DA, Cymbaluk NF, Schott HC, et al. Clinical, biochemical, and hygiene assessment of stabled horses provided continuous or intermittent access to drinking water. Am J Vet Res 1999; 60:1445–1450.

196. Welford D, Mills D, Murphy K, Marlin D. The effect of changes in management scheduling on water intake by the Thoroughbred horse. The role of the horse in Europe. Equine Vet J Suppl 1999; 28:71–72.

197. Murphy K, Wishart S, Mills D. The acceptability of various flavoured solutions by Thoroughbred horses. The role of the horse in Europe. Equine Vet J Suppl 1999; 28:67.

198. Frape D. Equine nutrition and feeding, 2nd edn. Oxford: Blackwell Science; 1998.

199. Houpt KA. Equine welfare. In: Houpt KA, ed. Recent advances in companion animal behavior problems. Ithaca, NY: International Veterinary Information Services; 2001. A0810. 1201.

9

Eliminative behavior

DEVELOPMENT OF ELIMINATIVE RESPONSES

As a reflection of the changing nature of water balance from neonate to juvenile and the concurrent change in diet, the frequency of urination decreases as that of defecation increases with maturity (Fig. 9.1). By 5 months of age, defecation has plateaued from approximately twice per day in the first week of life so that it occurs every 3–4 hours.[1] Urination, on the other hand, declines from an hourly event to one that occurs about six times per day.[1] Perhaps because they can tolerate greater distensions of their bladders, filly foals are generally twice as old as colts when they first urinate (10.77 hours post-partum versus 5.97).[2]

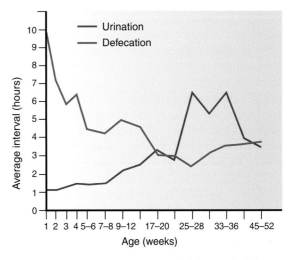

Figure 9.1   Frequency of urination and defecation in foals, expressed as the interval between eliminative behaviors. (Data from Tyler.[1] Redrawn, with permission, from Waring.[23])

DEFECATION

Horses can be prompted to defecate by the sight of feces or the action of another horse defecating. Drinking is also thought to provide a stimulation to dung,[3] possibly via a gastro-colic reflex.[4] Arousal in the form of both fear and excitement can also stimulate horses to defecate,[5] sometimes to the extent of intestinal hurry, as manifested by the presence of undigested grain.

Horses tend to show considerable care in the selection of defecation sites since they return repeatedly to areas that are not used for grazing. Fecal material makes the grass in latrine areas less appealing, even though the grass itself is readily consumed if presented to horses without the fecal material.[6] This response, which develops in foals as they mature and become less attached to their dams,[7] prompts the development of so-called latrine and lawn areas.[1] The tendency to defecate in soiled areas means the main body of pasture carries fewer parasites. This strategy is appropriate for free-ranging horses that have a virtually unlimited range but in smaller fenced grazing areas it behoves management to institute rotational grazing to break the lifecycle of endoparasites.

The vestiges of dunging strategy are sometimes evident in stabled horses that show an attempt to select sites. As noted by Mills et al,[8] when given the choice between two bedding substrates in looseboxes joined by a passageway, horses defecated in the passageway more than in either box. This could reflect the association between movement (between boxes when exercising choice) and hindgut motility, but should prompt further investigation into the aversiveness felt by horses to fecal material and the extent to which welfare may be compromised by making horses stand in close proximity to their own excrement for extended periods, as is the case in standard husbandry. Certainly, pastured horses tend to move forward after defecation.[7] Porcine studies have provided a possible model by demonstrating the olfactory threshold of the pigs for concentrations of ammonia in the air.[9] Since urine and fecal material may be offensive, not least because of their ammonia content but also because they attract flies, compounds such as sodium bisulfate that have been shown to decrease ammonia levels and behavior typical of horses being bothered by flies should be integrated in the stable hygiene routine.[10]

Some owners who note that their horses (often geldings rather than mares) repeatedly defecate in feed buckets, sometimes interpret this behavior as a form of protest. A more likely explanation is the establishment of a habitual dunging pattern that coincides with relatively little space and therefore few alternatives other than that in which the receptacle is routinely placed. Hanging the haynet over the favored site (and ensuring that plenty of hay is contained within it) is usually effective in keeping the horse oriented appropriately and capitalizing on the innate equine tendency to move away from a foraging site prior to defecation. Despite such efforts, some horses do seem to target their food and water receptacles and repeatedly compromise their own ingestive activities as a result. Intriguingly, it appears that Thoroughbreds are more likely to perform this behavior than other breeds.[11] Ethologists note that the response is seen mainly in buckets that are placed on the wall next to the stable door and suggest that barrier frustration may contribute to the etiology.[11]

Despite the rarity of territories, stallions indicate their presence by piling their feces. About 25% of interactions between stallions occur in the vicinity of fecal piles (see Ch. 6).[12] Regular marking by stallions and dung-pile rituals are effective means of avoiding fighting and confrontation between stallions. As a cardinal feature of such interactions, a behavioral sequence that includes defecation is performed by them, either in succession or in unison.[13] It has been suggested that the dominant stallion is usually the last to defecate on the pile.[14] The culmination of these rituals is mutual passive withdrawal, pushing of the subordinate away, or a full-scale fight. The sequence of behaviors targeted on the pile runs as follows:

1. approach
2. olfactory investigation
3. flehmen
4. pawing
5. pivot around or step over

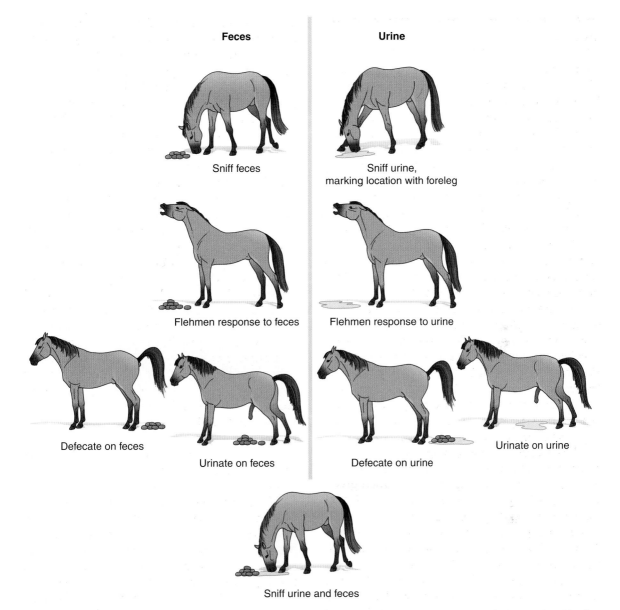

Feces | **Urine**

Sniff feces

Sniff urine,
marking location with foreleg

Flehmen response to feces

Flehmen response to urine

Defecate on feces

Urinate on feces

Defecate on urine

Urinate on urine

Sniff urine and feces

Figure 9.2 The elimination/marking sequence of harem stallions involves voiding feces and urine after the olfactory investigation of urine and feces recently voided by harem members. (After McDonnell SM. *A Practical Field Guide to Horse Behavior – The Equid Ethogram*. Lexington, KT: The Blood Horse Inc; 2003.)

6.   defecate
7.   pivot around or step over.

The entire sequence, or elements within it, are repeated.

In the free-ranging state, dung piles may serve as orientation marks for stallions. Domestic stallions often accumulate fecal piles beside fence-lines because this is the nearest they can get to conspecifics.[15] Occasionally, geldings create fecal piles,[7] but greeting rituals involving them have not been reported. Whereas stallions usually move over fecal material and defecate or urinate on top of it (Fig. 9.2), mares and, to a lesser extent, geldings tend to sniff feces within latrine areas and defecate without much movement. This has the effect of spreading the area of rank grass[6,16,17] and the resultant repugnance and lack of close cropping facilitates the growth of weed species, including thistle (*Cirsium* spp.) and ragwort (*Senecio jacobaea*).[6,18]

URINATION

As with defecation, horses prefer to visit latrine areas to urinate. However, movement toward latrine areas occurs less reliably prior to urination than it does prior to defecation.[7] The number of urinations per day is related to water intake but, because of water loss through sweating, it is also negatively correlated with exercise.[3]

Generally mares and stallions adopt a similar posture before urinating. The croup is lowered and the tail is raised, with the hindlegs abducted and extended posteriorly. Both colts and fillies are sometimes seen urinating on top of fecal material.[1] While this trait disappears in females as they approach puberty, it becomes more obvious in males. When a stallion encounters a mare's dung, he urinates on it, apparently in a bid to mask its odor.[19] After being turned-out, some stallions mark with their urine as a priority ahead of greeting conspecifics.[6]

Spurting of urine by mares is sometimes seen, for example, in combination with kick threats when herded by stallions. Urination in mares becomes elaborate when they are in estrus, since they maintain a straddled stance for longer periods than when in anestrus and often tilt their hindtoes until one no longer bears weight (Fig. 9.3). This stance may act as an inviting visual signal for stallions since they have been observed rushing excitedly toward urinating mares.[1] In pony mares the tail is generally not held to one side as it is by horse mares.[20] The clitoral winking that occurs in all mares after urination is far more frequent when they are in estrus. In estrus, mares also pass less urine at each urination.[20] Urination often occurs as a spontaneous solicitation and in response to teasing.[21]

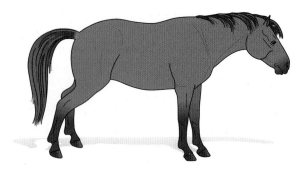

Figure 9.3 Estrous mare urinating with characteristic posture.

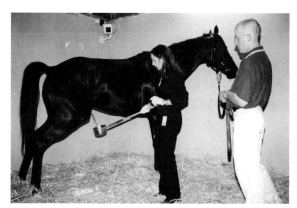

(a)

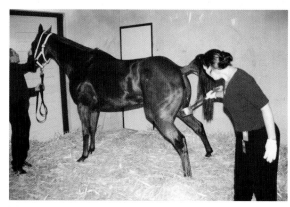

(b)

Figure 9.4 (a) Gelding and (b) mare providing post-race urine samples. Familiar bedding materials and whistling are used as classically conditioned stimuli for urination in racehorses. Anecdotal evidence suggests that females are less easy to train to urinate on cue than males.

In an apparent bid to avoid having their legs splashed by their own urine, horses select soft substrates on which to urinate. This is thought to be the origin of straw being a classically conditioned stimulus for urination in stabled horses. The association is routinely used to aid urine collection in performance horses (Fig. 9.4). Removal of bedding from stables during the day is often undertaken for the purposes of hygiene or economy. While laudable if used only as a means of drying the stable floor while the horse is at pasture, this intervention can have unwelcome consequences if the horse remains in the stable without bedding since it deters both recumbency and urination. The growing trend towards the use of rubber matting in place of traditional bedding substrates may have similar effects and merits investigation. A similar impediment to comfortable urination is thought to apply to urban horses, such as draft animals used in cities for tourism.

Increased frequency of urination has been noted as an indicator of social distress in isolated horses.[22] Although it may reflect urinary calculi and cystitis,[23] polyuria is usually a consequence of polydipsia that can be organic or psychogenic in origin (see Ch. 8). The usual presenting sign is an excessively wet bed. Determination of water intake is an important step in defining the extent of the problem, and direct observation of the horse's drinking and eating behavior can help to identify contributing behavioral anomalies such as excessive use of salt licks.

SUMMARY OF KEY POINTS

- Urination and defecation are influenced by age and sociosexual factors.
- The distribution of feces and urine can affect grazing behavior at pasture.
- Urine may be used to mask olfactory stimuli left by other horses.

REFERENCES

1. Tyler SJ. The behaviour and social organization of the New Forest ponies. Anim Behav Monogr 1972; 5:85–196.

2. Jeffcott LB. Observations on parturition in pony mares. Equine Vet J 1972; 4:209–213.

3. Schafer M. The language of the horse, London: Kaye & Ward; 1975.

4. Ganong WF. Review of medical physiology, 14th edn. California: Lange Medical Publications; 1989.

5. Houpt KA, Hintz HF, Pagan JD. Maternal-offspring bond of ponies fed different amounts of energy. Nutr & Behav 1983;1:157–168.

6. Kiley-Worthington M. The behaviour of horses – in relation to management and training. London: JA Allen; 1987.

7. Ödberg FO, Francis-Smith K. A study on eliminative and grazing behaviour – the use of the field by captive horses. Equine Vet J 1976; 8(4):147–149.

8. Mills DS, Eckley S, Cooper JJ. Thoroughbred bedding preferences, associated behaviour differences and their implications for equine welfare. Anim Sci 2000; 70(1):95–106.

9. Jones JB, Wathes CM, Persaud KC, et al. Acute and chronic exposure to ammonia and olfactory acuity for n-butanol in the pig. Appl Anim Behav Sci 2001; 71(1):13–28.

10. Sweeney CR, McDonnell S, Habecker PL, Russell GE. Effect of sodium bisulfate on ammonia levels, fly population and manure pH in a horse barn. Proc AAEP 1996; 42:306–307.

11. Perry PJ, Houpt KA. Aetiology of faecal soiling of buckets by horses. In: Overall KL, Mills DS, Heath SE, Horwitz D, eds. Proceedings of the Third International Congress on Veterinary Behavioural Medicine. UK: UFAW; 2001:139–141.

12. Miller R. Male aggression, dominance and breeding behaviour in Red Desert feral horses. Z Tierpsychol 1981; 64:97–146.

13. McDonnell SM, Haviland JCS. Agonistic ethogram of the equid bachelor band. Appl Anim Behav Sci 1995; 43:147–188.

14. McCort WD. Behaviour of feral horses and ponies. J Anim Sci 1984; 58(2):493–499.

15. McDonnell S. Reproductive behavior of stallions. Vet Clin North Am Equine Pract: Behav 1986; 535–555.

16. Carson K, Wood-Gush DGM. Equine behaviour, ii: A review of the literature on feeding, eliminative and resting behaviour. Appl Anim Ethol 1983; 10:179–190.

17. Rees L. The horse's mind, London: Stanley Paul; 1984.

18. Edwards PJ, Hollis S. The distribution of excreta on New Forest grassland used by cattle, ponies and deer. J Appl Ecol 1982; 19(3):953–964.

19. Kimura R. Volatile substances in feces, of feral urine and urine-marked feces of feral horses. Can J Anim Sci 2001; 81(3):411–420.

20. Asa CS. Sexual behavior of mares. Vet Clin North Am Equine Pract: Behav 1986; 519–534.

21. Fraser AF. The behaviour of the horse. London: CAB International; 1992.

22. Strand SC, Tiefenbacher S, Haskell M, et al. Behaviour and physiologic responses of mares to short-term isolation. Appl Anim Behav Sci 2002; 78:145–157.

23. Waring GH. Horse behavior: the behavioral traits and adaptations of domestic and wild horses including ponies. Park Ridge, NJ: Noyes; 1983.

10

Body care

GROOMING

In addition to maintaining the health of the integument, grooming behaviors can contribute to the affirmation of social bonds not least by reinforcing affiliations and sharing odors.

MUTUAL GROOMING

Mutual grooming not only allows horses to reach areas that defy self-grooming strategies, but also facilitates the exchange of odors[1] and has been shown to reduce heart rate when conducted in certain parts of the mane and withers.[2] Grooming of the withers by humans has a similar calming effect.[3] The effects on cardiac function are particularly striking in foals, with a mean reduction of 14% in heart rate being reported when preferred areas were scratched by humans.[2] This phenomenon is regularly harnessed by personnel who want to reward horses of any age without using food.

Mutual grooming can begin in the first week of life[4,5] but peaks in the second and third months of life,[6] a period during which foals seem to find physical contact intensely gratifying. In the first instance the foal's mutual grooming partner is its dam, who may dismiss other grooming partners if her foal solicits her attention by attempting to allogroom.[4] Although some mature horses never allogroom, most regularly indulge in reciprocated activity of this sort with favored affiliates for periods of about three minutes at a time.[7] Broadly speaking, regardless of their age, females spend more time mutually grooming than males.

223

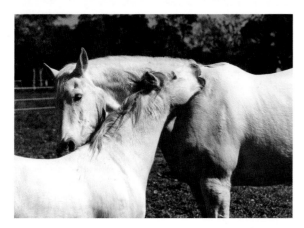

Figure 10.1   Mutual grooming helps equids to develop and maintain pair bonds. (Photograph courtesy of Sandra Hannan.)

Mutual grooming partners are usually preferred associates that are close in social rank.[8] In a natal band, mares and their offspring mutually groom kin rather than unrelated conspecifics.[9] The absence of a stallion seems to bring with it some liberation in that grooming partners are preferentially from same sex-age groups.[10] The stallions in multi-stallion harems will mutually groom one another.[11]

Mutual grooming often starts at the cranial neck and proceed to the withers (Fig. 10.1), the shoulders and then to the tail-head, sometimes with changing of sides (see Fig. 2.14).[12] While youngsters often attempt to begin allogrooming, such overtures are rarely reciprocated by unrelated adults.[4] As discussed in Chapter 5, there is equivocal evidence for the role of rank in the commencement of a bout of mutual grooming.[4,10] Recent reports indicate that low-ranking individuals groom more and initiate more groomings and that allogrooming may have a role in appeasement.[11] However, most bouts are ended by the departure of the higher-ranking member of the dyad.[4] Mutual grooming between foals is often observed before or after a bout of play.[13]

The frequency of mutual grooming is subject to daily and seasonal variation, with predictable troughs that coincide with recumbency.[14] The shedding of the winter coat and the seasonal peak in idling behavior account for annual peaks in mutual grooming (i.e. April and July in northern hemisphere studies[4]). When allowed to interact freely with other horses after 9 months of social deprivation, colts stabled singly showed significantly more social grooming than colts stabled in groups, which may reflect a build-up of motivation (a post-inhibitory rebound effect).[15]

SELF-GROOMING

Self-grooming brings out a great deal of resourcefulness in horses as they use their hooves, their mouths and objects in their environment to relieve irritation (Fig. 10.2). The frequency of self-grooming peaks at 12.3 times per hour in weeks 5–8 of a foal's life.[16] The relative proportion of body parts and the innate flexibility of foals both help to explain their relatively enhanced ability to self-groom and may account for the decline in the frequency of self-grooming to 1.2–2.2 times per hour in adults.[16] While their dams focus self-grooming on rolling and rubbing against the forelimbs, conspecifics or inanimate objects, foals are more frequently found scratching anteriorly with their hindlimbs or nibbling posteriorly.[16]

Along with appetite and growth, pelage cycles are related to the duration of the photoperiod.[17] Therefore the amount of grooming required is subject to seasonal flux and tends to peak with the shedding of the winter coat.

Scratching by humans can act as a highly valuable primary reinforcer, so an appreciation of the pleasure that grooming may bring can help to consolidate the horse-human bond. However, grooming by humans must take account of the variable sensitivity of different individuals and breeds.[1] The need to have a clean horse has been over-stated by some horse care manuals. Further, the perceived need to pull manes and tails undoubtedly irritates many horses and possibly compromises the horse-handler bond.

Rolling

Because the preferred substrates are sand, fine dry soil and occasionally mud, horses at pasture tend to select bare patches on which to roll, often beside gates or water troughs.[18] Some feral horses

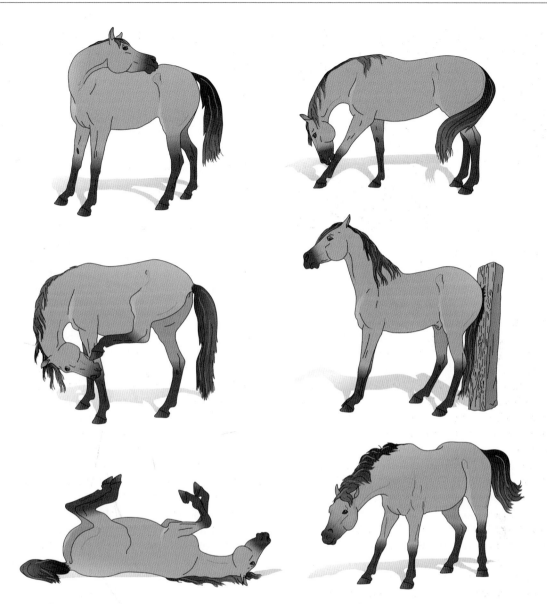

Figure 10.2   Grooming styles used by horses include rolling, shaking, rubbing, scratching and nibbling (of both the back and forelegs). (Redrawn, with permission, from Waring.[12])

have been observed to roll preferentially in water.[7] With more than 80% of rolling occurring where another horse has rolled,[1] its function is believed to include the opportunity to deposit scent over the body. The fact that horses, especially males,[19] smell chosen sites before and after rolling appears to support this view.

The head and neck help to propel the horse laterally while rolling (Fig. 10.3).[12] Similarly, lateral flexion of the vertebral column and thrashing of the hindlegs seems to help the horse to balance itself on the dorsal midline.[12] Rolling horses usually return to the same side they started lying on but often repeat the roll before rising.[12]

Apart from some foaling boxes, the space on the floor of most stables and many custom-built sand rolls is less than the width of most natural rolling sites. This helps to explain why we should

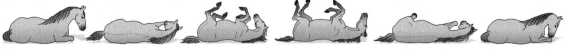

(a)

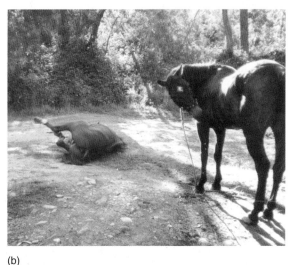

(b)

Figure 10.3 (a) Sequence showing horse rolling. (Redrawn, with permission, from Waring.[12]). (b) After a bath horses seem more itchy than normal and enjoy rolling, especially in dusty substrates.

be pleased that more horses do not get cast (stuck against the walls of stables or upside down in their stables). The use of anti-casting rails is a measure believed to help inverted horses to right themselves when stuck against the side of a stable. These rails are set about one meter from the floor, although their height should strictly speaking depend on that of the occupant. They work by providing some purchase against which the horse can push in a bid to move itself away from the wall.

Bedding materials such as straw that lend themselves to being banked up against the side of the stable wall are likely to reduce the risk of casting. Whatever bedding is selected must be managed carefully to maintain air hygiene. Beds that drain readily are less likely to be accompanied by high ammonia levels or allow humidity to rise to levels that increase the viability of fungal spores implicated in lower-airway disease.[20] Bedding preference studies suggest that the appeal of straw depends on its being deep and is linked to its alternative use as a source of dietary fiber.[21,22]

Shaking

Shaking is frequently seen after untacking, rolling and recumbency. It involves coordinated contraction of the superficial musculature that travels caudally from the head leading to vibration and rotation of the skin on the body. The neck is lowered prior to shaking,[12] and a wide placement of the forelegs is assumed. Males and non-estrous females often shake after urinating.[12]

Head and neck involvement is variable. Nodding and shaking the head can send the mane in different directions in a bid to dislodge insects. Before rectal palpation became established as a means of pregnancy diagnosis, folklore maintained that after having had water squirted into their ears, mares would not shake their heads if pregnant.

Rubbing

Rubbing can involve fixed objects or the muzzle.[12] The latter is used to reach places, such as

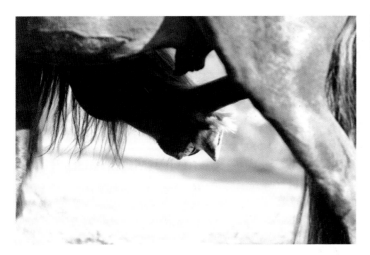

Figure 10.4 Horses sometimes use their mouths to groom the hindlegs. (Photograph courtesy of Francis Burton.)

the barrel and forelegs, that are hard to rub against fixed objects. Foals may rub target areas, such as the head, neck, croup and buttocks, on objects for as long as 15 minutes at a time.[12] Less frequently horses are observed using low branches to rub their backs and may sometimes even straddle vegetation on which they rub their ventral surface by walking forwards and backwards.[12] Rubbing of the vulva, tail and buttocks has been recorded in mares,[12] with accompanying signs of pleasure, such as lip quivering, highly suggestive of masturbation.[4]

Scratching

After turning its head and neck to the rear, a horse can use its hindlimbs to scratch parts of the cranial and anterior cervical region. More common in foals than in adults,[16] this response is thought to be retained by more ponies than horses.[12] Indeed some lice-ridden ponies may go on to insert a pastern into the mouth and proceed to mumble on the limb.[23]

Nibbling and licking

The use of the teeth in body care varies from a rhythmic scratching action by the upper incisors, to small bites. While the areas that can be reached by the teeth include the sides and loins (see self-mutilation in Ch. 11) and even the hindlegs

(Fig. 10.4), the forelegs seem to receive especially detailed attention that incorporates considerable licking. This is a means of removing bot eggs from the hairs that effectively facilitates their ingestion. Although licking seldom occurs as part of mutual grooming[12] the licking of a neonate by its dam is probably the most important instance of a horse using its tongue during grooming a conspecific. This can last for 30 minutes and, as well as consolidating the mother-infant bond, it provides tactile stimuli that may have a role in stimulating responses such as standing. Licking by a stallion as part of courtship is a means of tasting rather than grooming.

PEST AVOIDANCE

Flies bite and spread diseases, such as conjunctival infections, and proteins in the saliva of *Culicoides* spp. are the stimuli responsible for the often grotesque self-mutilation of sweet itch (Queensland itch, summer itch, summer eczema). Apart from ill-advised excoriation, horses have developed adaptive behavioral responses to combat pests. For example, in foals, the percutaneous invasion of the third-stage larvae of *Strongyloides westeri* is reported to cause repeated episodes of frenzied behavior lasting about 30 minutes.[24] The energy expended in motor responses such as tail-swishing to reduce irritation of insect origin may be considerable, and movement to areas (such as cooler parts of the home range) that provide respite may therefore be seen as forms of energy conservation.[25] Tabanid flies drive free-ranging Camargue horses to change their time-budgets and their use of their home ranges, apparently in a bid to capitalize on the prevailing winds in key areas.[26] Similarly, Assateague ponies have been noted to use inshore water and snow patches as refuges from tabanids.[25] For horses, insects are not the only airborne pest. Avoidance measures have also been demonstrated in response to the vocalization of vampire bats.[27]

With pliable, mobile skin and extensive subcutaneous muscles, horses are among the best skin-twitching animals. The sensitivity of horse skin, for example, to alighting flies as they stimulate the panniculus response, should serve to remind riders how little pressure is needed for signaling. Riding instructors who find themselves telling their pupils to kick their mounts should consider the lesson they are providing for both rider and horse. While stamping, kicking and shaking of the whole body or head are all employed to dislodge insects, the forelock and the tail can act both as screens and swats in combating fly problems. The effectiveness of mutual tail-swishing as a means of reducing the harm caused by flies is reflected by there being demonstrably fewer bites per horse in animals that live in large groups.[28] Horses frequently swing their heads in the direction of flies on their flanks in a motor pattern similar to an agonistic head threat that occasionally includes a consummative nip at their own skin.[12] Along with pawing, tail-swishing increases with ambient temperature in horses while being prepared for work.[29] Since this effect is not a function of fly numbers, it has been suggested that such comfort behaviors may be useful indicators of irritation in horses, especially where ambient temperatures are high.[29]

The use of other horses' tails in helping to reduce the frustration of flies on the face is established in foalhood as foals frequently rest within the shelter of their dams' swatting tails.[6] The solitary housing of horses denies them this facility and should oblige owners to provide such animals with some form of screen. The importance of the tail in body care is implied by reports of horses with docked tails occasionally using sticks to scratch their sides.[30] Veterinarians who prioritize the welfare of animals in their care recognize the function of the tail as a source of comfort and therefore do not dock horses for cosmetic reasons.

BEHAVIORAL THERMOREGULATION

Horses often surprise owners with their reluctance to use field shelters. This rejection of enclosed space relates to their dislike of confinement and reduced surveillance and visual contact with conspecifics. Having said that, horses are often seen using shaded areas, natural windbreaks, sun-baking and even wading in water to regulate their body temperature. Evaporative heat losses are thought to be increased by the sprinkling effect of tail-swishing while standing in water[31] and by the occasional instances of nose-dunking in water (Fig. 10.5). Thermoregulation is often made difficult by rugs, especially in warm weather when rugs are sometimes used to prevent sun-bleaching. Discomfort caused by overheating, skin disorders and generally badly fitted rugs may prompt some horses to become rug chewers. Other horses, especially youngsters, may adopt this response as a form of object play.

REST AND SLEEP

Fraser[32] identifies four resting states: idling, resting, drowsing and sleeping. He also gives a detailed account of pandiculation (stretching) elsewhere.[33]

Idling is adopted as a passive waiting style between more animated activities and involves stationary standing with some limb-shifting and positional changes. It can occur as a group activity, in contrast to recumbent sleep, which is rarely undertaken by all the members of a group at one time.[33] Seasonal peaks in resting behaviors occur in the summer[4] when forage is relatively plentiful and there is pressure to seek shade and avoid

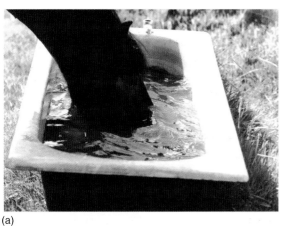 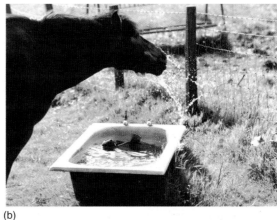

(a)   (b)

Figure 10.5   In an apparent attempt to refresh themselves, horses will occasionally dunk their noses in water. (Photographs courtesy of Francis Burton.)

insects. Common sites are usually selected for lying, a behavioral mechanism thought to help produce a group odor.[1] Elevated sites are often selected since they provide refuge from heat and flies.[34] Resting occurs in the standing or recumbent position and in the wakeful periods between sleep and drowsing. Generally, light horses spend less time standing to rest than draft mares.[35] Drowsing and sleep are discussed below.

DROWSING

A drowsing horse stands with its eyelids partly opened and its head hanging at a medium height (Fig. 10.6). The flexion of a single hindlimb is facilitated by the reciprocal apparatus in the hindlimb, which means that movements of the stifle joint drive those of the hock.[36] Thus, once the stifle is fixed in position, the hock is obliged to follow suit. In combination with the stay apparatus found in the forelimb as a means of supporting the fetlock, this allows the horse to remain upright with a minimum of muscular effort. The advantages of remaining standing include the ability to achieve a quick escape if threatened, but also avoidance of the cardiorespiratory compromise that comes with recumbency. Interestingly, the adoption of certain postures for rest has been shown to have familial tendencies.[37]

SLEEP

The distinction between drowsing and sleep necessitates an understanding of the different physiological characteristics of various states of wakefulness. In adult horses, sleep occupies 3–5 hours per day, while drowsing consumes a further 2.[38]

Postural changes tend to accompany certain states – for example, although the eyes remain partly open, the head gradually descends as the horse goes from drowsing to sleep.[34] Animals may rest without sleeping and while the distinction between drowsiness and sleep is reasonably subtle, since they may appear very similar externally, electrophysiological studies of animals in various stages of sensitivity to their environment have helped to unpick the differences. Although such measurements require some restraint of the subjects, we can assume that the same differences apply in unrestrained horses. Using data extrapolated from restrained subjects, inferences can be made from the posture of horses indulging in various rest behaviors.

The two types of sleep clearly defined in horses are slow-wave sleep (SWS) and rapid eye movement (REM) sleep (also known as deep or paradoxical sleep).[38] The electroencephalogram (EEG) waves of SWS, as the name suggests, are characterized by a low frequency, a feature that disappears as the horse drifts into REM sleep.

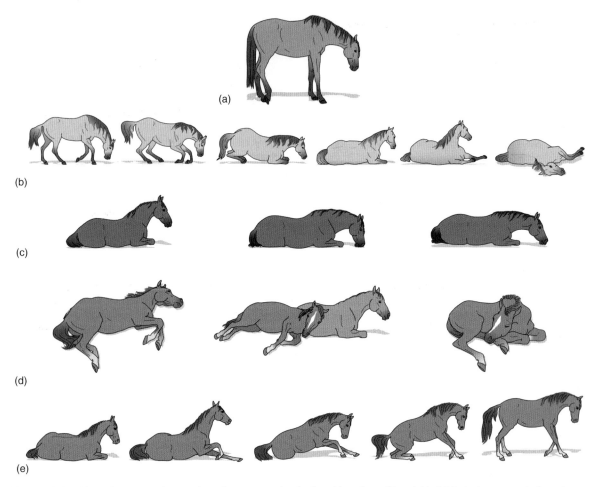

Figure 10.6 A horse's posture changes in various states of activation: (a) resting with weight distributed among only three legs; (b) lying down; (c) recumbent resting attitudes; (d) arising. (Redrawn, with permission, from Waring.[12])

Some muscular tone is retained in SWS, even when the head is resting on the ground during sternal recumbency. It is the only form of sleep that occurs in standing horses. Although it may increase in horses that are unable or reluctant to lie down, SWS cannot compensate for lost REM. This is illustrated by post-inhibitory rebound in REM sleep after periods without recumbency.[38] Along with the suggestion that horses do not lie down unless they are confident about their surroundings,[33,38] this accounts for some of the concerns for the welfare of horses that do not or cannot lie down.[39]

REM sleep was dubbed paradoxical because, while its EEG is similar to that of wakefulness (Fig. 10.7a), it has the highest arousal threshold. Cardiac and respiratory rates decrease in all forms of sleep.[40] REM sleep is peculiar in that it involves the absence of postural tone (and therefore the eyes are shut). It occurs entirely during recumbency and is marked by the greatest degree of variability in cardiac and respiratory frequencies of any state, including wakefulness. As its name implies, REM sleep is also often accompanied by rapid eye movements. During REM sleep during lateral recumbency, limb movements, especially of the upper limbs, may occur.[12]

In studies of adult horses, REM sleep has not been observed to occur without a preceding period of SWS, and this gives rise to the term

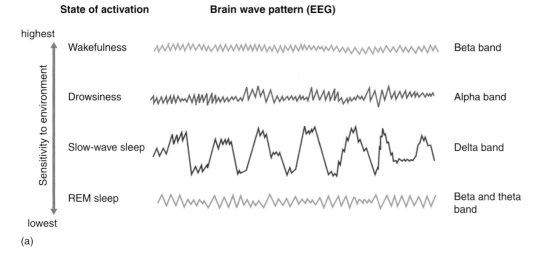

State of activation

Brain wave pattern (EEG)

highest

Wakefulness — Beta band

Drowsiness — Alpha band

Slow-wave sleep — Delta band

REM sleep — Beta and theta band

lowest

Sensitivity to environment

(a)

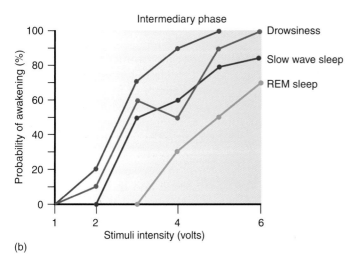

Intermediary phase

Drowsiness

Slow wave sleep

REM sleep

Probability of awakening (%)

Stimuli intensity (volts)

(b)

Figure 10.7 (a) Brain wave patterns vary in amplitude and frequency in various states of activation in mammals. (After Dallaire.[38]). (b) Variations in arousal threshold from drowsiness to REM sleep. (After Dallaire.[38])

'sleep cycle' (SC). Horses, like most non-primates, are polyphasic sleepers in that they sleep in more than one phase throughout the 24-hour period, with one or more SCs occurring in each phase. During the night, horses have about six sleep phases within which the mean duration of sleep cycles is 15 minutes and the mean duration of SWS and REM sleep they contain are 6.4 and 4.2 minutes, respectively.[38] The balance comprises drowsing within a sleep cycle and a third type of sleep labeled the intermediary phase.[38] Although it has an EEG pattern similar to that of drowsiness, intermediary sleep is characterized by an arousal threshold closer to that of wakefulness than that of drowsing (Fig. 10.7b).[38] Found in almost 30% of SCs, the intermediary phase may provide a protective punctuation of sleep that helps to prompt extra surveillance before deep sleep.[38]

Time spent lying increases in horses when they are exercised,[41] and good deep bedding may therefore help to keep performance horses in peak condition by facilitating adequate rest. While the mean time spent in continuous sternal recumbency is 23 minutes,[33] twice as much time is generally spent in lateral recumbency. In sternal

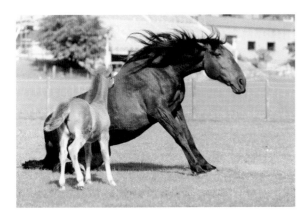

Figure 10.8 The main muscular effort used in standing after a period of recumbency comes from the hindquarters. (Photograph courtesy of Francis Burton.)

recumbency horses lie asymmetrically with their hindquarters rotated so that the lateral aspect of the lower limb is on the ground. Rising from this position, once the upper foreleg has been extended, is achieved chiefly by a thrust from the hindquarters (Fig. 10.8).[33] In lateral recumbency the importance of the upper limb in rising quickly is demonstrable in that it is almost always anterior to the lower limb, which is usually flexed to some extent.[33] As with rolling, it seems probable that horses demonstrate laterality in their preferred side for recumbency.

The timing of sleep is important, since management schedules sometimes interfere with innate rhythms that facilitate sleep. Although most sleep occurs between 2000 and 0500 hours, horses also often sleep in the first 2 hours after midday.[38] It is therefore good practice to keep activity in a stable yard to a minimum during the early afternoon.[33]

The restorative functions of sleep have been compartmentalized by Dallaire,[38] who proposes that during SWS sleep the brain is resting, whereas during REM sleep the absence of muscle tone suggests that the muscles are resting. Fraser[33] proposes that during REM sleep the brain consolidates long-term memory traces and the forebrain is functionally disconnected so that the brainstem must be responsible for any accompanying limb movements.

The effect of environment

While domestic horses tend to rest in sheltered areas, Przewalski horses when released into extensive enclosures have been noted to rest in the highest parts of the available terrain.[42]

Horses at pasture show slightly less total sleep and more drowsiness than those kept in separate stalls (Fig. 10.9).[38] Drowsing at pasture studied in a small number of ponies occurred only while they were standing. These data may suggest that the external environment may require the deployment of more surveillance than the stable. However, a similar trend toward an increase in the proportion of SWS is reported in sensory-deprivation studies on ponies, which implies that a barren environment may be sufficient to modify sleep patterns, regardless of any concurrent perception of security.[43]

The weather may also influence rest behavior. For example, in especially hot weather, perhaps because of the prevalence of flies and the resultant need for mutual tail-swishing, horses may rest only in the standing position.[44] The standing position is also favored for rest during the colder months of the year,[45] perhaps because it involves less heat loss through convection. Daylength, via the action of serotonin and thus melatonin, can influence sleep patterns, and it is reported that tryptophan, a precursor of serotonin, may be used clinically to induce sleep.[33]

The effect of rank and group size

Resting postures are subject to individual preferences.[38] However, the standing position is adopted for rest preferentially by adult mares more than males or youngsters.[45] Among adults, the highest-ranking member of a band is often the first to lie down.[46] Furthermore, it is believed that the effects of a novel environment in making horses that are unfamiliar with an enclosure reluctant to lie down may be diluted if a resident horse is present to offer an example.[38] There are data suggesting that as group size rises within a population, time spent resting in the standing position increases at the expense of time spent in recumbency (Fig. 10.10).[45]

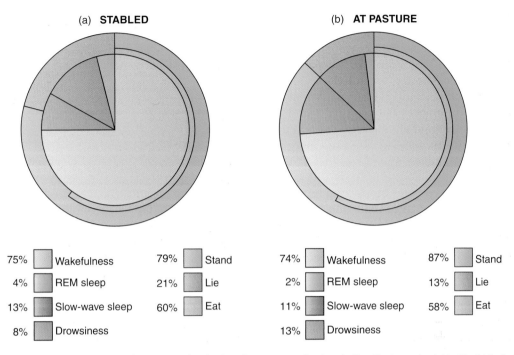

(a) **STABLED** (b) **AT PASTURE**

75%	Wakefulness	79%	Stand
4%	REM sleep	21%	Lie
13%	Slow-wave sleep	60%	Eat
8%	Drowsiness		

74%	Wakefulness	87%	Stand
2%	REM sleep	13%	Lie
11%	Slow-wave sleep	58%	Eat
13%	Drowsiness		

Figure 10.9 The distribution of the four states of activation change according to whether the horse is stabled individually (n = 5) or kept at pasture (n = 2).

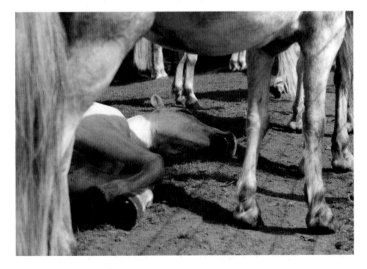

Figure 10.10 A horse lying in lateral recumbency close to standing companions. Horses may have a heightened sense of security in a group, but recumbency is unlikely to occur as a group activity. (Photograph courtesy of Francis Burton.)

The effect of age

Compared with adults, foals have a greater need for sleep and are less capricious about recumbency, so they often rest in groups.[33] Both SWS and REM sleep occur in foals, but their proportions differ.[6] With their mothers nearby, newborn foals spend about a third of their time recumbent. When they lie in lateral recumbency, they enter REM sleep and their limbs may move as if running.[6] It may be that learning is consolidated during these periods.[47] It has been suggested that because it is associated with a reluctance to lie down and therefore may jeopardize sleep patterns and possibly even learning, extended episodes of road transit could be highly undesirable for foals.[6]

Interesting differences between colts and fillies in the amount and characteristics of recumbent rest in the first week of life are emerging. Fillies have been noted spending 42% of their time in recumbent rest while for colts this is only 20%. Furthermore colts rested upright more and stood more (20% and 28%) than fillies (4% and 23%, respectively) (Machteld van Dierendonck, personal communication 2002). After a peak of the daily time budget spent in recumbency that occurs in the first week of life,[48] the need for rest declines as a foal matures, with a striking shift occurring at about 3 months of age (Fig. 10.11).

At this time, foals generally become more social with their conspecifics and especially their peers, if any are present.[4] Because of their attachment to their dams, who must graze for extended periods to meet the nutritional demands of lactation, foals do most of their resting in lawn areas.[18] They are more likely to rest either upright or recumbent if the dam is resting upright.[48] Foals spend only 3.5% of their time resting upright in the first week of life but, as time spent recumbent falls, this steadily increases to a peak of 23% in week 13.[48] Meanwhile, nursing mares reach a peak of 32.5% of their time resting upright in week 13 post-partum.[48]

PLAY

Activities involving a sense of pleasure and elements of surprise but apparently no immediate function are broadly characterized as play.[49] The benefits of play (apparent or otherwise) must outweigh the costs in terms of energy and associated risks.[50] One of the immediate rewards of play may well be pleasure, but this is difficult to study. Often initiated by grooming bouts and oral snapping actions, play may establish or strengthen social bonds within a pair or a group.[51] The value of play is illustrated by the way in which bachelor groups can draw colt foals towards them, with the opportunity to play appearing to be the chief attractant.

Most of the galloping and fast twists and turns used in anti-predator behavior are incorporated into play activities by foals. Sexually dimorphic play-fighting preferences reflect adult agonistic responses, with fillies tending to fight by kicking with their hindlegs as a mare does, while colts prefer to rear, bite and chase each other.[11] By practicing these actions before they are required in a serious situation, the foal develops its neuromuscular pathways, the activity becomes learned and so may be executed when needed with ease or flair. Play promotes and regulates developmental rates and therefore contributes to the development of physical strength, endurance and skill.[51]

Fraser[33] argues that the urge to play is derived from a basic need to have optimal blood flow to the muscles. This may provide a mechanism to explain post-inhibitory rebound in locomotory responses after confinement.[15,39] Other than its physiological functions, play may be a form of training that offers problem-solving opportunities and experience that can yield specific information. This is likely to give young animals tactical and behavioral flexibility to fight, find mates and escape predators as adults.[50] Play in

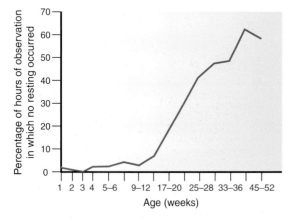

Figure 10.11 The changing percentage of daylight hours that New Forest foals *do not* spend resting. (After Tyler.[4] Redrawn, with permission, from Waring.[12])

adult horses, which usually takes the form of object or locomotory play,[6] may be a luxury afforded by domestic circumstances and occur as evidence of post-inhibitory rebound or a response to lack of stimulation at other times.

Play is greatly reduced during periods of extreme ambient temperatures, food scarcity, and other occasions of physiological or psychological stress.[12] While animals that have not had their basic food and water requirements met do not play, a low play drive can also be indicative of ill health or poor nutrition. The range of play behaviors may also be limited by a dearth of playmates.

Prospective studies may demonstrate links between features of play and neuromuscular development, social rank and competitive performance. Rees[52] suggests that a horse's personality as manifested by its mannerisms during play, may be an indication of what to expect when the same horse is under saddle, especially when presented with an unfamiliar or unsettling situation. Indeed, Fraser[33] pursues this idea by advocating that we examine horses' personalities before assigning their work, or that we even attempt to create play responses in work situations because, he proposes, this will maximize the horse's willingness to complete the task. For example, a horse that often displays flamboyant paces when playing may experience a play response to the challenges of dressage.[33] This is supported by studies of play responses of 698 horses (representing 16 breeds and 13 types) that showed type, rather than breed or gender, was the major influence on free operant responses.[53]

Playfulness may affect the human-horse bond. For example, Fraser[33] endeavored to explain most equestrian pursuits in terms of game theory,[54] suggesting that horses learned rules of games when they were being schooled. However, the validity of this approach has been questioned by those who propose that equestrian activities such as jumping easily-avoided obstacles or moving repeatedly in circles must appear rather pointless to the equids involved.[52,55]

Play can be considered under three broad divisions: locomotory play, interactive play and manipulative play.

LOCOMOTORY PLAY

Locomotory play begins within a few hours after birth and takes the form of exaggerated or vigorous physical activity, with the foal moving in circles close to the dam, and exhibiting actions such as spinning, and kicking.[32] Other labels used to describe locomotory play include frolic, run, chase, buck, jump, leap and prance.[13] Solitary running and bucking is noted more frequently in fillies than in colts.[56] The lengths of locomotory play bouts can be related to the increasing courage of the foal as it gradually moves farther away from the dam. Williams[57] notes that locomotory play often seems unfinished, since it is often ended by some form of distraction, such as spotting a shadow. Rather than being unconsummated, bouts of locomotory play may end this way for sound reasons that currently elude us. All age groups of domestic horses will indulge in this form of play without conspecific company.[6]

INTERACTIVE PLAY

If opportunities are available, interactive play occurs among horses of various ages (Fig. 10.12) and its nature seems to depend on the age of the participants. Characterized by repeated physical

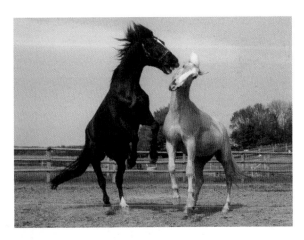

Figure 10.12 Play fighting is recognized among adult companions as they become familiar with one another, especially in bachelor groups. (Photograph courtesy of Francis Burton.)

contact between participants, it often mimics combat between harem stallions but lacks the characteristic vocalizations, persistent ear-pinning and heightened risk of injury.[6] It is possible to subdivide interactive play as play fighting and play sexual behavior,[13] but in the current text interactive play is considered in the light of the partners involved. Play partners can be adult horses or other foals.

Play between foals and adult horses

During the month of dependence[6] the focal point of the foal's life is its dam. In the first week of life the foal will spend 56% of its time by itself or with its mother.[4] She allows it to play on or around her, showing considerable tolerance (Fig. 10.13). Types of play behaviors include nibbling and chewing the mane and tail of the mare, biting and bumping her legs and sides, and attempting to climb over or jump the mare when she is lying down.[6] At first this play is rough and there is little the mare can do other than tolerate it. But after 2 weeks or so, as the foal becomes more gentle, his dam will have the opportunity to teach him the benefits of mutual grooming.[52] Play between the mare and her foal decreases as the foal spends an increasing amount of time with its peers. Although time spent playing does not differ between fillies and colts, the types of games and, therefore, the energy consumption do.[56] For example, interactive play bouts of colts are longer than those of fillies.[56]

Play between foals and a mare other than their mother is rare. Mares will often threaten foals that are not their own, while young and barren mares may show more tolerance. Colts engage in this form of interaction more often than fillies.[56] Snapping is usually exhibited before and during these interactions, especially when the adult is a stallion.[32] Free-ranging stallions allow foals (again, more commonly colts than fillies[4]) to investigate or play with them and are generally careful in their treatment of youngsters, often withdrawing from play fights rather than responding agonistically.[4] This gentle attitude may continue to be displayed until the foals reach puberty, at which point they often begin to be treated as competition, if male, or with relative indifference, if female. Kiley-Worthington[1] notes that the stallion may ultimately eject both colts and fillies from the natal band, but more common causes of natal dispersal are considered in Chapter 5.

Play among foals

A neonatal foal's social interactions with other foals gradually increase in frequency so that at 3–4 weeks of age the average number of solitary play bouts matches the average number of bouts of social play (Fig. 10.14).[4]

Invitations to play often begin with staring, tentative sniffing and head-tossing approaches that initially amount to no more than the touching of muzzles followed by galloping retreats

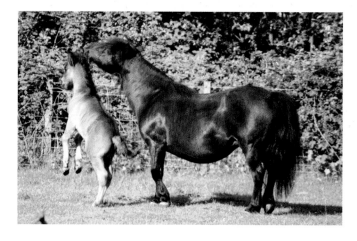

Figure 10.13 Pony foal playing with its dam. (Photograph courtesy of Francis Burton.)

and flamboyant bucking (Fig. 10.15).[32] Colts are more proactive than fillies in using these invitations to initiate play with their peers.[35]

Possibly because they often get variable responses from adults other than their dams, foals tend to associate more often with other foals.[58] Foals tend to affiliate and play with one other foal regularly (Fig. 10.16). The nature of the play within these dyads differs according to the sex of the combination, most notably after the first month of life. Tyler[4] indicates that 50% of play involves a colt and a filly, 34% involves two colts and 16% involves two fillies. In the first 8 weeks of life, colts are generally more active and graze less than fillies.[59] Colts attempt to mount their peers or, for that matter, their dam about seven times more often than do fillies,[4] who are seldom seen mounting after the first month.[12] The peak of mounting by all foals coincides with the foal heat. Mounting by foals is tolerated by mares and stallions alike.[56]

The pair-bonds that form between fillies may be lifelong.[1] While pairs of fillies engage in locomotory play and mutual grooming,[52] mock fights are more prevalent and indeed rougher among pairs of colts. Mock fighting includes inhibited biting on the head and neck of the opponent and attempting to unbalance the opponent by

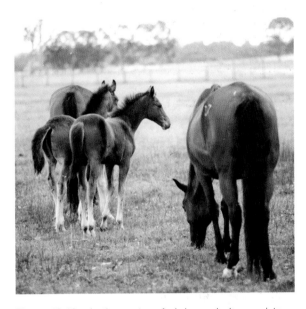

Figure 10.16 As they mature, foals increasingly associate with other foals. (Photograph courtesy of Michael Jervis-Chaston.)

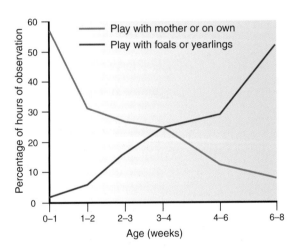

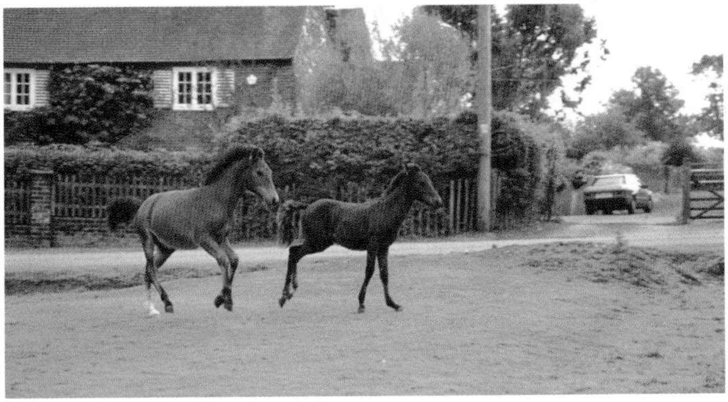

Figure 10.14 The changing complexion of play with age over the first 8 weeks of the foal's life. (After Tyler.[4] Redrawn, with permission, from Waring.[12])

Figure 10.15 Locomotory play is commonly seen among foals.

pushing against him. Interactive play of this sort may be regularly interrupted by bouts of mutual grooming,[12] occasional mounting[6] and regular flehmen-like responses.[60] It has been suggested that mock fights end with the subordinate player offering a final rear that prompts the higher-ranking player to give chase.[9] Mock fighting also occurs in mixed-sex pairs but it is readily curtailed by outright aggression on the part of the filly if it becomes too rough.[6] It is likely that play between sexes is the natural forum in which colts learn about tactful courtship.[6] Colts that have bonded with colts rather than fillies will sometimes approach fillies, apparently for mutual grooming.[12] Occasionally, the colt will begin to nibble a filly's hindquarters and sometimes then attempt to mount her. This usually elicits aggression from the filly.

MANIPULATIVE PLAY

Manipulative play involves nosing, sniffing, licking, nibbling or biting at objects, from stones and sticks to the manes and tails of other horses, and may progress to pulling, lifting, carrying or apparent attempts at throwing.[6] The feet may also be used in manipulation, e.g. when pawing at water or kicking at an object on the ground. Object play seen in foals[56] often follows a repetitive pattern of advancing upon and retreating from the object, with the integration of some locomotory activity. So objects, including other horses, may be the focus of locomotory play as foals circle them and run to and from them.[13]

It has been suggested that, in the absence of conspecifics, the provision of objects to foals isolated at the time of weaning may improve their welfare.[61] Paddocks give weanlings the opportunity to play, and this may help to explain why they are associated with more normal time-budgeting than stables.[62] In their relative isolation, stabled horses often learn to occupy themselves by manipulating objects in their restricted environment. Water, haynets, chains and bedding provide serviceable playthings.[52] Nipping and nibbling are classic play actions, and horses often chew at wooden rails when confined and on lead ropes when tied-up. Through manipulative play, some horses learn

self-reinforcing responses, such as opening stable doors (see Fig. 1.10) and untying themselves.

The social environment of foals influences object play in that foals without peers tend to manipulate objects for longer than socially kept foals.[63] Kiley-Worthington[1] proposes that horses deprived of visual contact with conspecifics may interact with items in their stable to make noise in a bid to keep in touch with others. When owners provide horses with stable toys, they should bear in mind that there is little or no research to confirm their effectiveness in enriching the environment, that the novelty value of such devices can rapidly dwindle and that horses require several toys that can be alternated.[55]

BEHAVIORAL ANOMALIES IN MAINTENANCE BEHAVIOR

UNMANAGEABLE PLAY

Owners sometimes complain about behaviors that, while emerging from a motivation to play and perform vigorous exercise, are nonetheless dangerous. While examples in ridden horses include bucking and pulling at the gallop, similar problems on the ground include pulling away at the time of turn-out, and rearing in hand. Horses that are fed too much grain are prime candidates for exuberant locomotory displays. This trend is compounded by their being the horses that generally spend most of the day confined. Fortunately, the managers of stable yards in which play gets out of hand are beginning to appreciate the need for relatively more forage in diets and the provision of a recreation area for affiliated inmates.

It is important to remember the role of learning in these responses. Very often they appear in experimental situations and are allowed to be reinforced. For this reason, thoughtful riders never allow horses to begin to find rewards in pulling but instead respond to playful bucking by reducing the pace and returning to the spot where the buck occurred in a bid to show the horse that it is not effective as a means of progress. Horses that are allowed to pull under saddle rapidly habituate to bit pressure and soon become horses that can bolt. This is one of the reasons some racehorses are difficult to re-educate as safe riding animals for leisure. Therefore, the racing industry should recognize that heavy hands make horses lean on the bit, and are responsible for considerable wastage. Grading-up to a more severe bit is a very short-term solution to the problem, which lies not so much in the horse's mouth as at the other end of the rein. With consistency at its core, retraining as discussed in Chapter 13 is the best means of preventing the escalation of battles between horse and rider.

Interactive play under saddle can cause horses to use agonistic responses when jostling for position as they begin vigorous exercise – for example, at a place in a familiar route that has become associated with faster gaits. The danger here is that because communication between such horses is compromised by human intervention, injuries to both horses and riders may occur. The safest approach to this contingency is to keep ridden horses at least one body length apart and to keep higher-ranking horses that may be more likely to kick if they are inadvertently challenged, at the back of the group.

Because they are impressionable and can quickly find reinforcement in locomotory play, youngsters should always be handled by experienced personnel. Prevention of inappropriate responses not only involves elimination of inappropriate learning opportunities, but also the institution of a routine in husbandry techniques. For example, prior to turn-out, it is excellent practice to turn all horses round to face the gateway through which they have just passed. With this routine in place, youngsters learn that they must change direction before being released and this has a tempering effect on the speed with which they pass through the gateway, and older horses, which may kick out simply as a form of post-inhibitory rebound after confinement, are always released facing in a direction that is safe for personnel.

REFUSAL TO LIE DOWN

While a horse that shows increased resting should be examined for other evidence of illness,[33] less recumbency than normal is also a cause for concern. Refusal to lie down has been listed among 'vices and bad habits'.[64] It was unwelcome because it was often associated with a lack of musculoskeletal rest, and a resultant abbreviation of the horse's working life. The popularity of standing stalls may have contributed to the prevalence of this complaint. When 16 mares were confined in standing stalls for 6 months, 9 were not observed in recumbency on videotapes that recorded each horse for 24 hours every week, suggesting that horses with no previous experience of such confinement may be reluctant to lie down.[39] Thirteen of the mares dropped to their knees at least once during the 6-month observation period, a response attributed to their being in REM sleep while standing.[39] (Readers are directed to Ch. 3 for a consideration of narcolepsy.)

Although horses spend 90% of their time standing and when they lie for longer than is typical there may be a welfare problem,[62] it is important that provision be made for them to lie down whenever they wish.[65] While reluctance to rise is associated with musculoskeletal disorders and most commonly lower limb pain (most notably laminitis),[12] reluctance to lie down may occur through:

- neophobia, for example, in a new stable
- confinement and perhaps fear of becoming trapped in a particularly small stable
- inappropriate substrate, for example, lack of bedding for a stabled horse or lack of dry surfaces for a horse at pasture
- pain – for example, an arthritic horse may be disinclined to lie down because lying down and, more especially, standing up may be associated with pain.[33] Pain is also the reason for horses showing reluctance to lie down as a feature of peritonitis and purpura haemorrhagica.[12]

INAPPROPRIATE RESPONSES TO BEING GROOMED

While some horses enjoy being groomed to the extent that they attempt to return the favor and in so doing inadvertently hurt, or more frequently alarm, their grooms, others find the intervention ticklish, distressing or even painful.

Hand-reared foals and single foals that attract the status of pets are more likely to regard humans as suitable mutual grooming partners. Key trigger spots are the part of the neck and withers in which foals find grooming most gratifying (for physiological reasons discussed in Ch. 2). The unwelcome consequences of early learning of this sort should be considered before misguided personnel are permitted to indulge a foal's attempts to reciprocate. Occasionally, owners actively encourage this form of bonding in juvenile and mature horses, despite horses having powerful jaws that can cause inadvertent damage to human skin[52] (Fig. 10.17) but the majority find it inappropriate and seek to eliminate the response. Direct punishment by hitting the muzzle is inadvisable, since it frequently makes the recipient head-shy. To shape the behavior more appropriately handlers should apply negative punishment by stopping the reinforcing stimulation of these premium areas when the horse turns its head toward them. The horse quickly learns

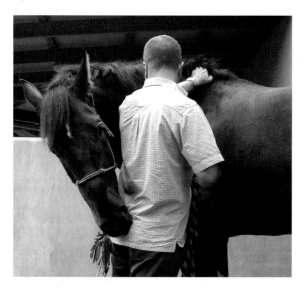

Figure 10.17 Mutual grooming between horse and human. When they have their withers scratched, many horses will attempt to reciprocate as a form of mutual grooming. In most cases this is discouraged because people are fearful of being bitten. (Photograph courtesy of Sandro Nocentini.)

that to receive more of the preferred attention it must face away from the groomer.

Breed and individual differences in the sensitivity of the skin through different parts of the body should be accommodated by the selection of brushes and modification of the brushing technique so that minimal reaction is evoked.[1] The alternative to this considerate, adaptive approach is to simply persist in tickling and annoying the horse, which is likely to signal its frustration with tail-swishing. If this signal is ignored, the behavior may mature to kick threats and eventually kicks. This effectively lowers the horse's threshold to kick and makes it generally more dangerous to be around. Since sensitivity, especially in the groin, is innate, it requires extensive innocuous stimulation before any habituation occurs and, moreover, it is a feature likely to return after a period without stimulation.

Sensitivity in the girth region has been considered part of the so-called cold-back syndrome, an abiding equine enigma that seems related more to somatic pain than wilful disobedience or a desire to avoid work. While it is certainly possible to modify aspects of the evasive strategies learned by horses that seem to suffer such pain, therapy should focus on controlling or eliminating the pain.

Many horses find some husbandry techniques, such as tail and mane pulling, distressing. The repeated use of the twitch to accomplish routine procedures in such horses does nothing to reduce their anticipation of the distress caused by the intervention and, indeed, handling is often made yet more difficult when the horse learns to evade the twitch. Instead of struggling intermittently with a distressed animal and teaching it to struggle more the next time, or waiting for learned helplessness to occur, stable managers aiming for long-term success gradually combine small tolerable exposure to stimuli associated with the procedure before the arrival of meals as the first step in a counter-conditioning program.[66]

Another management technique that can present problems is the trimming of ear hair. Ear hair is something that some humans find unacceptable. Its function seems related to the prevention of foreign bodies and therefore its removal is difficult to justify for purely esthetic reasons. Occasionally a build-up of wax on the aural hair can be removed with the judicious use of scissors, but the pulling of such hair is inhumane and the proximate pain involved has the potential to teach the recipient of such attention to be head-shy after remarkably few lessons.

SUMMARY OF KEY POINTS

- Grooming plays a major role in maintaining health.
- Stabling can compromise a horse's ability to perform many normal maintenance responses.
- Mutual grooming facilitates social bonds.
- The quantity and quality of sleep can be influenced by age, rank, group size, diet and environmental stimuli.
- Prior to 1 month of age, play is more likely to be solitary or with the mother.
- After 1 month of age, play is more likely to be with peers.
- Play is important in physical and social development.

CASE STUDY

A 12-year-old Thoroughbred mare had learned to nip her owner when having her girth tightened and to do so very deftly and with little warning. She had learned to get her head out of the way very quickly to avoid punishment but at the same time she was becoming tense and rather head-shy during this part of the tacking-up process.

Before the mare's behavior could be modified the eliciting causes were investigated. The mare was highly reactive to palpation in the girth region. The unusual sensitivity and muscular guarding was ameliorated only slightly by a short course of non-steroidal anti-inflammatory drugs, and the hyper-reactivity of the girth region was considered to be a chronic condition that could be managed (in conjunction with the use of long-term analgesics) rather than cured. Management of the condition involved the purchase of some new saddlery and the institution of a novel girthing routine:

- The saddle was re-fitted so that it gave a great deal of clearance over the withers.
- The existing girth was replaced with a sheepskin-covered cushioned girth with 10–15 cm of elastic at either end.

To overcome the context-specific elements in the mare's response, she was moved to a new part of the yard at the start of the new routine. Palpation of the pectoral region and the thoracic region medial to the elbows was conducted in conjunction with counter-conditioning. If the mare kept looking forward and did not swing her head when touched in these areas she was rewarded with scratching of the lower neck and withers or premium food items.

It was important to implement control of the head movements with consistent commands from the handler. Using the pressure-release system detailed in Chapter 13, the head was turned by pressure on the head-collar to teach the mare that it was appropriate to turn on command. She was rewarded for these turns with rubbing on the forehead and then the head was manually turned back, followed by more rewarding. This palpation program was applied twice daily for 1 week before any girthing.

In a bid to break down learning from previous episodes, the girth was fastened from the off-side. The horse was led around the yard three or four times before the forelegs were stretched to smooth the skin under the girth and were held in the stretched position for 30 seconds before being returned to the ground. In addition to mounting from each side, mounting from a block or some other support became obligatory regardless of the weight of the rider. Once mounted, the rider gradually tightened the girth with one hand while scratching the lower neck and withers with the other.

Two months after presentation, the biting had stopped completely. The mare could best be described as tolerant of the girth. The search for a more substantial cure for her primary girth pain continues.

REFERENCES

1. Kiley-Worthington M. The behaviour of horses: in relation to management and training. London: JA Allen; 1987.
2. Feh C, de Mazieres J. Grooming at a preferred site reduces heart rates in horses. Anim Behav 1993; 46:1191–1194.
3. Normando S, Haverbeke A, Meers L, et al. Heart rate reduction by grooming in horses (Equus caballus).

Havemeyer Workshop on Horse Behaviour and Welfare, Holar, Iceland, 2002:23–25.

4. Tyler SJ. The behaviour and social organization of the New Forest ponies. Anim Behav Monogr 1972; 5:85–196.

5. Blakeslee JK. Mother-young relationships and related behavior among free-ranging Appaloosa horse. Thesis, Idaho State University, Pocatello, 1974.

6. Crowell-Davis SL. Developmental behavior. Vet Clin North Am Equine Pract: Behav 1986; 573–590.

7. Feist JD, McCullough DR. Behaviour patterns and communication in feral horses. Z Tierpsychol 1976; 41:337–371.

8. Houpt KA. Equine maintenance behavior: feeding, drinking, coat care and behavioral thermoregulation. Havemeyer Workshop on Horse Behaviour and Welfare, Holar, Iceland 2002; 92–95.

9. Wells SM, von Goldschmidt-Rothschild B. Social behaviour and relationships in a herd of Camargue horses. Z Tierpsychol 1979; 49:363–380.

10. Clutton-Brock TH, Greenwood PJ, Powell RP. Rank and relationships in Highland ponies and Highland cows. Z Tierpsychol 1976; 41:202–216.

11. Feh C. Relationships and communication in socially natural horse herds. Havemeyer Workshop on Horse Behaviour and Welfare, Holar, Iceland 2002; 84–91.

12. Waring GH. Horse behavior: the behavioral traits and adaptations of domestic and wild horses including ponies. Park Ridge, NJ: Noyes; 1983.

13. McDonnell SM, Poulin A. Equid play ethogram. Appl Anim Behav Sci 2001; 78 (2–4):263–295.

14. Keiper RR, Keenan MA. Nocturnal activity patterns of feral ponies. J Mammal 1980; 61:116–118.

15. Christensen JW, Ladewig J, Sondergaard E, Malmkvist J. Effects of individual versus group stabling on social behaviour in domestic stallions. Appl Anim Behav Sci 2002; 75(3):233–248.

16. Crowell-Davis SL. Self-grooming by mares and foals of the Welsh pony (Equus caballus). Appl Anim Behav Sci 1987; 17(3/4):197–208.

17. Fuller Z, Cox JE, Argo CM. Photoperiodic entrainment of seasonal changes in the appetite, feeding behaviour, growth rate and pelage of pony colts. Anim Sci 2001; 72(1):65–74.

18. Ödberg FO, Francis-Smith K. A study on eliminative and grazing behaviour–the use of the field by captive horses. Equine Vet J 1976; 8(4):147–149.

19. Saslow CA. Understanding the perceptual world of horses. Appl Anim Behav Sci 2002; 78 (2–4): 209–224.

20. Clarke AF. Stables. In: Wathes CM, Charles DR, eds. Livestock housing. Wallingford, Oxon: CAB International; 1994:379–403.

21. McGreevy PD, Cripps PJ, French NP, et al. Management factors associated with stereotypic and redirected behaviour in the Thoroughbred horse. Equine Vet J 1995a; 27:86–91.

22. Mills DS, Eckley S, Cooper JJ. Thoroughbred bedding preferences, associated behaviour differences and their implications for equine welfare. Anim Sci 2000; 70(1): 95–106.

23. McGreevy PD. Why does my horse …? London: Souvenir Press; 1996.

24. Dewes HF. The association between weather, frenzied behaviour, percutaneous invasion by Strongyloides westeri larvae and Rhodococcus equi disease in foals. NZ Vet J 1989; 37(2):69–73.

25. Keiper RR, Berger J. Refuge-seeking and pest avoidance by feral horses in desert and island environments. Appl Animal Ethol 1982; 9(2):111–120.

26. Hughes CF, Goodwin D, Harris PA, Davidson HPB. The effect of social environment on the development of object play in the domestic horse foals. Havemeyer Workshop on Horse Behaviour and Welfare, Holar, Iceland, 2002:21–22.

27. Delpietro HA. Case reports of defensive behaviour in equine and bovine subjects in response to vocalisation of the common vampire bat (Desmodus rotundus). Appl Anim Behav Sci 1989; 22(3–4):377–380.

28. Duncan P, Vigne N. The effect of group size in horses on the rate of attacks by blood-sucking flies. Biol Behav 1979; 5:55–60.

29. Kasper M, Beck AM. Effect of environmental temperature on the behaviour of Clydesdales during preparation time before athletic performances. Equine Pract 1997; 19:25–28.

30. Lawick-Goodall JV. Tool-using in primates and other vertebrates. In: Lehrman DS, Hinde RA, Shaw E, eds. Adv Study Behav 1970; 3:195–250.

31. Boyd L, Keiper R. Behavioral ecology of feral horses. Havemeyer Workshop on Horse Behaviour and Welfare, Holar, Iceland, 2002:70–73.

32. Fraser AF. Curious idling. Appl Animal Ethol 1983; 10:159–164.

33. Fraser AF. The behaviour of the horse. Wallingford, Oxon: CAB International; 1992.

34. King SRB. Home range and habitat use of free-ranging Przewalski horses at Hustai National Park, Mongolia. Appl Anim Behav Sci 2002; 78(2–4):103–113.

35. Flannigan G, Stookey JM. Day-time time budgets of pregnant mares housed in tie stalls: a comparison of draft versus light mares. Appl Anim Behav Sci 2002; 78(2–4):125–143.

36. van Weeren PR, Jansen MO, ven den Bogert AJ, Barneveld A. A kinematic and strain gauge study of the reciprocal apparatus in the equine hindlimb. J Biomech 1992; 25:1291–1301.

37. Wolff A, Hausberger M. Behaviour of foals before weaning may have some genetic basis. Ethology 1994; 96(1):1–10.

38. Dallaire A. Rest behavior. Vet Clin North Am Equine Pract: Behav 1986; 591–607.

39. Houpt KA, Houpt TR, Johnson JL, et al. The effect of exercise deprivation on the behaviour and physiology of straight-stall confined pregnant mares. Anim Welfare 2001; 10(3):257–267.

40. Parmeggianni PL. Behavioral phenomenology of sleep (somatic and vegetative). Experientia 1980; 36:6–11.

41. Caanitz H, O'Leary L, Houpt K, et al. Effect of exercise on behaviour. Appl Anim Behav Sci 1991; 31(1–2):1–12.

42. van Dierendonck MC, Bandi N, Batdorj D, et al. Behavioural observations of re-introduced Takhi or Przewalski horses in Mongolia. Appl Anim Behav Sci 1996; 50:95–114.

43. Dallaire A, Ruckebusch Y. Sleep patterns in the pony with observations on partial perceptual deprivation. Physiol Behav 1974; 12:789–796.

44. Boy V, Duncan P. Time-budgets of Camargue horses, I: Developmental changes in the time-budgets of foals. Behaviour 1979; 71:187–202.

45. Duncan P. Time-budgets of Camargue horses, II: Time-budgets of adult horses and weaned sub-adults. Behaviour 1980; 72:26–49.

46. Ruckebusch Y. The relevance of drowsiness in the circadian cycle of farm animals. Anim Behav 1972; 20:637–643.

47. Fischbein W, Gutwein BM. Paradoxical sleep and memory storage processes. Behav Biol 1977; 19:425–464.

48. Crowell-Davis SL. Daytime rest behavior of the Welsh pony (Equus caballus). Appl Anim Behav Sci 1994; 40(3/4):197–210.

49. McFarland D. The Oxford companion to animal behaviour. New York: Oxford University Press; 1987.

50. Bekoff M. The essentials of good play. BBC Wildlife 2000; 18(8):46–53.

51. Fagen R. Animal play behaviour. Oxford: Oxford University Press; 1981.

52. Rees L. The horse's mind. London: Stanley Paul; 1984.

53. Hausberger M, le Scolan N, Bruderer C, Pierre JS. [Temperament in the horse: factors in play and practical implications] Le temperament du cheval: facteurs en jeu et implications pratiques. 24 Journée de la Recherche Equine, Institut de Cheval, Paris, 1998:159–169.

54. Maynard-Smith J. Evolution and the theory of games. Cambridge: Cambridge University Press; 1982: 263–297.

55. Goodwin D, Hughes CF. Horse play. Havemeyer Workshop on Horse Behaviour and Welfare, Holar, Iceland, 2002:102–105.

56. Crowell-Davis SL, Houpt KA, Kane L. Play development in Welsh pony (Equus caballus). Appl Anim Behav Sci 1987; 18(2):119–131.

57. Williams M. Horse psychology. London: JA Allen; 1976.

58. Crowell-Davis SL, Houpt KA, Carini CM. Mutual grooming and nearest neighbor relationships among foals of Equus caballus. Appl Anim Behav Sci 1986; 15:113–123.

59. Duncan P, Harvey PH, Wells SM. On lactation and associated behaviour in a natural herd of horses. Anim Behav 1984; 32(1):255–263.

60. Schoen AMS, Banks EM, Curtis SE. Behavior of young Shetland and Welsh ponies (Equus caballus). Biol Behav 1976; 1:199–216.

61. Mills DS, Nankervis KJ. Equine behaviour: principles and practice. Oxford: Blackwell Science; 1999.

62. Heleski CR, Shelle AC, Nielsen BD, Zanella AJ. Influence of housing on weanling horse behavior and subsequent welfare. Appl Anim Behav Sci 2002; 78(2–4):297–308.

63. Hughes RD, Duncan P, Dawson J. Interactions between Camargue horses and horseflies. Bull Entomol Res 1981; 71(2):227–242.

64. Hayes MH. Veterinary notes for horse-owners. London: Stanley Paul; 1968.

65. Houpt KA. Equine welfare. In: Houpt KA, eds. Recent advances in companion animal behavior problems. Ithaca, NY: International Veterinary Information Services; 2001. A0810. 1201.

66. Gough MR. A note on the use of behavioural modification to aid clipping ponies. Appl Anim Behav Sci 1999; 63(2):171–175.

11

Behavior of the stallion

FREE-RANGING HAREM-MAINTENANCE BEHAVIOR

Observations of free-ranging horses have provided numerous examples of the ways in which we restrict the behavior of managed stallions, restrictions that can lead to reduced fertility, libido and behavioral compliance.

Herding is usually employed to move the family group away from a single stallion or another group. Free-running stallions typically herd together a harem of mares as a relatively stable social unit. They tend to recruit and retain mares most effectively when 6–9 years of age.[1] The upper limit on the size of harems relates to the fact that if a stallion monopolizes too many mares he loses the ability to dissuade other males from performing sneak matings.[1] Sometimes juvenile males, old stallions and, more occasionally, mares cooperate with the harem stallion in his herding activities. This herding behavior can be used to tighten a band or to move interlopers out of or, occasionally, non-member females into the group. The behavior is also seen during courtship, its aim being to transiently distance the mare from the harem for copulation.[2] Vigilant herding is most evident after a harem mare has foaled. At this time the stallion works to maintain a greater than usual distance from other bands, perhaps because this helps him to capitalize on the fact that free-ranging mares are highly fertile during the foal heat.[3] Additionally, cohesion of the group contributes directly to biological fitness because, for example, invasion by non-member stallions can induce abortion and bring mares into season for subsequent mating by invading males.[4]

Sometimes low-ranking males, notably the sons of low-ranking mares, form lifetime alliances in which both stallions have mating rights and cooperate to defend their mares from intruding males.[5] The balance of the pair is rarely equal, with the subordinate stallion siring approximately one quarter of the harem's brood. This compares favorably with the success of sneak matings that represent the only alternative for non-alpha males.[5] However, reciprocal altruism and mutualism do not occur in multi-stallion groups. Linklater & Cameron[6] reported a positive relationship between aggression by the dominant stallion toward subordinate stallions and the subordinates' effort in harem defense, which was negatively correlated with the extent to which these stallions were seen to consort with harem mares. Perhaps because they undergo more social flux than single-stallion groups, multi-stallion groups are associated with more aggressive interactions and reduced foaling rates – hence, the suggestion that there is selection pressure for single-stallion groups.[7] The various agonistic responses that arise between stallions appear in Table 11.1.

The harem stallion exhibits characteristic, even ritualistic, responses to urine and feces of harem members. It is believed that olfactory characteristics of these materials inform the stallion of the reproductive status of the mares while his responses to them serve to maintain the harem. Stallions are more responsive to olfactory stimuli from conspecifics than are mares and geldings.[8] Contact with urine, feces or vaginal fluids during courtship and copulation occurs and forms an important part of the mating behavior, resulting in a flehmen response by the stallion.[2] Pawing, sniffing and flehmen are followed by the deposition of small amounts of feces or urine on top of the previously voided material.[9,10] The stimuli offered by fecal material are discussed in detail in Chapters 6 and 9.

DEVELOPMENT AND MAINTENANCE OF SEXUAL BEHAVIOR IN FREE-RANGING STALLIONS

From the first weeks of life colts demonstrate mounting attempts, mainly on their dams. These attempts are rarely accompanied by pelvic thrusting. Erections have been observed in colts as young as 3 months of age but these are of minimal import to a herd since the mature stallions monopolize estrous females and, in any case, spermatozoa are not found in testes before 12 months of age. Spermatogenesis lags behind hormonal maturity. Fertility does not increase significantly until the colt is approximately 2 years old with the histological transition from the pre-pubertal to the post-pubertal stage occurring at a mean age of 27.8 months (n = 28).[12]

Most colts leave the natal band and join bachelor groups around the time of the birth of their siblings.[13] For example, in one study of Misaki feral horses in Japan, 17 of 22 colts left their natal bands at this time.[13] Scarcity of resources is also regarded as a common cause of voluntary separation.[14] So, as colts become steadily bolder with age and playmates disperse, they may gravitate toward bachelor groups in search of recreation.[15] Beyond the age of 3 years, remaining young males may be forced to leave the harem group during the breeding season as a result of increased aggression by the harem stallion.[2,14]

The behavior of young stallions can then be considered in two stages. The first is a developmental stage in which the colts that have just dispersed from the natal band (between 0.7 and 3.9 years of age in Misaki horses) engage more in social play than agonistic behavior, while the second is a pre-harem formation stage which involves departure from the bachelor group.[16] The separation of the highest-ranking stallion from the subordinate males has significant behavioral and physiological consequences.

The status of the stallion is broadly correlated with androgen levels. Testosterone concentrations increase with the age of stallions until they form their own harems.[15] Furthermore, for individual stallions, testosterone concentrations are correlated with harem size.[15] So, in a harem stallion, sexual and aggressive behavior, accessory sex-gland activity, testicular size and semen quality are enhanced by the dispersal of potential challengers. Meanwhile, stallions becoming bachelors undergo changes in the opposite direction[3,11] and may show signs of concurrent depression

Table 11.1   Features of the agonistic ethogram (as described for bachelors[11]) that are particularly common among and between stallions

Response	Description
Boxing	Two stallions in close proximity simultaneously rearing and striking out with alternate forelegs toward one another
Defecate over	Defecation on top of fecal piles in a characteristic sequence: sniff feces, step forward, defecate, pivot or back up, and sniff feces again
Circling	Two stallions closely beside one another head-to-tail, pivot in circles, usually biting at each other's flanks, groin, rump and/or hindlegs. With prolonged circling, the stallions may progress lower to the ground until they reach a kneeling position or sternal recumbency, where they typically continue to bite or nip one another
Dancing	Two stallions rear, interlock the forelegs and shuffle the hindlegs while biting or threatening to bite one another's head and neck
Erection	Fully extended and tumescent penis. Observed during mildly and moderately aggressive encounters. Bachelors will mount one another with an erection and anal insertion has been observed
Flehmen	Head elevated and neck extended with the eyes rolled back, the ears rotated to the side and the upper lip everted exposing the maxillary gums and incisors. The head may roll to one side or from side to side. Typically occurs in association with olfactory investigation of feces
Head-bowing	A repeated rhythmic flexing of the neck such that the muzzle is brought toward the point of the breast. Head bowing usually occurs synchronously between two stallions when they first approach each other head to head

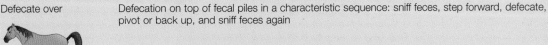

(contd.)

Table 11.1 (*Contd.*)

Response	Description
Head bump	A rapid toss of the head that forcefully contacts the head and neck of another stallion. Usually the eyes remain closed and the ears point forward
Head on neck, back or rump	The chin or entire head rests on the dorsal surface of the neck, body or rump of another horse. This often precedes mounting
Herding	Combination of head threat and ears laid back with forward locomotion, apparently directing the movement of another horse. When lateral movements of the neck occur, the horse is said to be snaking
Kneeling	Drop to one or both knees, by one or both stallions engaged in face-to-face combat or circling with mutual biting or nipping repeatedly at the head and shoulders and knees
Masturbation	Erection with rhythmic drawing of the penis against the abdomen with or without pelvic thrusting. This is a solitary or group activity
Mount	Stallion raises his chest and forelegs onto the back of another horse (be it a mare in a breeding context or another male in a bachelor group) with the forelegs on either side. Also seen primarily in bachelor groups are prolonged partial mounts, typically with lateral rather than rear orientation and often with just one foreleg across the body of the mounted animal. In a behavior similar to the initial mount orientation movements (termed head on neck, back or rump) the forelegs will not actually rise off the ground. Mounts and partial mounts may occur sequentially or independently of one another
Neck wrestling	Sparring with the head and neck that may involve one or both protagonists dropping to one or both knees or raising the forelegs
Parallel prance	Often seen immediately prior to aggressive encounters, two stallions move forward beside one another, shoulder-to-shoulder with arched necks and heads held high and ears forward, typically in a high-stepping low cadenced trot (passage, in dressage terminology). Rhythmic snorts may accompany each stride. Solitary prancing also occurs
Posturing	Posturing describes a suite of pre-fight behaviors that includes head-bowing, olfactory investigation, stomping, prancing, rubbing and pushing, all with neck arching and some stiffening of the entire body
Sniff faeces	Approach and sniff a pile of feces or a fecal pile, usually as a part of a fecal pile display. Often associated with some pawing, this is almost always followed by defecating over the feces and again sniffing the pile

(Sue McDonnell, personal communication 2002). Paradoxically, some domestic stallions may redevelop their libido when another stallion is brought to the breeding area, and some slow-breeding novice stallions seem to increase their arousal when given the opportunity to watch other stallions copulate.[9]

It is worth noting that despite low androgen levels, agonistic behavior, including mock and serious fighting, is a conspicuous characteristic of bachelor groups.[11] Continued studies of bachelor groups could serve to further challenge the traditionally held view that stallions are innately aggressive and somehow deserving of isolation.[17]

FREE-RANGING MATINGS

Prolonged pre-mating interactions are the norm for all free-ranging equids. Harem stallions discriminate among mares, according to their maturity and length of residency in the harem. As evidenced by the increased frequency of flehmen responses, olfactory stimuli help to identify estrous mares, but they are supported by visual and auditory cues from the mare.[18,19] Always favoring mature harem mares, the harem stallion will often ignore estrous young mares (from both his and other harems) and actively chase away mature mares from other harems.[20] Free-running stallions usually interact with sexually active mares or their excrement for many days before copulation. Often these encounters can be counted in hundreds per day.[20] Because stallions can differentiate the sex of a horse on the basis of its feces (not its urine), it has been suggested that sampling of feces is extremely informative for a stallion when monitoring the cyclicity of females in his harem.[10]

When he has located an estrous mare, or she has located him, the harem stallion will often attract her attention by whinnying from a distance and then pawing the ground, prancing and nickering as he approaches. Once these preliminaries have taken place, the mare actively contributes to pre-copulatory behavior.[21] By way of illustration it has demonstrated that 88% of sexual interactions that lead to successful copulation begin with the mare approaching the stallion.[20] An important trigger

of the stallion's physical sexual arousal seems to be the head-to-head approach by the mare toward him, followed by moving forward or the swinging of her hips towards his head.[20]

A stallion's method of determining a mare's receptivity is to nuzzle and push her hindquarters. Pre-copulatory behavior demonstrated by the stallion includes sniffing, nuzzling, licking and nibbling or nipping of the head, shoulder, belly, flank, inguinal and perineal regions of the mare (Fig. 11.1).[2,20,22] These prompts may elicit a mildly aggressive display by the mare, despite her being in full estrus. However, as this aggression subsides, the mare tolerates closer approaches by the stallion. Further arousal results when positive feedback is received from the mare.[23]

Pre-copulatory behavior continues until the mare's stationary 'sawhorse' posture cues the stallion to mount. Mounting may occur without erection. Studies have shown that mounting without an erection is common and has been demonstrated among highly fertile pasture-breeding horses.[2] The number of mounts without erection is typically 1.5–2 times the number of mounts with erection.[2] In free-ranging equids, mounting with erection almost always leads to insertion and ejaculation. While young inexperienced stallions typically mount laterally and then adjust their position, mounting by mature males is usually achieved by an approach from the rear. Although they may ejaculate sooner than their more experienced peers, colts take significantly longer to achieve an erection (after first seeing an estrous mare) and to mount.[24] Once he has mounted correctly, the stallion grasps the mare's iliac crests with his forelegs while his head leans against her neck, and he often nips or grasps her mane with his teeth.[2]

Free-ranging pony stallions achieve intromission during the first mount in 55% of copulations.[25] Successful intromission (see Fig. 11.1) during subsequent attempts is facilitated if the mare remains stationary. Intromission is generally accomplished after one or more seeking thrusts and is often marked by the stallion closely coupling up to the mare and paddling his feet as if attempting to ensure that they are on a firm surface.[2] An average of seven pelvic thrusts[26] occur

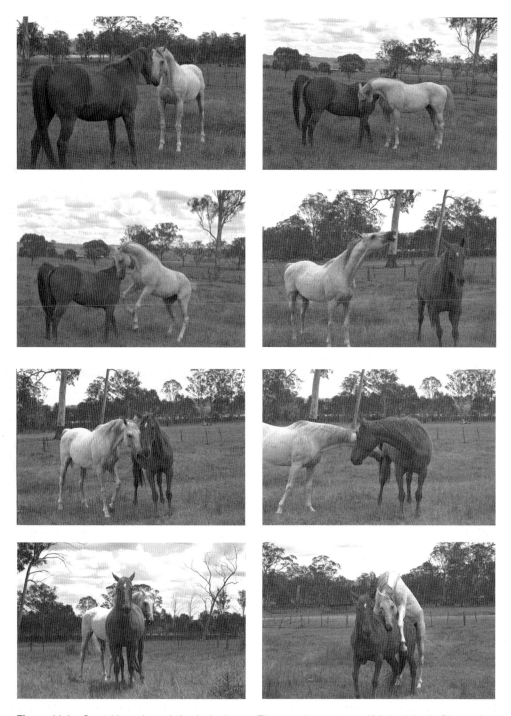

Figure 11.1 Courtship and copulation in the horse. (Photographs courtesy of Michael Jervis-Chaston.)

before ejaculation, which is characteristically indicated by:

- flagging of the tail (associated with transient shrinkage of the urethral lumen and six to nine spurts of ejaculate)[27]
- rhythmic contractions of the muscles of the hindlegs
- an increase in respiratory rate
- drooping of the stallion's head against the mare's mane.

The period from intromission to ejaculation is usually 10–15 seconds, with young males tending to take less time.[23] After ejaculation, the stallion often appears dazed as he relaxes on the mare's back and his penis becomes flaccid. Once the stallion has regained his alertness, the mare steps forward, easing the stallion's chest over her hindquarters, so that he lands gently on his front feet.[27] The mean interval between the end of ejaculation and the start of dismount is eight seconds (Table 11.2).[23]

The stallion's post-copulatory behavior often includes sniffing of the mare's vulva, as well as the spilled ejaculate or urovaginal secretions of the mare, and this typically prompts the flehmen response.[28] After ejaculation, the stallion and mare generally part company within 3–15 seconds, with the mare being first to move away in 60% of cases and the stallion in 26%, although occasionally the mare follows.[25]

Mares and stallions will often separate from the harem group during courtship and mating. Although the pre-copulatory interactions with mares may last several days, the copulatory interactions themselves frequently last for less than a minute. While breeding rates as high as 18 per day have been recorded,[2] the daily mean for adult stallions is 11.[23] The refractory period after ejaculation appears to be shorter in free-running stallions than in their intensively managed counterparts.[20]

SEASONALITY

Stallions possess an endogenous circannual reproductive cycle that is responsive to photoperiod.[29] Timed to synchronize with the emergence of mares from winter anestrus, the responsiveness of stallions to sexual cues increases in spring and is maintained until the beginning of autumn but never completely disappears. The seasonality in testosterone concentrations[15] is reflected in semen quality and can also influence the number of mounts per ejaculation, latency to achieve intromission, frequency of biting and striking.[30] The prevalence of spontaneous erections in masturbating stallions also increases with day length.[31]

The artificial breeding season that starts in late winter for many breeds (such as the Thoroughbred, Standardbred, Quarter Horse and Arabian) may contribute to reports of low sexual vigor. The physiological season can be brought forward in young and middle-aged stallions by placing them under artificial lights, which can increase testicular size and sperm output.[32] It is interesting to note that no deleterious effects on fertility have yet been reported in shuttle stallions that work two seasons per year by being shipped between northern and southern hemispheres.[32]

Table 11.2 Typical frequency and latency of copulatory behaviors by young and adult domestic stallions

	Typical value	Range
Frequency of responses		
Sniff or nuzzle	3	0–80
Lick	0	0–20
Flehmen response	2	0–10
Nip or bite	0	0–25
Kick or strike	0	0–10
Vocalization	3	0–35
Number of mounts	1	1–3
Number of thrusts	7	2–12
Latency of responses (seconds)		
Time to erection	10	0–500
Time to first mount with erection	15	10–540
Time from mount to insertion	2	1–5
Time from intromission to first emission	15	8–20

After Waring et al[24] and McDonnell.[2]

TRADITIONAL STALLION MANAGEMENT

The value of many stallions and the risk of injury through fighting are the principal factors that drive their owners to stable them and minimize unsupervised contact with other horses. By clipping out elements of the harem stallion's socio-sexual behavioral repertoire, hands-on stallion management can leave the entire male equid with the opportunity to perform only brief pre-copulatory interactions (Fig. 11.2).[20] The resultant arousal and thwarted motivation can contribute to the handling difficulties some stallions present.

Domestic breeding stallions are generally maintained in physical isolation, either stabled alone or near other stallions.[33] Breeding farms with more than one breeding stallion often stable all the stallions together, away from the mares, in a stallion barn. This management regime has the potential to impose some characteristics of the bachelor group on some occupants of the barn. McDonnell[20] found that the bachelor status of stallions could be effectively reversed by housing them in a barn with mares or in a paddock adjacent to mares. Regardless of the season, libido, testosterone levels, testicular volume and efficiency of spermatogenesis increase once the trappings of bachelor status are removed.[3]

While most stallions over 20 years of age retain their libido, few maintain competitive sperm counts. The decline of this fertility parameter begins at approximately 10 years of age. Testosterone concentrations 36 hours before and after injection of human chorionic gonadotropin (HCG) may help in the detection of declining reproductive function in aged stallions.[34]

Domestic stallions are generally permitted to copulate in three situations:

- pasture mating
- in-hand breeding (Fig. 11.3)
- semen-collection (for artificial insemination).

While pasture mating usually follows the template of free-ranging horse behavior discussed above (except that stallions are sometimes

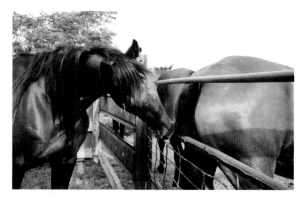

Figure 11.2   A stallion testing olfactory stimuli from an estrous mare.

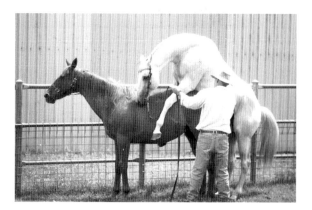

Figure 11.3   If the mare has been properly teased and is truly receptive, minimal restraint is required for in-hand breeding. (Photograph courtesy of Michael Jervis-Chaston.)

separated from their mares during anestrus), in-hand breeding and semen-collection involve some radical departures from the normal ethogram.

Compared with equids breeding at liberty, in-hand breeding stallions show lower rates of sexual vigor and fertility and higher rates of sexual behavior dysfunction. This may be because the selection of breeding animals adopts inappropriate criteria and perhaps favors stallions that would not achieve harem stallion status in a free-ranging context. Stallions at pasture are generally capable of breeding nine times (every 2.5 hours) throughout the day and night with sustained fertility, while in-hand breeding stallions show diminished rates of fertility when bred more than once or twice daily.[20,22,35]

Ginther[36] found that a stallion will copulate with one estrous mare repeatedly, even when more than one mare is in estrus. Stallions breeding at liberty have been observed to copulate twice with the same mare during a 7-minute period, while other stallions have copulated three times with two mares during a 2-hour period.[2] While free-ranging equids are able to interact year-round on a moment-to-moment basis, domestic stallions are typically allowed minimal contact with mares other than brief limited pre-copulatory interactions immediately before copulation.[20] McDonnell[20] concludes that it is remarkable that stallions denied these interactions are considered to have a normal breeding career. Human success in maintaining a stallion's performance under these conditions relies on the ability of most stallions to respond to suboptimal stimuli, either naturally or as a result of conditioning.

Vesserat and Cirelli[37] found that the conception rates of in-hand breeding were in the range 55–60%, while with pasture-bred horses conception rates per cycle were 75–85%. This is largely due to the performance of more matings at pasture than is expected with in-hand mating.[22] Pasture-bred pregnancy rates at the end of the breeding season can reach 100%,[38] but the management of the herd has to be optimal. The best foaling rates (in Icelandic ponies) on pasture are achieved when no more than 15 fertile cycling mares per stallion are run for one heat cycle, or a maximum of 20 fertile cycling mares per stallion if they remain as a group for two heat cycles (6 weeks).[39]

FACTORS AFFECTING SEXUAL RESPONSES IN THE STALLION

The quality of sexual responses in domestic stallions may vary considerably because it is under the influence of a number of factors, including previous experience and current stimuli.

INDIVIDUAL PREFERENCES

Occasionally, stud owners report a stallion's preference for small mares. In these cases, it pays to conduct a thorough examination of the musculoskeletal system before assuming that this is a learned response. Intriguing color preferences have also been reported. For example, there is a report of a stallion selecting and running with only buckskin (dun) mares.[28] One must remember, however, that the affiliation between mares and their filly daughters is often very strong indeed and the effect this has on the color distribution of a natal band may offer an alternative explanation for the apparent preference.

VISUAL STIMULI

In most stallions, an overtly estrous mare will elicit a stronger sexual behavioral response than a breeding dummy or ovariectomised mare.[2] Movement of the receptive mare as she turns from a head-to-head to hips-to-head presentation can have a strong arousing effect on stallions.[20] It is likely that restraint of the mare reduces the extent to which she can send solicitous expressive movements.

Typically the receptive mare urinates frequently and takes longer than normal to step out of the urination straddle. With her tail raised and slung to one side (most notably if she is a horse, rather than a pony) she winks her vulva repeatedly to deliver a flashing signal. A stallion responds to all of these cues by approaching and starting to tease her, which elicits further visual cues that signify receptivity in his prospective mate. Hostile signaling by a non-receptive mare includes laying back of the ears, tail-swishing, kicking and biting. This is usually accompanied by squealing. A receptive mare is largely passive once she is in a hips-to-head position, but may actively present herself with a raised tail in response to the stallion's nuzzling.

OLFACTORY STIMULI

The odor of an estrous mare's genital region and her urovaginal discharges contributes significantly to a stallion's arousal.[40] This accounts for the use of such fluids in the training of stallions for semen collection. The fluids cause a generic rather than specific response, since although stallions have been shown to discriminate between the urovaginal secretions of individual mares,[8] olfaction appears to contribute to sexual arousal less than vision.[41]

LEARNING

Sexual behavior of domestic stallions is clearly influenced by experience and learning (Fig. 11.4),

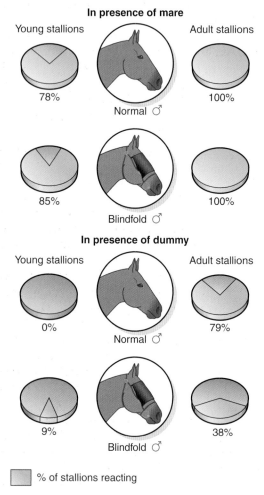

In presence of mare

Young stallions   Adult stallions

78%   Normal ♂   100%

85%   Blindfold ♂   100%

In presence of dummy

Young stallions   Adult stallions

0%   Normal ♂   79%

9%   Blindfold ♂   38%

☐ % of stallions reacting

Figure 11.4 Stimuli affecting the sexual responses of naïve and experienced stallions (after Wierzbowski[42]). Stallions visually assess mares (and dummies) as they approach to mount. Without the benefit of learning, naïve stallions may be more likely to mount when blindfolded because they are unaware of visual stimuli that are discouraging to them (e.g. threats in the case of mares) or simply inadequate (in the case of a dummy).

with breeding stallions learning by classical conditioning (see Ch. 4) to respond sexually to non-sexual stimuli associated with breeding. For example, in stallions bred in-hand, the service bridle, the service area and even key personnel can become conditioned stimuli that can cause arousal and erection.[9] The importance of voyeurism in educating novice stallions should not be overlooked (see Fraser Darling effect in Glossary) since many free-ranging colts show keen interest when the harem stallion copulates.

Stallions used for semen collection are expected to show sexual responses to a dummy. While occasional stallions will respond immediately to the dummy, most require the supportive effect of a transitional stimulus mare as an adjunct to several ejaculations with the dummy before reliable conditioning takes place. Teasing the stallion with a mare across the rear of the dummy is a particularly useful technique for developing the correct association.

Well-trained stallions distinguish themselves in the breeding shed by their tolerance of human interventions such as penis washing, while remaining responsive to conditioned commands used in the service area. The strength of innate responses and the role of learned associations have been quantified by comparing the responses of naïve and sexually experienced stallions when presented with a variety of stimuli.[42] Sometimes libido becomes dependent on such conditioned stimuli and a program of generalization (see Ch. 4) is required to break down the association between such discriminative cues and sexual outcomes. While weaning these stallions off their discriminative stimuli, changes in routine have to be introduced very slowly.

Learning applies equally in the development of abnormal sexual responses. Many stallions that learn to associate the breeding area with negative experiences (such as harsh discipline) will eventually become problem breeders and will require retraining.[30] As a result of inadvertent and inappropriate conditioning, fertile stallions may show minimal libido, so sexual responses are not reliable indicators of fertility.

Sometimes a change of service area can be sufficient to overcome context-specific reluctance to mount.[9] Simple changes to management practices that allow greater mobility of the mare and less alteration of her normal estrous posture, seem to make her more attractive and enhance the sexual responsiveness of the stallion.[3]

Safety concerns are paramount when dealing with breeding stallions and mares, but modification of sexual congress in domestic equids to resemble more closely that of their free-ranging counterparts has been shown to increase sexual arousal and to reverse sexual dysfunction.[2]

PHARMACEUTICALS

Descriptions of the effects of numerous pharmaceuticals on stallion behavior appear elsewhere in the literature.[35] Having said that, relatively little is known about endocrine control of reproduction in the stallion, but gonadotropins are considered pivotal in the regulation of libido and spermatogenesis. This is supported by the effects of Antarelix, a potent GnRH antagonist that reduces libido and plasma concentrations of gonadotropins, testosterone and estradiol within 48 hours of administration.[43] Gonadotropin and testosterone secretion can be stimulated by GnRH analogues, but chronic treatment can impose a reversible drop in sperm production and libido.[44] It has been suggested that because exogenous testosterone propionate implants reduce spermatogenesis, they may be of use in controlling fertility, for example, in feral horses.[45]

Anxiolytics may reduce fearfulness in stallions that have developed negative associations with breeding.[46] The stimuli that are most commonly responsible for reduced libido are linked to the presence of humans.[46] However, the use of anxiolytics in the absence of behavior modification is not recommended.

Some pharmaceuticals have side effects that may profoundly compromise the usefulness of breeding stallions. For example, reserpine has been associated with penile paralysis and paraphimosis, when used repeatedly (5 mg s.c. every 2 weeks for 2 months) to control unmanageable behavior.[47] Other agents, such as trimethoprim-sulfamethoxazole and pyrimethamine, may affect the pattern and strength of ejaculation (for example,

by altering lumbar flexibility or reducing coordination).[48] Anabolic steroids depress luteinizing hormone concentrations and hence libido and semen quality,[49] while sometimes causing a simultaneous increase in aggression.[9]

CASTRATION

In some senses it is possible to consider geldings as domestic analogues of bachelor stallions (e.g. in terms of their testosterone profiles and behavior towards mares).

Most castrations occur between 3 months and 2 years of age, and behavior manipulation is cited as the most common reason for the procedure.[50] Because early castration increases carpal and tarsal measurements,[51] it would be interesting to explore the consequences of pre-pubertal castration on morphology of the brain.

The social rank of geldings correlates with the age at which they were castrated. This suggests that experience in male horses prior to neutering influences the behavior afterwards.[52] But surprisingly, delaying castration until a stallion matures has been demonstrated not to increase the risk of stallion-like behavior after castration.[53] Castration reduces the intensity of normal male sexual behavior by reducing testosterone concentrations.[54] Houpt[55] states that the testosterone concentration of a gelding should be <0.2 ng/ml. Geldings are more responsive to the pacifying effects of progesterone than are stallions. Approximately 90% of mature stallions show low sexual activity within 8 weeks of castration.[56] That said, experienced adult stallions can maintain normal sexual responses for more than a year after castration.[53] McDonnell[20] estimates that up to 50% of geldings show some stallion-like behavior to mares. Indeed we should not expect castration to eliminate all traits that may be considered characteristic of a harem stallion. After all, some sexual behaviors, including teasing, mounting and performance of elements of the elimination marking sequence (see Ch. 9), are frequently observed in foals and adolescents of both sexes.[57] Occasionally, geldings in their teens, with normal estrone sulfate and testosterone concentration and no history of use as studs, achieve intromission.[58]

Such animals may become more libidinous in response to stilboestrol.[59]

Although the possibility of supplementary hormones generated by the adrenal gland has been raised, aggressive masculine behavior after castration is not usually dependent on hormones.[53,56,58] These significant outliers in the distribution of sex-related responses demonstrate that the brains of male horses are masculinized before birth.[55] Agonistic responses reinforced prior to castration may also contribute to some of the aggression seen in geldings.[60]

There is no evidence for the traditionally held belief that epididymal remnants perpetuate sexual responses after castration.[61] Because castration of cryptorchids can be difficult, it is possible that some testicular tissue and therefore testosterone production can remain after surgery.[62] Plasma estrogens are useful in discriminating between cryptorchids and geldings.[63] In horses over 3 years of age, estrone sulfate concentration is significantly greater (>10 000 pg/ml) where castration is incomplete than in geldings (<10 pg/ml).[64] For horses under 3 years of age, a single assay of estrone sulfate is not sufficient to make a definitive discrimination. Instead, blood samples for testosterone levels must be taken before and 2 hours after the administration of HCG (10 000 IU i.v.).[55] Cryptorchids typically have concentrations >2000 pg/ml, whereas geldings have concentrations <500 pg/ml.[55]

Chemical castration, for example using GnRH super agonists to down-regulate the pituitary-gonadal axis, is being developed. The transient castration of horses is likely to increase the flexibility with which potential breeding animals can be managed.

MASTURBATION

Many horse breeders traditionally consider masturbation to be an abnormal behavior. However, studies have shown that all free-running male equids, regardless of age, sociosexual environment and harem status, display frequent erections and penile movements (including the penis being bounced against the abdomen) referred to as masturbation, once every 1–3 hours.[2] The extent to which penile engorgement and movement are gratifying in a directly sexual sense is questionable. Either way, spontaneous erection and masturbation are now considered normal responses.[65] Furthermore it is now accepted that ejaculation is seen in only approximately 0.01% of such erections, thus dispelling the myth that masturbation leads to lower fertility rates.[31] Indeed, field and laboratory studies confirm that the levels of spontaneous erection and masturbation are not associated with loss of fertility. Observations of confined stallions have shown that there may be some association between masturbation and

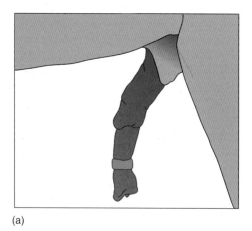

(a)

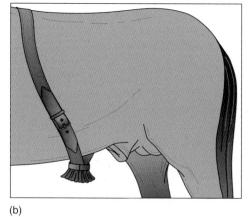

(b)

Figure 11.5 (a) Stallion ring; (b) brush. (After McDonnell.[2] Redrawn with permission of Sue McDonnell.)

REM sleep (see Ch. 10), which occurs only during recumbent rest.[66]

Despite reports that designate the behavior as normal and harmless, many devices exist for discouraging stallions from masturbation (Fig. 11.5). The multiplicity of devices suggests that none of them works universally. Most devices attempt to employ punishment to discourage masturbation. A stallion ring or a brush can be fitted. A stallion ring is a metal or plastic device that is placed on the shaft of the penis, inhibiting erection by physical restriction. The brush is a stiff-bristled brush that is strapped to the belly. These devices can cause abrasions and scarring of the penis (Fig. 11.6).[2] It is not surprising to learn that electric shocks have also been employed to modify erections. Anti-masturbation devices rarely reduce spontaneous erection and penile movement, but in many cases increase the frequency and duration of episodes and often cause penile injury.[20]

Conversely, while arousal may be unwelcome in most horses that are not currently required to mount a mare, it is actively encouraged in teasers. Circumcision of the prepuce and the penile epithelium with subsequent suturing is still practiced in parts of the world to create teasers.[67,68]

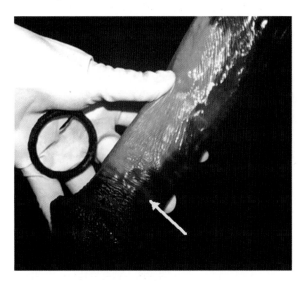

Figure 11.6   A stallion ring (in hand) and penis with a mild circumferential lesion (arrow) caused by abrasion. (From McDonnell[2]. Photograph by Sue McDonnell reproduced with permission.)

SEXUAL BEHAVIOR OF MALE DONKEYS

Male donkeys are more likely to be found alone than in an organized social unit.[69] They show courtship of a similar duration to that of *E. caballus* stallions but within a territorial sociosexual structure.[70] They also demonstrate significantly more vocalization and posturing (Fig. 11.7) as a prelude to copulation and seem to rely on more overtly active involvement of the female than horses do.[71] Several periods of sexual interactions interspersed with periods of male withdrawal from the female's company are typical.[71] It is a characteristic of male donkeys to take their time to mate. Experienced donkey breeders note that this is a delay that can be extended when the jacks detect novel stimuli. Such apparently innocuous differences as the presence of strangers or even particularly strong wind can cause procrastination for hours.[72]

In some populations, groups of donkeys include subordinate males that are allowed to mate with some of the jennies within the territory of a dominant jack, but this usually takes place only after mating by the dominant jack.[73] Subordinate jacks play a useful role in territorial defense and marking of excrement of the jennies.[73]

Typically jacks develop an erection only after mounting without an erection,[74] and as a normal feature of donkey sexual behavior this should be expected in managed matings. For some, erection is most frequently achieved when they stand at a distance from the jennies.[74] So experienced breeders of donkeys provide males with sufficient space and liberty to approach and retreat from their jennies during courtship.[74]

When selecting jacks for interspecies matings it is usual practice to separate them from other donkeys at weaning and rear them with at least one horse. Although requiring closer scientific scrutiny,[74] this is said to have a profound effect on their later choice of partner to the extent that it is common for a jack raised in this way to refuse to mate with a jenny.[72]

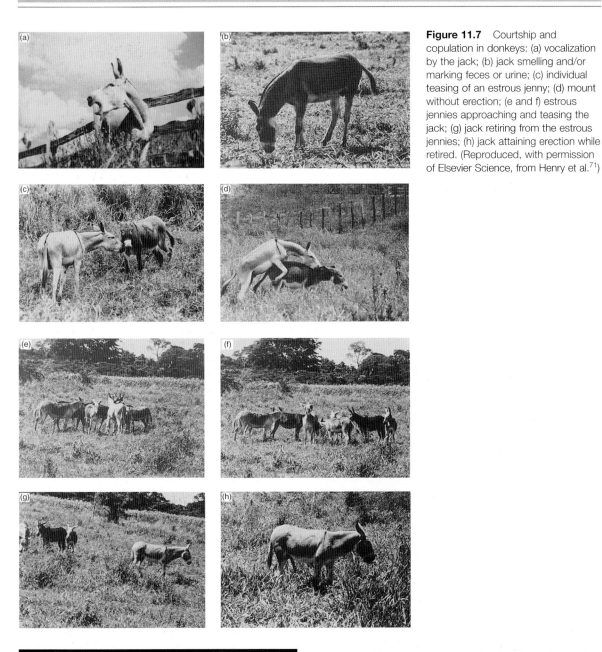

Figure 11.7 Courtship and copulation in donkeys: (a) vocalization by the jack; (b) jack smelling and/or marking feces or urine; (c) individual teasing of an estrous jenny; (d) mount without erection; (e and f) estrous jennies approaching and teasing the jack; (g) jack retiring from the estrous jennies; (h) jack attaining erection while retired. (Reproduced, with permission of Elsevier Science, from Henry et al.[71])

BEHAVIOR PROBLEMS IN THE STALLION

FAILURE IN REPRODUCTIVE BEHAVIOR

Broadly speaking, there are four aspects of failure to perform in the service area: libido, erectile, ejaculatory and coordination (Table 11.3).[75] Most classes of dysfunction involve both psychogenic and physical factors that must be addressed at the same time. An interesting technique to help distinguish between the psychogenic and physical causes of impotence is to observe the stallion for nocturnal bouts of masturbation because their absence may help to rule out extraneous impediments to performance such as fear of aversive stimuli in the service area.[72]

Table 11.3   An overview of the ways in which sexual behavior in the stallion may be compromised or mitigated

Problem	Approach
Reduced libido • Prior discipline for erection or masturbation during an earlier career as performance horse • Excessive use of stallion as a teaser • Isolation of stallion • Persistent presentation of a mare the stallion has rejected • Rough handling during matings • Exposure of a young stallion to hostile, unreceptive mares • Move to novel environment • Unstable dummy • Previous or current lesions on penis	• Eliminate any causative factors, including the presence of humans associated with negative stimuli • Behavior modification: gradual shaping of approach and arousal with positive reinforcement and tolerance of minor flaws in sexual response • If using an artificial vagina, increase stimulation of penis after identifying individual stallion's preferred liners, and temperatures within the artificial vagina • Expose stallion to receptive mare(s) • Develop ritualized breeding routine • Retain conditioned stimuli that are known to assist in arousal • Reduce distractions in breeding area
Erectile • Reluctance to approach and mount • Absence of erection • Failure to maintain erection • Abnormally prolonged refractory period	• Behavior modification as above • GnRH 50 μg Cystorelin s.c. 1 and 2 hours before breeding • Diazepam 0.05 mg/kg slow i.v.
Ejaculatory • Incomplete intromission • Inadequate pelvic thrusts after intromission • Failure to ejaculate • High threshold to ejaculate • Neurological lesions (e.g. in hypogastric and pudendal nerves)	• Behavior modification as above • Analgesics • Imipramine 500–100 0 mg/kg orally in concentrated feed (lowers threshold to ejaculate) • Imipramine 2.2 mg/kg i.v. (induces ejaculation when given to subjects standing quietly in the stall) • Xylazine 0.66 mg/kg i.v. • Prostaglandin F2α 0.01 mg/kg i.m. 10–15 minutes before breeding may help to induce smooth muscle activity in the accessory glands
Physical and coordination • Fatigue/poor condition/obesity • Physical trauma from kicks, stallion rings, priapism, paraphimosis • Current lesions on penis • Musculoskeletal disease • Reflected penis	• Analgesics • Modify dummy or mount mare's height • Weight loss and exercise • Lateral support of hips during mounting • Collect semen on ground

GnRH, gonadotropin-releasing hormone.
The doses are derived from reference material and should be modified according to veterinary clinical assessment. A number of the drugs have additional applications at different doses not discussed in this text.

The serum concentration of testosterone in normal and impotent stallions can be similar.[76] Because the causes are not always distinct from one another, there may be some overlap in treatment. In most cases, behavioral approaches are recommended with the occasional need for pharmacological support. As with all behavior manifestations, a clinical examination may reveal a somatic cause or contribution to the problem. For example, as a result of insufficient lubricant (a result of excessive washing or excessive smegma), a stallion that fails to draw may have a reflected penis that engorges within the sheath.[3]

The web site caltest.nbc.upenn.edu/behavior contains a tremendous amount of information and advice on the behavior and management of stallions. Before attempting to modify the sexual responses of stallions, e.g. for semen collection purposes, readers are advised to visit this site and study the research papers it offers.

AGGRESSION AND OTHER HANDLING PROBLEMS

Prancing and vocalization are normal responses made by a stallion that has seen a mare and should never be discouraged. Nipping and striking are less welcome and can be modified by negative punishment whereby the stallion is led away from the mare or the dummy as an immediate consequence of these responses.[77] Aggression by stallions during sexual congress is associated with freshness at the time of the first matings of the season[31] or failure to ejaculate.[36] Overuse at stud can also result in a stale attitude that manifests as aggression to both mares and handlers.[9] Having said that, offering stallions so many opportunities to mate that they become sated is one approach to the hyperlibidinous state. However, in modifying any unwanted behavior, it is especially important for the breeding stallion to retain desirable (sexual) responses.

When being handled in company (e.g. at a show) stallions are less likely to be aggressive to conspecifics if they are not allowed to sniff other horses' feces.[78] By the same token, the application of odor-masking substances to the nostrils of stallions is reported to make them more tractable under circumstances when stimuli from novel mares are being inadvertently presented.[78] When introducing mares to geldings as field mates, it pays to ensure they are not in estrus, since this occasionally precipitates stallion-like responses, including herding and aggression. Male sexual behavior can be reduced with oral (altrenogest) or injectable (medroxyprogesterone acetate) progestins.[61]

By retrieving straying youngsters and occasionally playing with foals and yearlings, stallions play a role in parenting especially after the first week of life.[79] Before then they allow the mare and foal to bond by reducing disturbances. However, although it seems unlikely to have any adaptive significance, infanticide has been reported in Przewalski stallions[80] and Camargue horses[81] as have isolated incidents of aggression toward foals by domestic stallions and even geldings.[61] This may have contributed to the perception that stallions are innately aggressive.[17] However, it is worth remembering that, in contrast to donkeys, in which the territorial adult males are dominant over all their conspecifics,[82] *E. caballus* stallions in the free-ranging state are generally not the dominant nor the most aggressive members of natal bands.[83] Despite this, the perception that stallions are inherently dangerous and therefore should be isolated prevails in many human traditions.[17] If aggression does emerge in the behavioral repertoire of a stallion, it is paradoxically preferable for personnel that he is consistently aggressive rather than being unpredictable.

Hyper-reactive and so-called frenzied stallions benefit from managemental changes that help to resolve fizzy riding horses. Turn-out and reduced grain intake are especially helpful when used in combination with behavior modification and are always worth trying before hormonal approaches, such as the use of progesterone or tranquilizers, are attempted.

SELF-MUTILATION

Frustration in stallions restrained from estrous mares can be directed towards personnel, anestrous mares, youngstock and even their own bodies. Self-mutilation shows some seasonality and is most commonly seen in stabled stallions and very occasionally in geldings, mares and foals.[61] For these reasons it is regarded as a product of thwarted motivation to be among a harem and also a redirection of agonistic responses. Physical restraint, such as the traditional neck cradle, is largely counterproductive[9] and while Shuster & Dodman[84] suggest that clomipramine (1.0 mg/kg p.o.) reduces self-biting attempts by approximately 50%, attempts to enrich the animal's environment are pivotal to successful therapy. The strategic presentation of ample forage in place of concentrated feed, the provision of company, preferably equine, and exercise should all be explored.

The combined use of stallions as breeding and performance animals has advantages and disadvantages. While helping to meet the behavioral needs of a stallion, exercise also enhances fertility and prolongs a stallion's working life by maintaining cardiovascular and musculoskeletal fitness.[38] By keeping the breeding stallion in ridden work, it may be possible to temper his explosive displays after periods of stabling and maintain his responsiveness to vocal commands. By contrast, there are some data to suggest that forced daily exercise can reduce libido in young stallions.[85] Despite the notable exception offered by several world-class stallions, many stallion handlers feel that such attempts to combine work can have deleterious effects on performance or fertility or both. It would be useful to identify the inter-relationships between fertility, biddability and competitive flare.

SUMMARY OF KEY POINTS

- Management regimes on studs should meet the behavioral and physiological needs of the stallion and the mare.
- In the free-ranging state, a harem stallion interacts with his mares almost continuously and the mare plays a pivotal role in the timing of copulation.
- The reproductive function of stallions is subject to social modulation.
- Free-ranging stallions protect foals in their natal band.
- If safety can be maintained, increased contact between mares and stallions can reduce the prevalence of unwelcome behaviors in stallions and improve herd fertility.
- Stallions can be allowed to mount without an erection. If it becomes necessary to force a stallion to dismount, this should be accomplished without aversive stimuli that can have unpleasant associations later.
- Allowing the mare to facilitate the stallion's dismount by walking forward reduces the risks of unwelcome associations with copulation.
- Masturbation is part of the normal ethogram of male horses.

CASE STUDY

A 10-year old Dartmoor x Shetland stallion, called Topper, showed a guarding behavior when placed with other horses, especially mares. The absence of good handling allowed this to become a dangerous default response to humans and other animals.

In the year before he arrived at his current home, Topper had killed four dogs as they were walked through his field. Poor fencing allowed him to wander from his paddock on many occasions. His visiting and guarding of other horses in his area had taken him out of his home paddock and this was causing tremendous disruption in the local village. He had been beaten repeatedly for displays of aggression but this had not

helped matters. On the day of his prehension at the request of the police, three experienced personnel and an RSPCA officer spent 6 hours driving him into a corral, then a further 2 hours in the pen with him before they caught him.

Topper was castrated 2 weeks before he arrived at his new home. On arrival at the new home Topper would not tolerate being touched. He was very aggressive when humans in his vicinity engaged eye contact with him, even if they were not approaching him. Rather than run away from such challenges he would, instead, charge straight towards the humans then rear and attempt to strike their heads.

After one month of passive habituation to the presence of humans, Topper would allow two key personnel to enter his yard as he watched suspiciously. He eventually discovered carrots and showed a tremendous liking for them. Carrots were therefore used first as lures that could be shown to him and then given to him if he approached. Soon Topper learned to look for carrots and to follow carrot-bearing humans while remaining a distance of a meter or so behind them. Clicker training (see Ch. 4) was used to shape desirable responses in the presence of humans. Using carrots as primary reinforcers, his responses were shaped so that he remained still with humans around him. Interestingly, because it was clearly rewarding for him, the departure of humans from a zone around him was also offered as reinforcement contingent on the sound of the clicker. This system is akin to the advance-and-retreat method used by many round-pen trainers. It gradually modulated his aggression and allowed him to develop an alternative response when overwhelmed by the proximity of humans: he learned to run away.

After one month Topper was safe with the two people who fed him, as long as they did not corner him. He would tolerate being touched as long as he was approached and handled very slowly. Although he would generally rather not be near people, aggression became extremely rare. However, his owners took the precaution of never allowing children into his box with him. Three years later, he still sounded very much like a stallion when he roared at mares in season in neighboring paddocks but gradually this response tended to occur only in early spring rather than the summer.

Whereas he was initially safe to groom only when tied up, now he can be groomed while standing loose in the stable. His owner notes that as long as Topper is shown each brush before it is used, he now seems to quite like being groomed although she remains convinced that he would prefer to be dirty. The vestiges of head-shyness remain, and handling the ears continues to be a problem.

Although Topper is content in the company of most horses and ponies he is persistently fearful of donkeys. He is kept with a gelding that he mutually grooms but does not guard. Through clicker training, Topper is used for demonstrations of liberty training in which he performs Spanish Walk (see Fig. 4.10) and jumps, bows and rears on command.

REFERENCES

1. Kaseda Y, Khalil AM. Harem size and reproductive success of stallions in Misaki feral horses. Appl Anim Behav Sci 1996; 47(3/4):163–173.
2. McDonnell SM. Normal and abnormal sexual behaviour. Vet Clin North Am: Equine Pract 1992; 8:71–89.
3. McDonnell SM. Stallion sexual behaviour. In: Samper JC, ed. Equine breeding and artificial insemination. London: WB Saunders; 2000.
4. Berger J. Induced abortion and social factors in wild horses. Nature 1983; 303(5912):59–61.
5. Feh C. Alliances and reproductive success in Carmargue stallions. Anim Behav 1999; 57(3):705–713.
6. Linklater WL, Cameron EZ. Tests for cooperative behaviour between stallions. Anim Behav 2000; 60(6):731–734.
7. Linklater WL, Cameron EZ, Minot EO, Stafford KJ. Stallion harassment and the mating system of horses. Anim Behav 1999; 58(2):295–306.
8. Marinier SL, Alexander AJ, Waring GH. Flehman behaviour in the domestic horse: discrimination of conspecific odours. Appl Anim Behav Sci 1988; 19(3–4):227–237.
9. McDonnell SM. Reproductive behaviour of the stallion. Vet Clin North Am: Equine Pract 1986; 2:535–556.
10. Stahlbaum CC, Houpt KA. The role of the flehmen response in the behavioural repertoire of the stallion. Physiol Behav 1989; 45:1207–1214.
11. McDonnell SM, Haviland JCS. Agonistic ethogram of the equid bachelor band. Appl Anim Behav Sci 1995; 43:147–188.
12. Melo MIV, Sereno JRB, Henry M, Cassali GD. Peripubertal sexual development of Pantaneiro stallions. Theriogenology 1998; 50(5):727–737.
13. Kaseda Y, Ogawa H, Khalil AM. Causes of natal dispersal and emigration and their effects on harem formation in Misaki feral horses. Equine Vet J 1997; 29(4):262–266.
14. Khalil AM, Kaseda Y. Early experience affects developmental behaviour and timing of harem formation in Misaki horses. Appl Anim Behav Sci 1998; 59(4):253–263.
15. Khalil AM, Murakami N, Kaseda Y. Relationship between plasma testosterone concentrations and age, breeding season and harem size in Misaki feral horses. J Vet Med Sci 1998; 60(5):643–645.
16. Khalil AM, Murakami N. Effect of natal dispersal on the reproductive strategies of the young Misaki feral stallions. Appl Anim Behav Sci 1999; 62(4):281–291.
17. Goodwin D. The importance of ethology in understanding the behaviour of the horse. The role of the horse in Europe. Equine Vet J Suppl 1999; 28:15–19.
18. Anderson TM, Pickett BW, Heird JC, Squires EL. Effect of blocking vision and olfaction on sexual responses of haltered or loose stallions. J Equine Vet Sci 1996; 16: 254–261.
19. Houpt KA, Guida L. Flehmen. Equine Pract 1984; 6(3):32–35.
20. McDonnell SM. Reproductive behaviour of stallions and mares: comparison of free-running and domestic in-hand breeding. Anim Reprod Sci 2000; 60–61:211–219.
21. Rees L. The horse's mind. Sydney: Stanley Paul; 1984.
22. Bristol F. Breeding behaviour of a stallion at pasture with 20 mares in synchronized oestrus. J Reprod Fert Suppl 1982; 32:71–77.
23. Waring GH. Horse behavior. Park Ridge, NJ: Noyes; 1983.
24. Waring GH, Wierzbowski S, Hafez ESE. The behaviour of horses. In: Hafez ESE, ed. The behaviour of domestic animals. 3rd edn. London: Baillière Tindall; 1975.
25. Tyler SJ. The behaviour and social organisation of the New Forest ponies. Anim Behav Monogr 1972; 5:85–196.
26. Asa CS, Goldfoot DA, Ginther OJ. Sociosexual behaviour and the ovulatory cycle of ponies (Equus caballus). Hormones Behav 1979; 13:49–65.
27. Kosiniak K. Characteristics of the successive jets of ejaculated semen of stallions. J Reprod Fert Suppl 1975; 23:59–61.
28. Feist JD. Behaviour of feral horses in the Pryor Mountain Wild Horse Range. PhD thesis, University of Michigan; 1971.
29. Clay CM. Influences of season and artificial photoperiod on reproduction in stallions. Diss Abstr Int B Sci Eng 1989; 49(8):2941.
30. Pickett BW, Voss JL, Squires EL. Impotence and abnormal sexual behaviour in the stallion. Theriogenology 1977; 8:329–347.
31. Tischner M, Tomica E, Jezierski J. Age and seasonal effects on sexual behaviour of stallions at rest. Anim Reprod Sci 1986; 12(3):233–237.
32. Umphenour NW, Steiner JV. Breeding of the Thoroughbred stallion. In: Samper JC, ed. Equine breeding and artificial insemination. London: WB Saunders; 2000.
33. McCarthy PF, Umphenour NW. Management of stallions on large breeding farms. Vet Clin North Am: Equine Pract 1992; 8:219–235.

34. Clement F, Plongere G, Magistrini M, Palmer E. Appreéciation de la fonction sexuelle de l'étalon. Le Point Veterinaire 1998; 29(191):343–348.

35. McDonnell S, Garcia MC, Kenney RM. Pharmacological manipulations of sexual behaviour in stallions. J Reprod Fert Suppl 1987; 35:45–49.

36. Ginther OJ. Sexual behaviour following introduction of a stallion into a group of mares. Theriogenology 1983; 19:877–886.

37. Vesserat GM, Cirelli AA Jnr. Stallion behaviour. Equine Pract 1996; 18:29–32.

38. Tischner M. Patterns of stallion sexual behaviour in the absence of mares. J Reprod Fert Suppl 1982; 32:65–70.

39. Steinbjkornsson B, Kristjansson H. Sexual behaviour and fertility in Iceland horse herds. Pferdeheilkunde 1999; 15(6):481–490.

40. Lindsay FEF, Burton FL. Observational urine testing on the horse and donkey stallion. Equine Vet J 1983; 15(4):330–336.

41. Anderson TM, Pickett BW, Heird JC, Squires EL. Effect of blocking vision and olfaction on sexual responses of haltered or loose stallions. J Equine Vet Sci 1996; 16(6):254–261.

42. Wierzbowski S. The sexual reflexes of stallions. Roczniki Nauk Rolniczych 1959; 73(B-4):753–788.

43. Hinojosa AM, Bloeser JR, Thomson SRM, Watson ED. The effect of a GnRH antagonist on endocrine and seminal parameters in stallions. Theriogenology 2001; 56(5):903–912.

44. Boyle MS, Skidmore J, Zhang J, Cox JE. The effects of continuous treatment of stallions with GnRH analogue. J Reprod Fert Suppl 1991; 44:169–182.

45. Kirkpatrick J, Turner JW Jr, Perkins A. Reversible chemical fertility control in feral horses. J Equine Vet Sci 1982; 2(4):114–118.

46. McDonnell S, Kenney RM, Meckley PE, Garcia MC. Novel environmental suppression of stallion sexual behaviour and effects of diazepam. Physiol Behav 1986; 37:503–505.

47. Memon MA, Usenik EA, Varner DD, Meyers PJ. Penile paralysis and paraphimosis associated with reserpine administration in a stallion. Theriogenology 1988; 30(2):411–419.

48. Bedford SJ, McDonnell SM. Measurements of reproductive function in stallions treated with trimethoprim-sulfamethoxazole and pyrimethamine. J Am Vet Med Assoc 1999; 215(9):1317–1319.

49. Squires EL, Todter GE, Berndtson WE, Pickett BW. Effect of anabolic steroids on reproductive function of young stallions. J Anim Sci 1982; 54(3):576–582.

50. Moll HD, Pelzer KD, Pleasant RS, et al. A survey of equine castration complications. J Equine Vet Sci 1995; 15(12):522–526.

51. Heusner GL, Pope JB, Crowell-Davis SL, Caudle AB. The effect of prepubertal castration on the growth and behaviour of colts. In: Proceedings of the 15th Equine Nutrition and Physiology Symposium, Fort Worth, Texas, 1997. Savoy, USA: Equine Nutrition and Physiology Society Publications; 1997:223–224.

52. Van Dierendonck MC, Devries H, Schilder MBH. An analysis of dominance, its behavioural parameters and possible determinants in a herd of icelandic horses in captivity. Neth J Zool 1995; 45(3–4):362–385.

53. Line SW, Hart BL, Sanders L. Effect of prepubertal versus postpubertal castration on sexual and aggressive behaviour in male horses. J Am Vet Med Assoc 1985; 186(3):249–251.

54. Thompson DL Jr, Pickett BW, Squires EL, Nett TM. Sexual behaviour, seminal pH and accessory sex gland weights in geldings administered testosterone and (or) estradiol-17 beta. J Anim Sci 1980; 51(6):1358–1366.

55. Houpt KA. Is there life after castration? In: Harris PA, Gomarsall GM, Davidson HPB, Green RE, eds. Proceedings of the BEVA Specialist Days on Behaviour And Nutrition, Newmarket, Suffolk, UK, 1999:15–16.

56. Berbish EA, Ghoneim IM, Mousa SZ, Attia MZ. Effect of castration on sexual and aggressive behaviour on male horses. Vet Med J Giza 1996; 44(2B):535–539.

57. McDonnell SM, Poulin A. Equid play ethogram. Appl Anim Behav Sci 2002; 78(2–4):263–295.

58. Cox JE. Behaviour of the false rig: causes and treatments. Vet Rec 1986; 118(13):353–356.

59. Lunaas T. Libidinous behaviour in gelding exacerbated by stilboestrol. Norsk Veterinaertidsskrift 1980; 92(2):116.

60. England G. Allen's fertility and obstetrics in the horse. 2nd edn. Oxford: Blackwell Science; 1996.

61. Crowe CW, Gardner RE, Humburg JM, et al. Plasma testosterone and behavioural characteristics in geldings with intact epididymes. J Equine Med Surg 1977; 1:387–390.

62. Trotter GW, Aanes WA. A complication of cryptorchid castration in three horses. Am J Vet Med Assoc 1981; 179:246–248.

63. Ganjam VK. An inexpensive, yet precise, laboratory diagnostic method to confirm cryptorchidism in the horse. In: Proceedings of the 23rd Annual Convention of the American Association of Equine Practitioners, Vancouver, BC 1977. C/o Dr FJ Milne, Ontario Veterinary College, Guelph, Ontario, Canada, 1978:245–248.

64. Ekmann A, Lehn-Jensen H, Fjeldborg J. [A systematic clinical examination method for diagnosis of presumed equine cryptorchidism] Systematisk klinisk undersogel-sesmetodik til diagnostik af formodede kryptorchide heste i klinisk praksis. Dansk Veterinaertidsskrift 2000; 83(21):6–14.

65. McDonnell SM, Henry M, Bristol F. Spontaneous erection and masturbation in equids. In: Equine reproduction V: Proceedings of the 5th International Symposium on equine reproduction. Journals of Reproduction and Fertility Ltd, Cambridge, CB5 8DT, UK; 1991:664–665.

66. Wilcox S, Dusza K, Houpt KA. The relationship between recumbent rest and masturbation in stallions. J Equine Vet Sci 1991; 11(1):23–26.

67. Silva LAF, Fioravanti MCS, Marques Junior, AP, Melo MIV. Evaluation of the sexual behaviour of Managalarga stallions circumcised to prevent extension of the penis. Revista Brasileira de Reproducao Animal 1994; 18(3–4):110–115.

68. Silva LAF, Carneiro MI, Fioravanti MCS, et al. Creation of stallion teasers by shortening of the penis by circumcision. Arquivo Brasileiro de Medicina Veterinaria e Zoootecnia 1995; 47(6):789–798.

69. Rudman R. The social organisation of feral donkeys (Equus asinus) on a small Caribbean island (St. John, US Virgin Islands). Appl Anim Behav Sci 1998; 60(2–3):211–228.

70. Henry M, McDonnell SM, Lodi LD, Gastal EL. Pasture mating behaviour of donkeys (Equus asinus) at natural and induced oestrus. J Reprod Fert Suppl 1991; 44:77–86.

71. Henry M, Lodi LD, Gastal MMFO. Sexual behaviour of domesticated donkeys (Equus asinus) breeding under controlled or free range management systems. Appl Anim Behav Sci 1998; 60(2–3):263–276.

72. Taylor TS, Matthews NS. Mammoth asses – selected behavioural considerations for the veterinarian. Appl Anim Behav Sci 1998; 60(2–3):283–289.

73. McCort WD. The behavior and social organization of feral asses (Equus asinus) on Ossabaw Island, Georgia. Unpublished doctoral dissertation, The Pennsylvania State University, State College, 1980.

74. McDonnell SM. Reproductive behavior of donkeys (Equus asinus). Appl Anim Behav Sci 1998; 60(2–3):277–282.

75. Klug E, Bartmann CP, Gehlen H. Diagnosis and therapy of copulatory disorders in the stallion. Pferdeheilkunde 1999; 15(6):494–502.

76. Wallach SJR, Pickett BW, Nett TM. Sexual behaviour and serum concentrations of reproductive hormones in impotent stallions. Theriogenology 1983; 19(6):833–840.

77. Hurtgen JP. Breeding management of the Warmblood stallion. In: Samper JC, ed. Equine breeding and artificial insemination. London: WB Saunders; 2000.

78. Saslow CA. Understanding the perceptual world of horses. Appl Anim Behav Sci 2002; 78(2–4):209–224.

79. McDonnell SM. The equid ethogram: a practical field guide to horse behavior. Lexington, KT: The Blood Horse; 2003.

80. Boyd L. Behaviour problems of equids in zoos. Vet Clin North Am: Equine Pract: Behav 1986; 653–664.

81. Duncan P. Foal killing by stallions. Appl Anim Ethol 1982; 8:567–570.

82. Klingel H. Observations on social organization and behaviour of African and Asiatic Wild Asses (Equus africanus and Equus hemionus). Appl Anim Behav Sci 1998; 60(2–3):103–113.

83. Houpt KA, Keiper R. The position of the stallion in the equine hierarchy of feral and domestic ponies. J Anim Sci 1982; 54:945–950.

84. Shuster L, Dodman N. Basic mechanisms of compulsive and injurious behaviour. In: Dodman NH, L Shuster, eds. Psychopharmacology of animal behaviour disorder. Malden, MA: Blackwell Science; 1998:185–220.

85. Dinger JE, Noiles EE. Effect of controlled exercise on libido in 2-year-old stallions. J Anim Sci 1986; 62(5):1220–1223.

12

Behavior of the mare

SEXUAL MATURATION

The onset of puberty and reproductive activity during a filly's first ovulatory cycle is affected by her season of birth. Spring-born fillies tend to ovulate during the late Spring when they are 12–15 months old, whereas late-born fillies show surges of luteinizing hormone (LH) and progesterone that allow some (but not all) of them to display estrus and ovulate at younger ages.[1] When planes of nutrition are marginal, such as in the free-ranging state, puberty may not occur until the filly's third Spring.[2] Although fillies show a characteristic seasonal pattern of plasma follicle-stimulating hormone (FSH) and LH fluctuations even when ovariectomized, probably as a result of secretions by the adrenal cortex,[3] their breeding season appears to be shorter than that of adult mares.[1] In their free-ranging state, fillies usually seek contact with bachelor stallions or with unfamiliar harem stallions. When seeking sexual activity with resident, and therefore familiar harem stallions, fillies are likely to be ignored, especially if more mature mares are concurrently receptive. This allows subordinate stallions to consort with these young females and perform so-called 'sneak matings' (which are associated with low conception rates).

In terms of their social integration with other horses, mares can be categorised as being loyal to a single stallion, part of a multi-stallion band or social dispersers (females in transit, so-called mavericks).[4] Interestingly, compared with the mares in single-stallion bands, the disperser mares have been shown to have a greater parasite burden and poorer body condition despite spending a similar amount of time feeding.[4] Compared with all other mares, they also have the lowest fecundity and the greatest offspring mortality rates. A mare is thus much more likely to pass on her genes if she retains the companionship of at least one stallion. Beyond that, the stability of the mare–stallion relationship in single-stallion bands, with its resultant containment of agonistic behavior, contributes considerably to reproductive success and therefore biological fitness.[4,5]

Mares will regularly interfere with other mares during courtship and mating. The behavior of a mare in response to seeing another mare having contact with her stallion depends on her rank and reproductive state, being most obstructive when she is in estrus.[6]

In general, mares become increasingly receptive towards stallions as they age and will continue to breed until their early twenties.[7]

REPRODUCTIVE CYCLES

Being seasonally polyestrous, mares show a cyclical active estrus[8] (7.1 ± 4.2 days) and quiescent diestrus[8] (16.3 ± 2.9 days) throughout the breeding season[8] (152 ± 50 days). Season lengths become more restricted as one travels nearer the Poles.[7] Of all ungulates, horses have the most variable cycle length[9] and for this reason variations in estrous cycle are completely unreliable as a means of diagnosing ovarian dysfunction. Cycles, of which there are a mean of 7.2 ± 2.0 per year,[8] vary in length and behavior, with some mares showing a shift in temperament from normally placid disposition to irritability and vice versa. More common in fillies than in mares, protracted estrous periods of up to 50 days have been reported,[10] while their contraction as a result of veterinary examinations per rectum has also been noted.[11]

The duration of estrus decreases at the height of the breeding season (Fig. 12.1), the trend being matched by reciprocal increases in diestrus duration that keep the length of the whole cycle relatively constant.

Rejection of advances by stallions and relative disinterest in their company occurs during

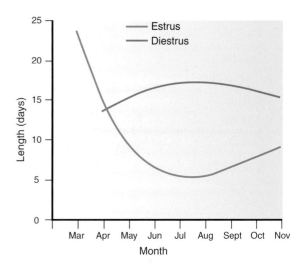

Figure 12.1 Variation of estrus and diestrus duration during the northern hemisphere breeding season. (After Ginther.[8] Redrawn, with permission, from Waring.[2])

diestrus and during periods of rising and high plasma progesterone concentrations.[12] A diestrous mare approached by a stallion becomes restless, switching her tail and flattening her ears as she threatens to kick, strike or bite (Fig. 12.2). Because behavioral responses associated with estrus may persist to varying extents in mares in anestrus,[13,14] it is important for stud personnel to take repeated measures of responses to teasing so that changes in frequency of responses, rather than the presence or absence of responses, can be monitored.

Even when a mare is receptive, squealing and strike threats may occur as a preliminary part of the nasal contact phase of a successful sexual encounter. Estrus in the mare is characterized by courtship behaviors such as abrupt halts during locomotion, approaching and following of stallions, lifting of the tail (before being mounted or after being mounted), clitoral winking (Fig. 12.3) especially during teasing, urinating (up to 21 urinations in an hour have been recorded[15]), and tolerance of the stallion's pre-copulatory behavior such as sniffing and nibbling. Depending to some extent on individual differences between mares, receptivity peaks 1–3 days prior to ovulation (although this has been disputed[16]). Above all, estrus in the mare is defined by her standing firmly with her tail up while being mounted.[13] Ovulation typically occurs

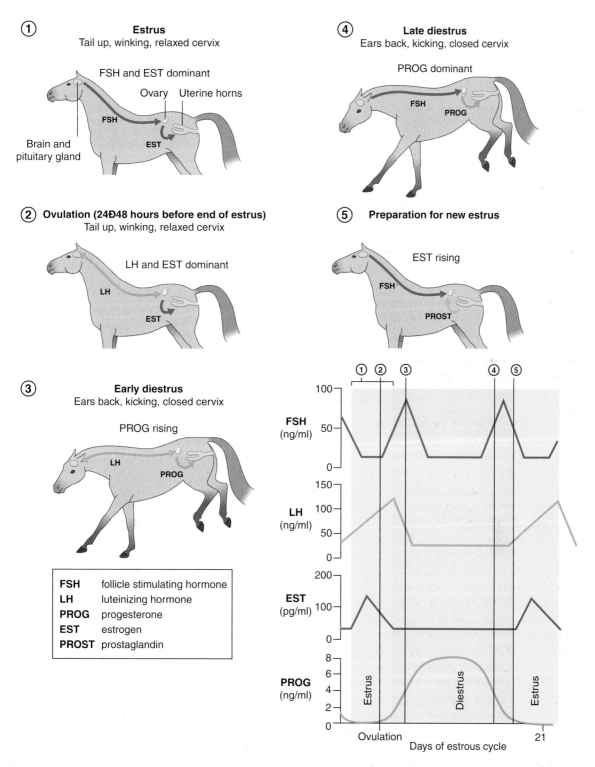

Figure 12.2 Illustration of the ways in which the mare's behavior changes throughout the estrous cycle. FSH, follicle-stimulating hormone; LH, luteinizing hormone; PROG, progesterone; EST, estrogen; PROST, prostaglandin. (After Noakes DE et al, eds; Arthur's veterinary reproduction and obstetrics; London: WB Saunders; 2001.)

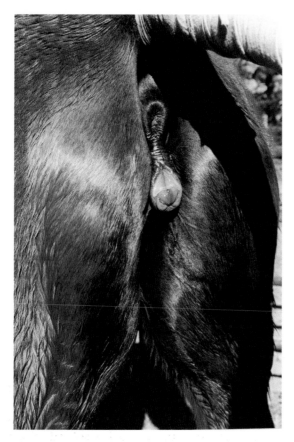

Figure 12.3 Clitoral winking in an estrous mare.

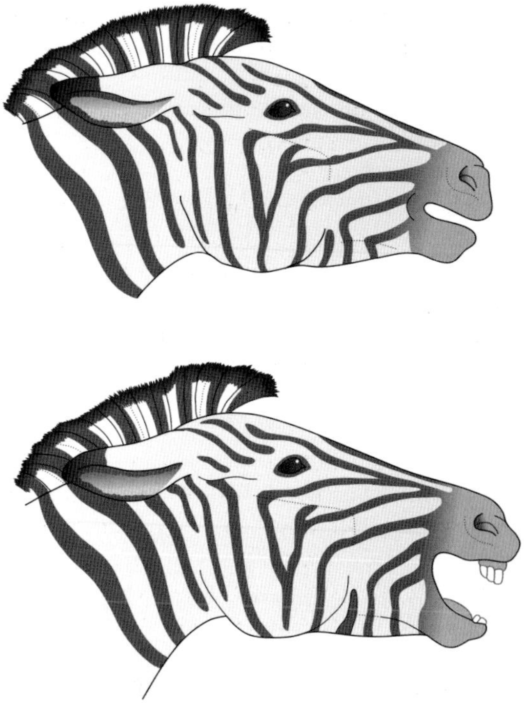

Figure 12.4 Drawing of two successive stages in the threatening *Rossigkeitsgesicht* response of a Grant's zebra (*E. burchelli boehmi*). (Redrawn from Waring GH, Wiersbowski S, Hafez EFE; The behaviour of horses; In: Hafez EFE, ed; Behaviour of domestic animals; 3rd edn; London: Baillière Tindall; 1975.)

36 hours before the end of estrus and is marked by the decline in the mare's receptivity.

Estrous mares frequently follow and place themselves in the vicinity of a stallion, especially if contact with him is intermittent.[6,17] If their solicitations are ignored they may display the estrous stance nearby periodically or, if this fails to attract the attentions of the harem stallion, they may disperse in search of other males. Occasional mares exhibit signs of colic during estrus to the extent that they are presented for bilateral ovariectomy.[18,19] There are also occasional instances of estrous mares mounting or being mounted by other mares.[2] Strangely, in Icelandic mares, this response is regarded as normal even when a stallion is present and is used by stud managers as an indication of early estrus. The estrous mares are almost always mounted, while the mounting is most usually performed by pregnant mares (Machteld van Dierendonck, personal communication 2002).

While prolonged tail-raising, the urination-like stance and clitoral winking in combination with the increased vascularity of the vaginal mucosae provide strong visual attractants for stallions, facial expressions in estrous mares have also been noted. Open mouths and bared teeth are common in the females of wild asses that adopt forced mating styles. Called 'Rossigkeitsgesicht' in zebras (Fig. 12.4), this accompanies the characteristic urination stance to contribute to the composite attractive signal to stallions.[20] The response is also seen in occasional mares,[21] with Standardbreds more likely to demonstrate it than Arabians.[22] Likened to the snapping response of juveniles in the presence of a threat, this response is interpreted by some observers as a sign of submission[2] or conflict[21] while others have demonstrated that it can elicit aggression from observing horses.[23]

Although pony mares have been described anecdotally as having more distinct ovulatory and anovulatory behaviors,[2] other data suggest that cold-blooded mares are more likely to have silent estrus than other breeds.[24] Meanwhile reduced antagonism to teasing when not in estrus and generally subdued manifestations of estrus are also reported in association with compromised thyroid function.[25] The average interval between the first signs of estrus and ovulation is 5.16 ± 2.65 days.[26]

Although they are irregular, estrous cycles are common in mules and the extent to which these hybrids are functionally infertile varies considerably.[27] Mules often have follicles that ovulate and luteinize but they generally lack oocytes (Lee Morris, personal communication 2002). Having said that, they do very occasionally bear live foals.[28]

The importance of auditory perception in eliciting typical estrous responses has been highlighted by studies of the relative effects on mares of audio recordings of the characteristic stallion nicker versus the presence of a stallion.[29] In response to these recordings, estrous mares, especially barren ones, showed overt estrous behavior including tail-raising, clitoral winking and abduction of the hindlegs. Maidens and mares with foals at foot exhibited some of these reactions but at a lower frequency. Although the usefulness of stallion vocalization recordings used in isolation in estrus detection has since been contested,[30] when used in combination with palpation of the inguinal region of mares this approach was reported to be 97% accurate.[31]

The length of courtship a mare receives from a harem stallion depends on her rank. A high-ranking mare may be courted by the harem stallion for several days before a series of matings takes place. Only then does she tolerate the stallion attending to other mares in the group.

During copulation the mare adopts a characteristic base-wide stance that helps her to balance. Although her neck is usually lowered, she remains very alert with her ears upright. She may look round slightly to monitor the stallion, especially

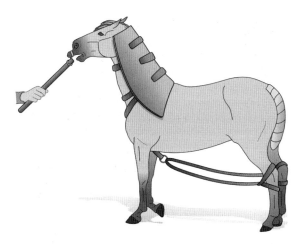

Figure 12.5 Restraint in the hand-bred mare often involves the use of a twitch and service hobbles which may alter her locomotory behavior and ability to signal. Meanwhile her appearance may be further affected by the use of a breeding cape to prevent her from being damaged by the stallion's teeth as they are used to grasp her neck, and by the use of tail wraps. It is not clear how much these interventions influence the mare's physiological stress response and the stallion's performance.

during ejaculation.[15] Dismounting is often assisted by the mare moving forward.[31] The couple remain reasonably close to one another after copulation and the mare continues to raise her tail and urinate until grazing and social interactions with others take priority.[32] In the free-ranging state, matings will occur approximately six times per heat in single stallion groups.[33] It is important that we recognize the many ways in which hand-breeding can so easily compromise a mare's ability to behave normally during courtship and copulation (Fig. 12.5).

ARTIFICIAL INFLUENCES ON THE BREEDING SEASON

It is broadly accepted that the breeding season imposed by humans on horses, most notably Thoroughbreds, is artificial and does not entirely coincide with most mares' maximal reproductive efficiency.[34] As a result, sexual receptivity without ovulation occurs during the early stages of the artificially advanced breeding season. The use of lights (not to mention GnRH, allyl-trenobolone or progesterone) to induce ovarian cycling is now commonplace and reasonably sophisticated but it necessitates the imposition of stabling and therefore may have deleterious effects on the social needs of mares. The imposition of artificial social groups is likely to have an effect on behavior since herd size is known to affect reproductive efficiency.[6]

The primary advantage of bringing mares into stables for exposure to 16 hours of artificial lighting is that it advances the onset of cyclicity early in the breeding season. In addition it facilitates supplementary feeding. Insufficient or inconsistent planes of nutrition may compromise sexual behavior and ovarian activity. [8,35,36]

It has been noted that a higher percentage of non-palpated mares conceive earlier in the breeding season compared with palpated mares,[11] but it is not clear whether a causal relationship exists or whether mares are more likely to be palpated because they are more likely to be failing to show behavioral manifestations of estrus. Follicular immaturity leading to behavioral estrus without ovulation (so-called 'spring estrus'), an ovarian dysfunction diagnosed in as many as 40% of infertile mares, is one of the most common causes of infertility in the horse and has been associated with unsatisfactory nutrition or management.[9] The most common cause of infertility is pregnancy loss.[37]

The length of estrous periods in a managed context is longer than in the free-ranging state, apparently because of the psychic effect of the separation of mares and stallions.[9] Data on herd mating activities suggest that stallions are twice as active sexually during 0600–0800 and 1600–1800 hours than during 1800–0600 and 0800–1600 hours.[38] Perhaps, as efforts are made to reduce the effects on horses of intensive management, the times of day at which stallions and mares are joined for breeding purposes should be brought into line with these times of peak natural activity.

While transportation induces hormonal and ascorbic acid responses indicative of stress,[39] it does not alter estrous behavior, ovulation, duration of the estrous cycle, pregnancy rate or preovulatory surges of estradiol and LH.[40] Artificial influences on fertility also include attempts at birth control, most notably in feral populations. Single inoculations with microspheres of porcine zona pellucida vaccine have reduced feral mares' reproductive rate to approximately 11%, a finding that offers support for alternatives to culling.[41]

FOAL HEATS

Characterized by their intensity as well as their association with diarrhea in the foal, foal heats occur on average 8 days after parturition[42] as a result of a decline in the blood progesterone: estradiol concentration ratio that begins at the time of parturition, and an initial surge followed by pulsatile releases of LH post-partum.[43] While free-ranging mares have been observed mating within hours of foaling,[2] most ovulate between 4 and 18 days post-partum. Similarly, mares display estrus 2–6 days after injections of exogenous prostaglandins (5 mg PGF2α, i.m.), given to induce abortions.[44] Daily progesterone injections have been used to delay the onset of foal heats.[45] Meanwhile the beta-blocker propanolol has been reported to increase the exhibition of foal heat and the pregnancy rate at this heat. The mechanism for this effect is thought to involve increased myometrial motility and enhanced uterine involution.[46]

SILENT HEATS

It is recognized that ovulation may occasionally occur without behavioral heat.[9] Approximately 6% of ovulations occur without overt signs of estrus.[8] Some mares are predisposed to such silent heats (also known as sub-estrus) without any disruption of their cyclicity. The role of social rank in mares' behavior at estrus is not as clear as that of cattle, but it appears that high-ranking mares may bully subordinates when in estrus. Mares that show no sign of cycling (see the case study at the end of this chapter) should have their diets investigated as part of a full clinical work-up that includes gynecological and endocrinological investigations.

SPLIT HEATS

When a mare exhibits behavioral estrus that is transiently interrupted by an uncharacteristically brief period of quiescence, she is said to have had a split heat. This phenomenon occurs with reasonable frequency (12% of ovulations[8]) and as such justifies at least daily teasing in commercial breeding operations. Meanwhile, the appearance of a prolonged estrus may arise in oliguric mares secondary to irritation caused by the persistent presence of urine.[2]

ANESTRUS

In late Autumn and Winter, most (but not all) mares become sexually dormant and are said to have entered anestrus (214 ± 50 days[8]). Entry into anestrus can be considered complete if a mare does not exhibit cyclic estrous behavior, has no follicles with a diameter of 25 mm or larger, and has progesterone at levels of <1 ng/ml for at least 39 days.[47] The transition into the breeding season occurs once a threshold in LH concentration within the anterior hypothalamus is reached.[48] Meanwhile, the onset of individual estrous cycles may be delayed by psychological influences over behavioral activity, spontaneously persistent luteal function, endometritis and granulosa cell tumours.[34]

THE INFLUENCE OF HORMONES AND EXOGENOUS FACTORS ON REPRODUCTIVE BEHAVIOR

Hormonal control of ovulation can be achieved by the use of exogenous steroids with or without prostaglandins.[49] Estrous displays can be induced by the administration of exogenous steroids.[49] For example, estradiol elicits soliciting behavior within 4 hours of injection, while progesterone usually results in the absence of sexual behavior.[3,50] Altrenogest can be given orally to regulate estrous behavior early in the year, and its withdrawal will synchronize estrus in cycling mares and those previously exposed to artificial light.[51] Conversely it has been suggested that endometrial edema as appreciated by ultrasonography may indicate the optimal time for coitus and provide an instant indication that the basal level of progesterone is <1 mg/ml.[52] But estrus is not purely a product of hormonal flux, since estrous behavior reflects a combination of other factors including the presence

of a stallion, social rank and duration of teasing. For example, when mares are stimulated by restrained teasers, their estrous display lengthens.[9] Similarly, failure of estrus can often be due to the absence of exogenous factors such as odors, sounds, sight and touch[9] that arise, for example, with appropriate attention from stallions.

PREGNANCY

The gestation period of the mare is approximately 11 months or 340 days, with generally slightly shorter periods in smaller breeds.[53] Gestation duration in a large study of Australian Thoroughbreds[54] (n = 522) ranged from 315 to 387 days (mean 342.3 days). The survival rate of Thoroughbred foals delivered at less than 320 days of gestation is approximately 5%.[55]

Factors that influence the duration of a mare's gestation include her plane of nutrition towards the end of her pregnancy and the sex of the foal. Howell & Rollins[56] found that mares on higher planes of nutrition tend to foal earlier than those on maintenance diets. In the free-ranging state, mares normally foal in mid to late Spring, a strategy that usually ensures sufficient feed is available for lactation. By showing that foals conceived in early Spring had longer gestations than those conceived in mid to late Spring, Hintz et al[57] confirmed the importance of seasonal effects on the biological fitness of foals (a similar trend was reported by Campitelli et al[58]). The sex of the foal contributes to the duration of gestation, in that fillies are generally born 1–2 days before colts.[54] Mares lose more condition prenatally when carrying a colt if they were originally in good condition at the time of conception, but more when carrying a filly if they were in poor condition.[59]

While some mares become actively aggressive to approaching stallions during pregnancy, others may remain friendly[60] and raise the suspicion that they are returning to estrus. After between 40 and 70 days of pregnancy, follicles are produced in response to eCG.[61] They are generally large in size and remain active, ovulating to form accessory corpora lutea. Estrogen produced from these follicles is thought to prompt some pregnant mares to consort with stallions and exhibit some estrous behavior during the first trimester of pregnancy. The response occurs more frequently in mares bearing female foals than in those bearing males.[62] Up to 35% of ovariectomized mares,[18] and also mares in an anovulatory period, show sexual responsiveness.[1,3] This suggests that mares' ability to dissociate sexual behavior from ovulation may persist even when they are pregnant. However, these manifestations (which may occur a mean 1.76 times per pregnancy[38]) are not all of the usual potency associated with ovulation. Asa[17] suggests that non-reproductive sex may serve to influence stallions to remain with their bands during the non-breeding season.

Asa et al[61] examined the effect of adding a stallion to an established group of 12 pregnant pony mares. After the experimental introduction of stallions into random harem groups, full estrous behavior was not observed. Instead, only weak signs of estrus were noted, with only four mountings recorded and only a single tail raised. Social interactions such as grooming between the mares increased, while the only approach between mares and the stallion was an initial ritual greeting early on in each exposure.

FOALING

Although the behavior of the mare does not change markedly in the months leading to parturition, significant differences arise immediately before foaling.[2,61] Shaw et al[63] examined mare behavior 2 weeks prior to parturition. A total of 52 pregnant mares in box stalls were observed at 30-minute intervals between 1800 hours and 0600 hours. In the 2 weeks before foaling, mares spent 66.8% of their time standing, 27% eating, 4.9% lying in sternal recumbency, 1% lying in lateral recumbency and only 0.3% walking. Challenging the notion that the mare reduces her ingestive activities immediately prior to parturition,[9,60] eating was the only behavior unaffected by the imminent foaling. On the night of foaling, mares spent less time (53.3%) standing and more time in sternal (8%) and lateral (5.3%) recumbency and walking (5.3%).[63]

This reflects the restlessness of mares when they are about to foal and the fact that they almost always choose to foal in a recumbent position (a phenomenon that led to the development of foaling belts that can detect recumbency).

In their free-ranging state, mares about to foal often become parted from the herd either by seeking relative isolation (sometimes accompanied by older offspring or another adult mare) or by being left behind. Along with the other peri-parturient behaviors, this strategy provides a nurturing environment for the foal and helps to avoid mis-mothering, in accordance with the 'binding theory' offered by Klingel.[64] Average time spent walking tends to increase on the day of birth (most notably the 30 minutes prior to parturition), with higher-ranking mares tending to try to separate themselves furthest from the herd, and maiden mares remaining reasonably close.[65,66] Mares confined in a box stall, on the other hand, may be required to foal within auditory, olfactory and visual contact of other mares. They are often described as being alert, uneasy and restless before parturition.[9] This may be due, at least in part, to the thwarting of their motivation to separate themselves by locomotion. While physiological changes include the swelling of the teats, distension of the udder and the softening of the cervix, behavior changes may also include swinging and rubbing of the tail against fixed objects as the vulva becomes relatively flaccid.[60]

It seems that regardless of the bond they may have with particular personnel, most mares prefer not to foal in the presence of humans and, perhaps in a bid to ensure isolation, may delay foaling by prolonging the initial stage of parturition.[2,63] When left undisturbed, most mares foal at night (e.g. in Shaw et al's study[63] 86% foaled between 1800 and 0600 hours), presumably as a means of avoiding daytime predators. Fraser[9] proposes that colts are born later in the night than fillies and rather unconvincingly suggests that this is for the 'good of the species' since fewer males are required for reproductive success of a group. There is evidence that the percentage of night births is higher in Spring than in Winter[58] although others report that seasonal daylength and onset of darkness have no effect on the mean time of foaling.[67]

Continual disturbance, especially at night may adversely affect the onset of foaling.[67] On many studs, laudable attempts to minimize human interference and reduce the imposition of unnatural delays include the use of one-way mirrors and video surveillance equipment. However, the avoidance response seen in most mares during foaling is by no means universal. Some mares even appear to seek human company at this time.[60] It would be interesting to see how attempts to 'imprint' fillies (see Ch. 4) affect their responses to humans when peri-parturient.

Immediately prior to parturition the behavior of the mare increasingly involves stretching, yawning, repeated recumbency and standing, walking, tail-swishing, kicking, looking at flanks, pawing at bed, crouching, straddling and kneeling. These responses all imply that the mare is undergoing abdominal discomfort[9] and may last from a few minutes to hours.[2] Patchy sweating on the flanks and girth area indicates that first-stage labor is about to commence. This and the persistent raising of the tail seen at this stage gave rise to the emergence of parturition detectors (e.g. as described by Bueno et al[68]).

Depending on their force and timing, contractions induce different responses in the mare.[60] With modest contractions the mare may swish her tail or stamp a hindleg. Larger, more powerful contractions cause her to become transiently tucked up in the flank or to lift her tail over her back and lean backwards onto her hindlegs.

The rupturing of the placenta and the escape of the allantoic fluid that indicate the second stage of parturition usually take place before the mare lies down (a response often accompanied by the greatest passage of fluid) in preparation for forceful and repeated straining. Some mares may investigate the fluid and consequently exhibit flehmen and occasionally nicker.[10] Sternal recumbency is commonly adopted but it is not unusual for the mare to stand and reposition herself repeatedly, especially if she is disturbed.[69] Vigorous rolling is also reasonably common and is thought to represent attempts to correctly position the foal. The foal's forelegs either side of or to one side of its head engage in the vagina, then may emerge from the vulva covered by a veil of amniotic membrane (Fig. 12.6).

Straining efforts, numbering between 60 and 100 (n = 5), are required especially to expel the foal's forequarters and head.[69] Data from Thoroughbreds suggest that compared with experienced brood mares, maidens spend slightly longer in second-stage labor (mean of 21 minutes for primiparae versus the mean of 18 for experienced mares[70]), while pony mares take an average of 12 minutes.[71] Foals from primiparous mares are considered to be at high risk of thoracic trauma.[72] The final expulsion is usually achieved with the mare in lateral recumbency with legs extended. Expulsive efforts may cause the mare's upper hindlimb to become raised. With the emergence of the foal's head, forelimbs and hips, the second stage of parturition is complete. Unless disturbed, the mare then usually remains in lateral recumbency, often with the foal's hindlimbs still in the vagina.

The third and final stage of parturition involves the transfusion of blood from the placenta to the foal during the post-partum pause and the passage of the placenta.[9] If parturition occurs without difficulty then, after the post-partum pause which allows blood to leave the placenta and reach the foal,[73] the foal will free itself of fetal membranes by raising its head and sever the foal's umbilical cord as it moves away from the mare.

Third-stage labor is marked by signs of abdominal discomfort, including looking at the flanks, sweating and pawing – behaviors that seem to have a stimulating effect on many observing neonates. Approximately 1 hour after delivery of the foal, the placenta is expelled, often as the mare rises from a bout of rolling. Mares typically show some olfactory investigation of the membranes, which elicit flehmen responses and occasionally some perfunctory nibbling. In the free-ranging state, the mare and foal leave the site of foaling soon after the placenta is discharged. This is thought to contribute to biological fitness by avoiding predators that may be attracted by the odors of the fluids and membranes passed during parturition. It also marks the mare's return to the relative safety of her herd, which may be seen moving towards the fresh dyad to investigate. High-ranking mares have been observed to take longer to rejoin their affiliates than subordinates.[65]

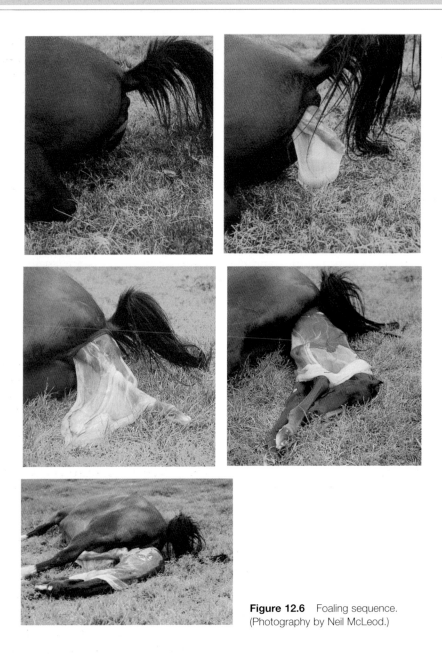

Figure 12.6 Foaling sequence.
(Photography by Neil McLeod.)

MATERNAL–INFANT INTERACTIONS

THE MATERNAL–INFANT BOND

Interactions between the mare and her newborn foal enhance the bond between them and contribute to biological fitness by facilitating the survival and full development of the foal. Bonding in the first few days is critical to the foal's survival because this is when mortality is at its highest.[74,75] The mare–foal bond seems to grow at the expense of the bond between the mare and her herd affiliates.[76] Indeed new dams put a distance between themselves and other adults, perhaps to reduce outside interference in

Behavior	Mean time after parturition (minutes)
Umbilical cord rupture	6.2
Suckling reflex	36
Standing	49[a]
First suckling	94[b]
Elimination of the meconium	127

[a]All foals stood up within 2 hours 23 minutes of parturition.[79]
[b]83% of foals suckled within 2 hours of parturition.[79]

the bonds they are forming with their offspring.[76] It is interesting to note that the attachment between primiparous mares and their male offspring (as estimated by the number of times colts return to their natal bands after dispersal) is significantly stronger than dam–filly combinations.[77]

Contact with the mare and urination along with various other behaviors listed in Tables 7.1. and 7.2 have been used to score foal health so that veterinary attention can be requested for those showing subnormal development or viability.[78] In addition the mean times taken by Thoroughbred foals[79] (n = 390) to perform key behaviors are shown in Table 12.1.

Soon after birth the mare begins to lick her foal, and any surface bearing amniotic fluid, and continues with some intensity for approximately 30 minutes.[2] This dries the foal, stimulates respiratory effort and blood flow and finally stimulates the foal to stand; it may also provide the mare with sensory information for later use via olfaction, allowing her to discern her foal from the others in the herd.[80] This function relies on the link between gustation and olfaction since horses do not lick one another during greetings, in contrast to many ruminants and carnivores. Having said that, the number of times a mare licks her foal is not an effective predictor of the quality of bonding between the two.[80] Once the mare has groomed the foal, removed the placental material and passed the placenta, suckling occurs. The mare assists the foal in locating the teats and may even push the foal towards them. The foal is innately driven to locate the teat and suckle – a response refined by learning. The suckling response can be stimulated by tactile stimuli around the muzzle and mouth, which cause the tongue to protrude. The foal displays this sucking behavior even before it stands.[81] Approximately 5% of foals need human assistance to suck[9] but intervention is scarcely warranted before 3 hours, since some foals, especially heavier ones, take this long to suckle naturally.[10]

Although the time the foal takes to stand is related to the time taken by the mare to expel the fetal membranes,[58] the physical interaction of the mare and foal begins immediately after parturition. Barber & Crowell-Davis[82] found that during the first day of life, upright foals and their mothers spent 96% of their time within 1 meter of each other. Ingestion of colostrum during the first few days of life is pivotal because the foal's intestine is capable of macromolecular uptake only until the foal is approximately 36 hours old.[83]

In the free-ranging state, it normally takes 2 weeks of close proximity and frequent interactions for the foal and mare to consolidate their bond.[80,84] The spatial relationship within the dyad can be characterized by the number of 'approaches' and 'partings' made by either member.[85] Although initially the mare's bond with the foal is much stronger than vice versa, foals do more work to maintain contact with their dams, but this tendency declines as they approach weaning age.[86]

The spatial distribution of the mare and foal is determined by the posture of the foal, in terms of whether it is recumbent or upright.[82] Until they reach 21 weeks of age, foals rest in a recumbent position for longer than adults do (this is possible because of their different ventilation:perfusion quotients), and this, among other features of foal behavior, influences the extent to which their dams are likely to move away during this time. For example, during the first week of life, foals spend approximately 32% of their time in recumbent rest,[87] and so dams tend to approach and remain with newborn foals more than with older foals. Perhaps because of its perceived vulnerability, a mare spends a greater amount of time near her foal when it is recumbent (Fig. 12.7) but seems to relax when it is in an upright position. Grazing behavior of the mare is seen mostly when the foal

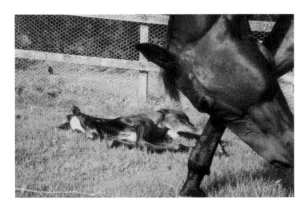

Figure 12.7 When a foal is recumbent its dam remains particularly close. (Photograph courtesy of Kate Ireland.)

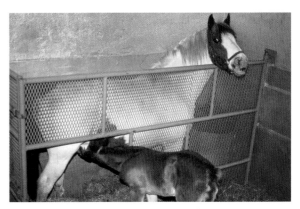

Figure 12.8 A fostering gate with hatch that can be closed to prevent overindulgence by hungry foals. (Photograph courtesy of Amanda Kelly McCreery.)

is standing; when the foal is recumbent the mare spends most of her time resting upright.

Generally, foals will return to their dams whenever they have encountered a novel or aversive stimulus. This allows them to maximize their safety and to feed in a bid to supplement energy expended during flight responses. The positive reinforcement that occurs when foals suckle after returning to their dams also helps to consolidate the bond necessary for success in follower species.[80] Additionally, the mare provides protection for the foal and will herd it away from disturbances that may interfere with the bond. Dams use the unique calls of their foal to locate them when the pair is parted.[84]

FOSTERING

Because a mare normally allows only her own foal to suckle, orphan foals must be introduced to surrogate mothers with tremendous tact. The bonding that occurs as a result of the licking and nuzzling in the first hours of life is tremendously important. If a foal is separated from its dam (for experimental hand-rearing) within a few hours of birth, the reunion with its mother several months later is significantly different to its interactions with other mares.[88] Rather than relying on chance to provide lactating mares that have lost their own foals, horse breeding centers are refining the process of nurse mare husbandry.

That said, this remains an area that merits considerable empirical study. Good nurse mares can rear up to three foals in a year, their first and own foal being removed after approximately 1 month.

To offer the mare some gratification from being suckled, the udder is allowed to become distended with milk by muzzling the mare's own foal. It is common to apply a blindfold to nurse mares before removing their own foals. The orphan can then be introduced and is encouraged to suckle. Once it has begun to drink, the blindfold can be removed. Scratching the mare's withers and feeding her are effective distractions during the introduction, while the safety of the foal can be optimized by the use of a fostering gate (Fig. 12.8), preferably one that the mare has previously come to associate with nursing her own foal and being fed.

The use of such a gate is not advised unless the mare has been thoroughly acclimatized. Some mares resist this level of confinement, and the ensuing struggle can be very dangerous for the mare, the foal and personnel. Furthermore some mares placed behind the gates become very preoccupied with getting out. A less obtrusive approach that is worth employing when the mare can be supervised is to place bales at the side of the mare to reduce the extent to which she is able to kick the foal. The potential for these adverse responses highlights the need for well-planned training programs for foster mares.

Regardless of the type of restraint used to render a foster or biological mother safe, it is advisable to habituate the mare to the apparatus before it is used to restrain her in the presence of a foal.[89] For mares that kick rather than bite, hobbles may be worth trying, but again the mare must learn that struggling is fruitless before such restraint is used in the presence of a foal. Deep bedding is obligatory whenever hobbles are used (see Ch. 14).

Foals use vision and olfaction to recognize their dams.[90] However, because olfaction is the chief sense a mare uses to recognize her foal, it is important, in the short term, to reduce a surrogate mother's ability to discriminate odors and to disguise the odor of the foal. The mare's use of vision to recognize her foal develops once the olfactory tags are in place, and therefore the visual cues offered by the foal are of secondary importance in the early stages of fostering.[91] If facilities are available, it is worth freezing the amniotic membranes from any foaling in case they are needed as an olfactory cue to be draped over the orphan for fostering. Often it is more practical to mask an introduced foal's odor by smearing it with the prospective surrogate dam's own milk and applying her own feces to its tailhead. Vaporous ointments are also sometimes applied to the nostrils of nurse mares prior to the removal of their own foals.

Probably because they are rewarded by the relief of udder pressure, mares accept foals within 1 to 12 hours of introduction, but it is not advisable to leave the pair unsupervised until they have been together for 3 days.[92] It is believed that, once it has passed through the foal's intestines, the characteristic odor of a mare's own digested milk is the key stimulant that mares must detect before the artificial maternal–infant bond is cemented.

Happily there are some mares who will readily nurse more than one foal. For example, some feral horses or Przewalski horses occasionally suckle their new-born foal and one or two older siblings. There are also accounts of mares that, having lost their foals, will suckle other foals (orphaned or otherwise) (Machteld van Dierendonck, personal communication 2002). Clearly these types of mares are more likely to accept a surrogate foal. At the other end of the spectrum, some ambivalent surrogate mothers and those that have been treated for the signs of rejecting their foals may merely tolerate their foals for a matter of weeks before relapsing into active aggression.[93] The responsibility to nurture the bond between mother and infant is not entirely the mare's. Foals that fail to show sufficient attachment to their dams may prompt reciprocal ignorance and ultimately rejection.[94]

Lactation can be induced in non-pregnant, non-parturient mares via a combination of estradiol, progesterone and a dopamine antagonist (sulpiride).[95] Fostering latencies can be shortened in mares treated with this hormone cocktail, if they receive two 3-minute periods of vaginal–cervical stimulation because, it is believed, a release of oxytocin is triggered by this manipulation.[95]

Cardinal signs of successful fostering bond include the mare standing over the foal when it is recumbent and protecting it from other horses. Interestingly the approach of a teaser seems to have the effect of consolidating the bond in some cases where the mare seems unconvinced of her attachment to the introduced foal.[92] The introduction of a large dog is said to have a similar effect in stimulating maternal defensiveness.[93]

SUCKLING

Time spent sucking is a poor indicator of milk intake in foals because some suckling may be non-nutritive.[96] When the availability and quality of milk is compromised (e.g. because of a reduced food intake by the dam) it is more likely to manifest itself in colts than in fillies.[97] Given that the interval between births increases after a mare has reared a colt, it would appear that it may be more costly to raise sons than daughters.[97] As described earlier, dams in better condition generally favor sons whereas those in worse condition favor daughters.[59]

Intriguingly the parity of a mare can influence her foal's future. For example, fascinating insights into the relationship between age of a dam and the racing success of her offspring have led to the radical suggestion that mares should be removed from stud once they pass their reproductive peak, i.e. at the age of about 12–15 years.[98]

The number of sucklings peaks at approximately 48 hours, with a concurrent increase in grazing.[99] In the first 8 weeks of life, colts spend 40% more time suckling than fillies, a strategy that presumably helps them to compensate for their performing significantly more locomotory activity and interactive play.[100] In early lactation, the foal usually adopts a position parallel to the dam for a concerted suckling session,[101] while any position may be adopted if the drink is brief. A mare will often nuzzle and groom the foal as it drinks. This affirms the bond between them in the long term but may also reduce the likelihood of the foal being disturbed by extraneous stimuli.

It has been stated that the time spent in each suckling bout does not vary significantly with age.[102] This may be because gastric volume increases at a similar rate to sucking strength and thus the volume that must be consumed for satiation can be consumed with appropriate speed (Fig. 12.9). The frequency of nursing bouts decreases rapidly from 7/hour during the first week of life and then continues to gradually decline until the 17th week (Fig. 12.9).[81,103] Generally, successful sucking bouts outweigh unsuccessful ones throughout the suckling period. Barber & Crowell-Davis[82] state that nuzzling with no attempts to suckle may act as a comforting behavior for both the mare and foal.

The teats of the mare can become extremely sensitive around the time of parturition, and this may make a dam transiently reluctant to allow her foal to suckle. Maternal aggression is seen when the foal is nudging at the udder before suckling. Once the foal begins to suck, the mare is rarely aggressive towards it. It has been suggested that mares employ a number of strategies to hinder suckling activity during weeks 2 and 3, perhaps because suckling is painful at this time.[81,82] Notwithstanding agonistic behavior during this sensitive period, the mare and foal show complementary behaviors that ensure the foal receives adequate nutrition. For example, mares appear to initiate nursing bouts by approaching the foal and standing nearby. A mare can also facilitate nursing by adopting a slouching stance with her hindlegs that tilts the udder to the side on which her foal is standing (Fig. 12.10).

Mild aggression by the mare during the post-suck portion of the bout is frequently associated with the nuzzling activity of the foal. Waring[2] notes that a mare, especially with offspring less than 1 week old, will terminate a nursing bout by rocking her hindquarters, an activity that seems to prompt the foal to move its head away.

Lactation compromises the body condition of mares, which in any case is generally poorer than that of stallions.[104] Especially in late lactation, mares play an active role in regulating the time spent suckling, by simply walking away from the foal.[100] As the foal matures, maternal aggression tends to increase and often initiates brief bouts of mother-directed foal aggression.[103]

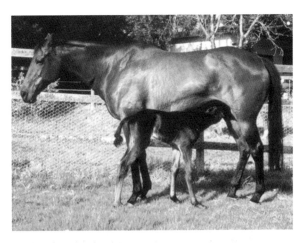

Figure 12.10 By resting the contralateral hind leg, a mare can help the foal locate the udder. (Photograph courtesy of Kate Ireland.)

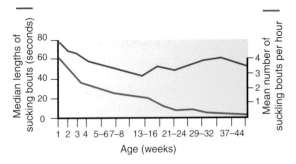

Figure 12.9 Changes with age in the length of sucking bouts and the number of bouts of nursing. (After Tyler.[32])

Waring[2] states that, in a box stall, the foal is more likely to nurse on one side of the mare than the other. However, the observation of preference is rarely recorded in the free-ranging state and has not been examined experimentally. It may be that the walls of the box prompt lateralization of the mare's behavior.

OTHER MATERNAL BEHAVIORS

There are frequent interactions between a mare and her foal during play. Initially the mare is the main focus of the offspring's activities.[2] The mare endures the nibbling, kicking and pawing antics of her offspring but shows little playful activity herself. The focus of the foal's activity shifts from its mother to other companions (especially peers) from approximately the first 7–8 weeks of life, and the time spent playing steadily increases over this same period (see Ch. 10). As the foal ages and becomes gentler towards the mare, she may respond to the foal's playful overtures by nibbling, often resulting in mutual grooming. Play between foals and mares (especially older ones) that are not their mothers is rarely seen.

WEANING

Individual mares show differing amounts of maternal aggression. Waring[2] noted that as foals age, the mares become more aggressive towards them. Maternal aggression seems to peak as the foal's primary source of nutrition shifts from mother's milk to grass (see Ch. 8). Aggression may negatively reinforce grazing behavior in the foal (see Ch. 4) and hence facilitate the change in diet.

Regardless of the sex of the foal, suckling occurs for 35–40 weeks in pregnant multiparous mares, with weaning usually taking place 15 weeks before the next foaling.[100] However, weaning may take place as close as 8 weeks to the next foaling.[105] Occasionally, suckling by the previous year's foal may be permitted even though a new foal is at foot.[106] Towards the end of the weaning process the mare may drive her foal away when it attempts to suckle. Primiparous mares lactate for longer and wean 5 weeks closer to the next foaling than multiparous mares.[100] In the free-ranging state, weaning is a gradual process characterized by dietary changes in the foal and the social dislocation of mother and offspring. Additionally, since weaning is usually followed shortly by the arrival of a new foal it is accompanied by an abrupt shift of the mare's attention and social activity away from her previous offspring. In a study of Misaki feral horses, 17 of 22 dispersing colts and 29 of 39 dispersing fillies left their natal groups around the birth of their siblings.[107]

The spatial separation of mare and foal at enforced weaning thwarts comfort-seeking and -giving responses by the dyad and therefore contributes to the behavioral and physiological stress response displayed by both the mare and her foal.[99] Behavioral changes associated with physical separation of the mare and foal may include an increase in vocalization, aggression and physical activity (e.g. walking around a stall, yard, paddock, etc.) as well as a reduction in appetite – responses that diminish with time post-weaning. The effects of weaning on ingestive behavior are considered in Chapter 8.

MANAGEMENT PRACTICES PRIOR TO WEANING

Handling and feeding practices prior to weaning have been developed primarily to reduce the effects of weaning and post-weaning stress.

Handling

Because horses of all ages can show signs of distress when separated from their group, a system that provides some form of habituation program that may help foals to avoid separation-related distress at weaning and in later life merits scientific investigation.

Pre-weaning handling regimes designed to ameliorate foals' flight responses in the presence of humans and increase the ease with which foals can be managed have had mixed results. Results have ranged from failing to have any effect[108] through to foals displaying a marked improvement in their manageability.[109] Similarly the optimal pre-weaning age at which to begin handling foals in order to enhance learning ability or manageability has yet to be determined (see Ch. 4).[108]

Feeding

An abrupt change of diet is thought to contribute to the distress of weaning. The behavioral response of anorexia and related increases in cortisol concentration may result in weight loss and possibly an increased susceptibility to disease. Post-weaning anorexia can even result in death.[110] Hence the appeal of pre-weaning creep feed and partial weaning that allows the foal to contact its dam through the fenceline.[110] The advantage of feeding concentrates to reduce weaning stress may be linked to their mineral contents. Thus supplementary concentrates may help foals meet increased requirements for phosphorus, iron and zinc. These elements are thought to help combat physical effects of fatigue, trauma and infection often associated with weaning.[111]

Foals accustomed to eating concentrates prior to weaning are more likely to maintain their feed intake throughout the early post-weaning period. Foals that have received a feed concentrate before undergoing weaning, in addition to the available pasture and mother's milk, have been observed exhibiting fewer stress-related behaviors at the time of weaning than foals that did not receive any concentrate before weaning.[112] Access to pre-weaning creep feed resulted in less activity than no pre-weaning creep feed, but no change in vocalization frequency.[113] This may be because, if it has been established as a relevant substrate, creep feed offered after weaning may allow the foal to redirect its oral behavioral needs so that it eats instead of trotting round in attempts to rejoin its dam. The persistence of vocalization, however, suggests that the motivation to rejoin the dam is similar to that of control foals that were not offered creep feed.

Using an adrenocorticotropic hormone (ACTH) challenge, Hoffman et al[111] monitored serum cortisol responses in foals on a pasture, hay and concentrate diet compared with foals fed a pasture and hay diet. Both diets had comparable energy and protein levels that exceeded maintenance requirements. Foals receiving the pasture and hay diet exhibited a poorer response to the challenge, possibly as a result of adrenal depletion arising from protracted distress. These foals also exhibited behavioral indications of distress, with more vocalization and less rest. However, despite its apparent appeal and the frequent need for supplementation because of poor pasture, caution should be used when considering the inclusion of concentrates in diets of youngsters before and after weaning (see Ch. 8). Sympathetic weaning should focus on providing a smooth transition from milk to grass and the tactful introduction of concentrated diets, preferably those least likely to precipitate problems of gastric acidity. Creep feeding has recently been identified as an important cause of oral stereotypies such as wind-sucking and crib-biting[114] and is likely to become less popular unless diets that counter associated gastrointestinal symptoms can be formulated.

MANAGEMENT PRACTICES AT WEANING

The practice of weaning is itself likely to cause profound stress that may compromise immune responses. Furthermore it seems likely that there could be long-lasting effects of weaning method and age at weaning on learning ability.[115]

Horses are commonly weaned at 4–6 months of age,[105] and Thoroughbred breeders tend to wean earliest. Best practice in weaning should aim to reduce distress in foals to avoid the consequent need for them to adopt coping styles that include stereotypic and overt redirected behaviors. Although some weaning techniques depend on there being a more than one mare–foal dyad, a number of approaches to artificial weaning exist. Foals can be isolated entirely, penned in pairs, or they can remain in a larger natal group that has mares gradually removed from it. A number of studies (referred to below) have attempted to measure the distress involved in these techniques.

Foals weaned abruptly show greater signs of stress than foals weaned more gradually.[105,111,113,116,117] Studies have shown that group weaning has clear benefits for the foals when compared with complete isolation.[113,118,119] A pre-weaning practice that uses familiarity rather than habituation to blunt the response to the final separation of mare and foal involves the abrupt removal of mares from foals when running in a herd situation.[120] In this system the foals are left together without their dams but in familiar surroundings.

When the behavioral developments of 218 foals were tracked for 4 years,[121] informal observations about the effects of isolation were confirmed. The risk of developing stereotypies was greater in foals weaned individually than in group-weaned foals.[121] While this study showed the prevalence of locomotory stereotypies such as box-walking and weaving to be similar to that found in previous surveys, it found twice as much crib-biting and wind-sucking as expected. Having said that, the median age of onset of weaning was 60 weeks, the median age of onset of crib-biting was only 20 weeks, i.e. before weaning. This indicated that the physical act of weaning had less impact than the change in diet from milk to solids. Additionally, at this age, a highly significant risk factor for the development of oral stereotypies was the feeding of concentrates. After weaning, foals given concentrate feeds were four times more likely to crib-bite than foals on grass-only diets (see Ch. 8).

Significantly, the study showed that many youngsters begin to weave after they have been sold from the stud to new homes.[121] Therefore we should recognize two discrete distressing episodes in the life of most young horses: the distress of nutritional weaning and the distress associated with dispersal.

WEANING METHODS

Confinement at the time of weaning is associated with a rise in the frequency of aberrant behaviors including pawing, bucking, rearing and kicking at the walls of the stable which may also be the target of licking and chewing behaviors.[119] These responses seem to reflect thwarted kinetic and foraging needs. Partial separation of the mare and foal that allows fenceline contact is associated with less vocalization and locomotion than total separation.[113] Abrupt separation is therefore losing favor in studs that can group mares and foals together and subsequently withdraw individual mares from the group. It would be good to see online liaison services that would allow small-scale breeders to employ the same system by putting them in touch with one another and thus allow them to coordinate weaning of their foals.

Because of the social attachments formed between foals within peer groups, it is believed a familiar companion will ease the stress associated with weaning.[2] For this reason foals are often weaned in pairs. Such paired foals have been observed displaying a lower frequency of vocalization compared with foals weaned into individual stalls.[111] This is considered helpful for the mare–foal dyad since a lower level of vocalization from the foal will elicit fewer vocal responses from the dam if she is located within hearing distance and reduce the chances of a vocal exchange contributing to an escalation of distress in the pair. However, the reduction in vocalization does not necessarily reflect passivity. Paired foals have been observed performing agonistic behaviors towards each other including ear-flattening, biting or threatening to kick each other.[111] This activity may take place despite the foals spending time together prior to weaning and suggests that for some breeders the possibility of injury to either foal may outweigh the benefits of companionship and certainly merits further investigation.

Aggression, along with pawing and non-nutritional sucking, is a normal consequence of frustration in freshly weaned foals. Non-nutritional sucking (i.e. of the other foal in a pair) starts within 2 hours of weaning and persists for up to 2 weeks.[113] It is suggested that a disadvantage of pair-weaning that is easily overlooked is the second episode of separation-related distress that occurs when the pair is eventually split[110] or when the foal leaves the stud of its birth.

Social problems may arise in barned situations because of the restricted environment and the imposition of new social groupings. Because the risk of bullying is increased indoors, Waters et al[121] recommend that foals are not box or barn-weaned but are turned out whenever possible. Since wood-chewing has been reported to accompany the withdrawal of exercise,[122] one would expect to see less of this behavior emerge in pastured horses. Hay replacers and concentrates should be introduced to the diet of youngsters gradually and in combination with ad libitum supplies of hay.

SEXUAL BEHAVIOR IN FEMALE DONKEYS

Some jennies show negligible signs of estrus unless approached by a jack.[123] Others may show marked changes in feeding and social behaviors that are especially apparent if other jennies exhibit estrus in synchrony.[123] Asinine estrus is characterized by lowering of the head with neck extended forward, ears pinning back the neck, hind legs splaying, standing with one foreleg slightly back and the other slightly forward, tail raising, and presentation of the perineum toward the jack (see Fig. 11.8).[124–127] However, perhaps the most conspicuous feature of the jenny's estrous display involves opening and closing of the mouth with the lips relaxed. These jaw movements make a characteristic sound that is audible to humans at a distance of up to several meters[128] and is known as jawing, yawing or clapping. They are usually accompanied by lowering of the head, extension of the neck, and pinning of the ears back against the neck (see Fig. 12.4).[128]

Some of the rituals of donkey courtship suggest ambivalence on the part of the female. For example, quick movement away from the jack tends to be followed by an abrupt stop and solid estrus stance, which is followed by mild tail swishing, abbreviated double hind-leg lifts (reminiscent of kick threats), and hip swaying.[128] It is proposed that the transition from muted non-receptive to clearly receptive behaviors may be pivotal in eliciting mounting by the jack.[128]

MATERNAL BEHAVIOR IN FEMALE DONKEYS

Jennies stay very close to their newborn foals but gradually approach them less frequently and

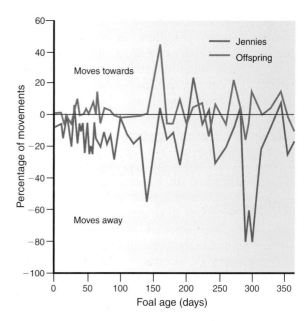

Figure 12.11 Spatial relationship between jennies and their offspring. The lines are composites of all the pairs and have been smoothed for clarity. They represent the number of approaches an animal made minus the number of times it left, and are plotted as a percentage of all movements the animal made during the hour's observation. Points above the x-axis indicate a net movement towards the other member of the pair. Points below the x-axis indicate a net movement away.[86] (Reproduced with permission from Elsevier.)

develop an overall tendency to move away, especially when their foals reach 10 months of age (Fig. 12.11).[86] The foals respond by moving towards their dams but are less persistent as they mature, regardless of their sex. In the free-ranging state this begins the process of weaning and allows for the possibility that they can become separated by some external event. Meanwhile in domestic contexts characterized by confinement, unlimited resources, and reproductive inactivity, the jenny–foal dyad does not dissolve at weaning. Instead their spatial relationship reverts to the close relationship seen between jennies and neonatal foals.[86] This largely reflects a shift in the jennie's behavior from leaving to approaching and, to a lesser extent, an increased number of approaches by the foal. The resultant pairings mean that related adult donkeys often stay very close together and are equally active in maintaining contact. Because it can lead to separation anxiety, this close relationship may prove undesirable for owners if the pair are parted, but it may provide many benefits including mutual grooming and the potential for the pair to develop a coalition for future support – for example, in mutual defense.[86]

REPRODUCTIVE BEHAVIOR PROBLEMS IN THE MARE

FOAL REJECTION

Persistence on the part of some newborn foals is often required for several hours before mares, especially maidens, will tolerate suckling. Mares sometimes squeal, bump and pivot their hindquarters, to avoid being suckled. While some use their stifles in rudimentary attempts to dislodge a foal as it approaches the udder, others even bite and kick. These responses that represent rejection of suckling (rather than rejection of the foal) and apparent fear of the foal are likely to subside in subsequent parities.

If mares do not lick their foals and vocalize towards them, they are more likely to reject.[129] Foal rejection is defined as the combination of refusal to allow sucking *and* of aggression towards the foal. Abnormal maternal behavior leading to the rejection of the foal occurs with varying prevalence between breeds.[93] Arabian mares seem to be more predisposed to foal rejection than Thoroughbreds, with the presence of one of two related sires being statistically more common in the pedigrees of rejecting versus non-rejecting mares.[130] Juarbe-Diaz et al[129] state that rejecting mares had not experienced more than three foalings, and that of 135 rejection cases, 75% of rejectors were primiparous mares. The beneficial aspects of past maternal experience may improve the mare's maternal performance. These findings need to be treated with care, because they could reflect the breeders' decision not to breed from mares with a history of foal rejection. Juarbe-Diaz et al[129] also found that, in a few extreme cases, the rejecting mares might injure or kill their foal. Mares that rejected foals exhibited less post-partum licking of foals and were less likely to show

protective behaviors towards them. The rejectors moved away from the foals as they approached and displayed threatening, squealing at, biting, chasing, or kicking behaviors. Three of 16 mares that rejected their foals injured or killed them within the first few days post partum.[129]

Periods of separation associated with veterinary intervention (e.g. for intensive care of the foal) can allow the mare to 'forget' her relationship with her foal, and for this reason veterinarians should provide neonatal care facilities with transparent partitions that allow dams to maintain visual contact with their offspring.[89] Other causes of foal rejection are not well understood. Hormonal priming with progesterone during pregnancy, estrogen and oxytocin, olfactory cues, exposure to neonatal offspring of other mares, and previous maternal experience have all been shown to play a role in the development of normal maternal behavior. When compared with normally behaving mares, the serum concentrations of progesterone in foal rejectors were lower immediately pre-partum.[129] Mares may have an innate predisposition to reject their foals that is elicited by as-yet unidentified concurrent stimuli. It has been speculated (Katherine Houpt, personal communication 1996) that this unhelpful genetic trait has been perpetuated in Arabians by the practice of hand-rearing. Although breeding from affected mares may be unwise, those that are predicted to be at risk of demonstrating poor maternal behavior may be treated with reserpine (2.5–5.0 mg orally s.i.d. to b.i.d.; see Ch. 3) 3–4 days before expected parturition.[131] Time spent habituating such mares to tactile stimuli in the inguinal region and counter-conditioning with food is well spent.

The presence of people at foaling was found not to have any effect on the rejection of foals by their mothers. However Juarbe-Diaz et al[129] state that there have been cases of mares redirecting aggression toward their foal – aggression that was originally aimed at another horse or human that had come too close to the mare and foal dyad. In a bid to mimic the peri-parturient mare's departure from the herd, it is therefore desirable to allow mares to see their group but to keep other horses beyond physical contact around the time of parturition. By the same token, if mares demonstrate aggression to personnel, human contact should be kept to a minimum.

While normal maternal and infant interactions are reasonably well understood, further studies, especially into hormonal concentrations around parturition, could assist in the understanding of foal rejection.

NYMPHOMANIA

Whereas it is used by many horse owners to describe excessive estrous manifestations during a normal estrus period, the term nymphomania is familiar to veterinarians as the behavioral outcome of truly cystic ovaries. Common in cattle, this disease process, characterized more by the length of the estrus than its intensity, is very rare in horses.[9] As long as debate and confusion about this term and what constitutes a normal ovarian rhythm prevails, overzealous intervention is a likely consequence.

In Sweden, treatment of racehorses with mild nymphomania using progesterone implants is permitted, with owners reporting good responses that last up to 5 months.[132] To prevent behavioral 'problems' during estrus in performance mares, a 15-day course of altrenogest ($0.044\,\mu g/kg$ p.o.) starting 3–4 days before competition will reduce the time spent in estrus.[133]

Mares are ovariectomized for various reasons, including behavioral modification and use as embryo-transfer recipients and dummy mares for semen collection.[18] Of 12 spayed mares used for performance events after ovariectomy, ten were judged by their owners to be competing at greater than pre-operative levels.[18] It would be useful to see an unbiased assessment of these mares' pre- and post-operative athletic performance.

Some interesting correlations between behavior and reproductive fitness have emerged from studies of free-ranging horses (e.g. Linklater et al[4]). Empirical studies have highlighted interesting relationships between the same parameters in domestic mares.[134] Mares classified retrospectively as less excitable produce significantly more foals in their breeding careers, with placid, mildly excitable and excitable mares having lifetime foal productions of 8.5, 7.2, 6.2 respectively. The relationship between these figures could be causal in that mares with more foals may be older and therefore less responsive to aversive stimuli. However, infertility showed a similar relationship, with 2.1% of placid mares, 2.2% of mildly excitable mares and 2.4% of excitable mares being infertile.[134]

MOUNTING

When a new mare arrives in a group, she may be mounted by resident mares.[135] Mares in heat may occasionally be mounted by estrous and non-estrous female companions, most notably in the absence of stallions. This has been described as a redirected behavior associated with frustration in some circumstances.[15] Other stallion-like traits such as snaking movements of the head and neck, herding, teasing, flehmen and trumpeting, which are associated with elevated plasma concentrations of steroids, including androgenic steroids, are a normal finding in some pregnant mares.[136] As with similar aberrations caused by anabolic steroid preparations (which can evoke more stallion-like responses in mares than stallions normally show), these signs may persist long after hormone levels have returned to normal.[137] It is usually recommended that mares being treated with these compounds are housed individually and not used for breeding.[138]

Although the normal value for plasma testosterone concentrations in mares is considered to be less than $50\,pg/ml$, natural elevations sometimes occur and are often associated with aggressive behavior.[139] Additionally, some granulosa cell tumors may cause mares to exhibit stallion-like behavior, especially when plasma testosterone concentrations exceed a nominal threshold of $100\,pg/ml$.[140] Since the same tumors can secrete progestins, estrogens and proteins, their effect on behavior is not isolated to masculinization.[141] Cases may present with abortion, erratic heats, continuous heats as well as physical changes that include the development of male secondary sex characteristics and abdominal distension.[142] Fortunately these neoplasms rarely metastasize, are most commonly unilateral and their removal brings about the return of normal behavior patterns and ovarian activity between 115 and 393 days.[140,143,144]

Investigations into the use of anabolic steroids for the creation of teaser mares for estrous detection suggest that such androgenized mares are of variable utility, with some studies showing an ability to elicit estrous responses in only one-third of estrous mares even when running with the group.[145,146] Intriguingly, true hermaphrodites with bilateral ovotestes are not reported to show stallion-like behavior. This implies that they are passive in the presence of normal stallions.[147] However, antisocial behavior towards stallions and geldings has been reported as a result of gynecological abnormalities such as uterus unicornis in combination with atresia of the tubular genital tract.[148]

AGGRESSION IN MARES

When not in estrus, mares may be aggressive to courting stallions, especially when first introduced. This is also a time when mares may show synchronous urination and kicking out with their hindlimbs in response to being herded (by stallions). Peri-parturient pain, including that associated with the passage of the placenta, is thought to predispose mares to acts of aggression by transiently lowering their pain threshold so that they respond agonistically.[93] Mares with foals at foot are also primed to defend their foals and may make aggressive responses when approached by an alien foal or unfamiliar adult. This is significant because aggression may be directed to personnel and the mare's own foal at these times. Mares that are fearful of their foals are sometimes misdiagnosed as foal rejectors because they use defensive aggression to keep the foal away from them. This sometimes abates if the dyad is presented with a threat such as the approach of another horse.

SUMMARY OF KEY POINTS

- Free-ranging mares can be categorized as either:
  - social dispersers (so-called mavericks)
  - loyal to a single stallion
  - part of a multi-stallion band.

- Normal courtship often involves the mare seeking the stallion and is characterised by:
  - nose-to-nose greeting
  - tactile and vocal communication
  - estrous display by the mare
  - eventual passivity on the mare's part
- The mare's behavior does not change markedly during gestation until immediately preceding parturition, when obvious changes include increased time spent walking and in recumbence.
- Some mares may exhibit estrous behavior during pregnancy as a result of high estrogen levels from accessory corpora lutea.
- Social attachments, such as the mare–foal bond, are the cement that holds social units together.
- Foals are chiefly responsible for determining proximity between mares and foals.
- Although the creep feeding of foals prior to weaning has been shown to reduce some forms of stress and optimize the post-weaning growth rate of the foal, it has been strongly linked with the emergence of oral stereotypies
- To reduce weaning stress in a herd situation the mares could be periodically and abruptly removed so that foals are left together in a familiar surrounding.
- Improper handling during pre-weaning and weaning can create undesirable behavioral characteristics.

CASE STUDY

A 5-year-old Thoroughbred mare with anorexia and weight-loss was presented, 4 weeks after the abrupt weaning of her first foal at 4 months of age. The results of a physical examination and hematological and serological profiles were normal. History included persistent running along the fenceline and daily episodes of aggression towards other mares in the paddock. The mare had not been in estrus since weaning.

The weight loss was attributed to the locomotory activity at the fenceline, an energy expense that was not supplemented with adequate nutrition. Uterine involution was satisfactory and, in the absence of ovarian abnormalities, the failure to cycle was considered a consequence of the weight loss and poor nutrition. The mare was diagnosed with separation-related distress. The aggression was a result of her agonistic responses to mares that were in the way when she was route tracing.

The therapeutic approach was designed to remove context-specific stimuli that were linked to the locomotory response and increase the mare's motivation to feed. She was kept with her original group but they were all moved to a different paddock several kilometers away. This seemed to help by breaking the association with the route that the mare had previously traced alongside the fence. The mare was brought in twice daily for supplementary feeds with her closest affiliate. The social facilitation of feeding and the competition offered by her companion helped to stimulate her to eat. The flushing effect of the nutritional changes brought her into estrus within 3 weeks. She was teased regularly throughout estrus and was served twice. After the season, her behavior returned to normal, although her attachment to the affiliate was the strongest of all the bonded pairs in the group. Her weight was maintained, pregnancy was diagnosed and no further symptoms were reported. The owners adopted a group weaning technique on their stud the following year and the separation of the mare's next foal was unremarkable.

REFERENCES

1. Wesson JA, Ginther OJ. Puberty in the female pony: reproductive behaviour, ovulation and plasma gonadotrophin concentrations. Biol Reprod 1981; 24(5):977–986.
2. Waring GH. Horse Behavior —Behavioral traits and adaptations of domestic and wild horses, including ponies. Park Ridge, NJ: Noyes; 1983.
3. Asa CS, Goldfoot DA, Garcia MC, Ginther OJ. Sexual behaviour in ovariectomised and seasonally anovulatory pony mares (Equus caballus). Horm Behav 1980; 14:46–54.
4. Linklater WL, Cameron EZ, Minot EO, Stafford KJ. Stallion harassment and the mating system of horses. Anim Behav 1999; 58(2):295–306.
5. Kaseda Y, Khalil AM, Ogawa H. Harem stability and reproductive success of Misaki feral horses. Equine Vet J 1995; 27(5):368–372.
6. Ginther OJ, Scraba ST, Nuti LC. Pregnancy rates and sexual behaviour under pasture breeding conditions in mares. Theriogenology 1983; 20(3):333–345.
7. Fraser AF. Reproductive behaviour in ungulates. London: Academic Press; 1968.
8. Ginther OJ. Occurrence of anestrus, estrus, diestrus, and ovulation over a 12-month period in mares. Am J Vet Res 1974; 35:1173–1179.
9. Fraser AF. The behaviour of the horse. Wallingford, Oxon: CAB International; 1992.
10. Rossdale PD, Ricketts SW. Equine stud farm medicine. London: Baillière Tindall; 1980.
11. Voss JL, Pickett BW. The effect of rectal palpation on the fertility of cyclic mares. J Reprod Fert Suppl 1975; 23:285–290.
12. Munro CD, Renton JP, Butcher R. The control of oestrous behaviour in the mare. J Reprod Fert Suppl 1979; 27:217–227.
13. Ginther OJ. Reproductive biology of the mare: basic and applied aspects. Cross Plaines, WI: OJ Ginther; 1979.
14. Back DG, Pickett BW, Voss JL, Seidel GE Jr. Observations on the sexual behaviour of nonlactating mares. J Am Vet Med Assoc 1974; 165(8):717–720.
15. Asa CS, Goldfoot DA, Ginther OJ. Sociosexual behaviour and the ovulatory cycle of ponies (Equus caballus) observed in harem groups. Horm Behav 1979; 13:49–65.
16. Witherspoon D. Nutrition and breeding management of problem mares. Modern Vet Pract 1977; 58(5):459–460.
17. Asa CS. Sexual behavior of mares. Vet Clin North Am Equine Pract: Behav 1986; 519–534.
18. Hooper RN, Tayor TS, Varner DD, Blanchard TL. Effects of bilateral ovariectomy via colpotomy in mares: 23 cases (1984–1990). J Am Vet Med Assoc 1993; 203(7):1043–1046.
19. McGreevy PD. Why does my horse … ? London: Souvenir Press; 1996.
20. Trumler E. Das 'Rosseigkeitsgesicht' und ahnliches Ausdrucksverhalten bei einhufern. Z Tierpsychol 1958; 16:478–488.
21. Woods GL, Houpt KA. An abnormal facial gesture in an estrous mare. Appl Anim Behav Sci 1986; 16:199–202.
22. Houpt KA, Kusunose R. Genetics of behaviour. In: The genetics of the horse. Wallingford, Oxon: CAB International; 2000:281–306.
23. Weeks JW, Crowell-Davis SL, Caudle AB, Heusner GL. Aggression and social spacing in light horse (Equus caballus) mares and foals. Appl Anim Behav Sci 2000; 68(4):319–337.
24. Singhvi CNM. Comparative studies on oestrus, oestrous behaviour and oestrous cycle in mares of different breeds under Indian tropical conditions. Indian J Anim Reprod 1992; 13(2):170–173.
25. Lowe JE, Foote RH, Baldwin BH, et al. Reproductive patterns in cyclic and pregnant thyroidectomized mares. J Reprod Fert Suppl 1978; 35:281–288.
26. Silva Filho JM, Fonseca FA, Carvalho GR, et al. [Sexual behaviour and ovulation in mares of undefined breeds] [Portuguese]. Anais, IX Congresso Brasileiro de Reproducao Animal, 22–26 de julho de 1991, vol II. Colegio Brasileiro de Reproducao Animal, Belo Horizonte, Brazil, 1991:273.
27. Zong E, Fan G. The variety of sterility and gradual progression to fertility in hybrids of the horse and the donkey. Heredity 1989; 62:393–406.
28. Ryder OA, Chemnick LG, Bowling AT, Benirschke K. Male mule foal qualifies as the offspring of a female mule and jack donkey. J Hered 1985; 76(5):379–381.
29. Veeckman J, Ödberg FO. Preliminary studies on the behavioural detection of oestrus in Belgian 'warm-blooded' mares with acoustic and tactile stimuli. Appl Anim Ethol 1978; 4:109–118.
30. McCall CA. Utilizing taped stallion vocalizations as a practical aid in estrus detection in mares. Appl Anim Behav Sci 1991; 28(4):305–310.

31. Tischner M, Bielanski W. Oestrus detection in mares using auditory and tactile stimuli [Polish]. Medycyna Weteryaryjna 1981; 37(5):300–301.

32. Tyler SJ. The behaviour and social organization of the New Forest ponies. Animal Anim Behav Monogr 1972; 5:85–196.

33. Steinbjornsson B, Kristjansson H. Sexual behaviour and fertility in Iceland horse herds. Pferdeheilkunde 1999; 15(6):481–490.

34. Allen WE. Abnormalities in the oestrous cycle in the mare. Vet Rec 1979; 104(8):166–167.

35. Belonje PC, van Niekerk CH. A review of the influence of nutrition upon the oestrous cycle and early pregnancy in the mare. J Fert Reprod Suppl 1975; 23:167–169.

36. Mintscheff P, Prachoff R. Versuche zur Ewrhohuung der Befruchttungsfahigkeitt der Stute durch Hungerdiat wahrend der Brunst. Zuchthyg. Fortpflstor Besam, Haustiere 1960; 4:40–48.

37. Morris LHA, Allen WR. Reproductive efficiency of intensively managed Thoroughbred mares in Newmarket. Equine Vet J 2002; 34:1,51–60.

38. Trillaud-Geyl C, Martin-Rousset W, Jussiaux M. La monte en liberte [Herd mating]. In: Le cheval: reproduction, selection, alimentation, exploitation. Institut National de la Recherche Agronomique, Paris, France; 1984:83–91.

39. Baucus KL, Ralston SL, Nockels CF, et al. Effects of transportation on early embryonic death in mares. Journal of Animal Science 1990a; 68(2):345–351.

40. Baucus KL, Squires EL, Ralston SL, McKinnon AO, Nett TM. Effect of transportation on the estrous cycle and concentrations of hormones in mares. J Anim Sci 1990b; 68(2):419–426.

41. Turner JW Jr, Liu IKM, Flanagan DR, et al. Immunocontraception in feral horses: one inoculation provides one year of infertility. J Wildlife Manage 2001; 65:235–241.

42. Matthews RG, Ropiha RT, Butterfield RM. The phenomenon of foal heat in mares. Aust Vet J 1967; 43:579–582.

43. Pope NS. The influence of season on estrus, ovulation and reproductive hormone secretions in barren and periparturient pony mares. Diss Abstr Int B Sci Eng 1985; 45(11):3437.

44. Rathwell AC, Asbury AC, Hansen PJ, Archibald LF. Reproductive function of mares given daily injections of prostaglandin F2α beginning at day 42 of pregnancy. Theriogenology 1987; 27(4):621–630.

45. Loy RG, Hughes JP, Richards WPC, Swan SM. Effects of progesterone on reproductive function in mares after parturition. J Reprod Fert Suppl 1975; 23:291–295.

46. Ingarden J, Dubiel A, Rauluskiewicz S. The effect of administration of a beta blocker in periparturient mares. Equine Clinical Behaviour. Equine Vet J suppl 1998; 27:19–20.

47. King SS, Neumann KR, Nequin LG, Weedman BJ. Time of onset and ovarian state prior to entry into winter anestrus. J Equine Vet Sci 1993; 13(9):512–515.

48. Silvia PJ, Squires EL, Nett TM. Changes in the hypothalamic – hypophyseal axis associated with seasonal reproductive recrudescence. Biol Reprod 1986; 35(4):897–905.

49. Loy RG, Pemstein R, O'Canna D, Douglas RH. Control of ovulation in cycling mares with ovarian steroids and prostaglandin. Theriogenology 1981; 15(2):191–200.

50. Asa CS. The effect of estradiol and progesterone on the sexual behavior of ovariectomized mares. Physiol Behav 1984; 33(4):681–686.

51. Squires EL, Stevens WB, McGlothlin DE, Pickett BW. Effect of an oral progestin on the oestrous cycle and fertility of mares. La Clinica Veterinaria 1981; 104(4):131–140.

52. Pycock JF, Dieleman S, Drijfhout P, et al. Correlation of plasma concentrations of progesterone and oestradiol with ultrasound characteristics of the uterus and duration of oestrous behavior in the cycling mare. Reprod Domest Anim 1995; 30(4):224–227.

53. Hendrikse J. Draagtijden van Nederlandse paarderassen. Tijdschr Diergeneesk 1974; 97: 477–480.

54. Ropiha RT, Matthews RG, Butterfield RM, et al. The duration of pregnancy in Thoroughbred mares. Vet Rec 1969; 84:552–555.

55. Leadon DP, Jeffcott LB, Rossdale PD. Behavior and viability of the premature neonatal foal after induced parturition. Am J Vet Res 1986; 47(8):1870–1873.

56. Howell CE, Rollins WC. Environmental sources of variation in the gestation length of the horse. J Anim Sci 1951; 10:789–796.

57. Hintz HF, Hintz RL, Lein DH, van Vleck LD. Length of gestation periods in Thoroughbred Mares. J Equine Med Surg 1979; 3:289–292.

58. Campitelli S, Carenzi C, Verga M. Factors which influence parturition in the mare and development of the foal. Appl Anim Ethol 1982; 9(1):7–14.

59. Cameron EZ, Linklater WL. Individual mares bias investment in sons and daughters in relation to their condition. Anim Behav 2000; 60:359–367.

60. Males R, Males V. Foaling. Sydney: Lansdowne Press; 1977.

61. Asa CS, Goldfoot DA, Garcia MC, Ginther OJ. Assessment of the sexual behaviour of pregnant mares. Horm Behav 1983; 17:405–413.

62. Hayes KEN, Ginther OJ. Relationship between estrous behaviour in pregnant mares and the presence of a female conceptus. J Equine Vet Sci 1989; 9(6):316–318.

63. Shaw EB, Houpt KA, Holmes DF. Body temperature and behaviour of mares during the last two weeks of pregnancy. Equine Vet J 1988; 20(3):199–202.

64. Klingel H. Reproduction in plains zebra, Iquus burchelli boehmii: behaviour and ecological factors. J Reprod Fertil Suppl 1969; 6:339–345.

65. Blakeslee JK. Mother–young relationships and related behaviour among free-ranging Appaloosa horses. Thesis, Idaho State University, Pacatello; 1974.

66. Collery L. The sexual and social behaviour of the Connemara pony. Br Vet J 1978; 125:151–152.

67. Newcombe JR, Nout YS. Apparent effect of management on the hour of parturition in mares. Vet Rec 1998; 142(9):221–222.

68. Bueno L, Tainturier D, Ruckebusch Y. Detection of parturition in cow and mare by a useful warning system. Theriogenology 1981; 16(6):599–605.

69. Rossdale PD, Mahaffey LW. Parturition in the Thoroughbred mare with particular references to blood deprivation in the newborn. Vet Rec 1958; 70:142–152.

70. Rossdale PD. Clinical studies on the newborn Thoroughbred foal, I: Perinatal behaviour. Br Vet J 1967; 123:470–481.

71. Jeffcott LB. Observations of parturition in crossbred pony mares. Equine Vet J 1972; 4:209–213.

72. Jean D, Laverty S, Halley J, et al. Thoracic trauma in newborn foals. Equine Vet J 1999; 31(2):149–152.

73. Neal FC, Ramsey FK. Cranial nerve injuries. In: Catcott EJ, Smithcors JF, eds. Equine medicine and surgery, 2nd edn. Wheaton, IL: American Veterinary Publications; 1974.

74. Berger J. Wild horses of the Great Basin. Chicago: University of Chicago Press; 1986.

75. Duncan P. Horses and grasses. New York: Springer; 1992.

76. Estep DO, Crowell-Davis SL, Earl-Costello SA, Beatey SA. Changes in the social behaviour of draft horse (Equus caballus) mares coincident with foaling. Appl Anim Behav Sci 1993; 35(3):199–213.

77. Khalil AM, Kaseda Y. Behavioral patterns and proximate reason of young male separation in Misaki feral horses. Appl Anim Behav Sci 1997; 54:281–290.

78. Bostedt H, Hospes R, Herfen K. Program zur fruhzeitigen erkennung von krankheitszustanden bei Fohlen in den ersten 24 Lebensstunden. Tierarztliche praxis, Ausgabe G, grosstiere Nutztiere 1997; 25(6):594–597.

79. Kurtz Filho M, Depra NM, Alda JL, et al. [Physiological and behavioural parameters in the newborn Thoroughbred foal] [Portuguese]. Revista da Faculdade de Medicina Veterinaria e Zootecnia da Universidade de São Paulo 1997; 34(2):103–108.

80. Houpt KA. Formation and dissolution of the mare foal bond. Appl Anim Behav Sci 2002; 78(2–4):325–334.

81. Carson K, Wood-Gush DGM. Behaviour of Thoroughbred foals during nursing. Equine Vet J 1983a; 15:257–262.

82. Barber JA, Crowell-Davis SL. Maternal behaviour of Belgian mares. Appl Anim Behav Sci 1994; 41:161–189.

83. Weaver LT. Milk and neonatal gut: comparative lessons to be learnt. Equine Vet J 1996; 18(6):427–429.

84. Carson K, Wood-Gush DGM. Equine behaviour: a review of literature on social and dam – foal behaviour. Appl Anim Ethol 1983b; 10:165–178.

85. Wolff A, Hausberger M. Behaviour of foals before weaning may have some genetic basis. Ethology 1994; 96:1–10.

86. French JM. Mother-offspring relationships in donkeys. Appl Anim Behav Sci 1998; 60(2–3):253–258.

87. Crowell-Davis SL. Daytime and rest behaviour of the Welsh Pony (Equus caballus) mare and foal. Appl Anim Behav Sci 1994; 40(3/4):197–210.

88. Cox JE. Some observations of an orphan foal. Br Vet J 1978; 126:658–659.

89. Houpt KA. The battered foal —mare rejection of the foal. In: Harris PA, Gomarsall GM, Davidson HPB, Green RE, eds. Proceedings of the BEVA Specialist Days on Behaviour and Nutrition; 1999:35–36.

90. Wolski TR, Houpt KA, Aronson R. The role of the senses in mare – foal recognition. Appl Anim Ethol 1980; 6(2):121–138.

91. Leblanc MA, Bouissou MF. Development of a test to study maternal recognition of young in horses. Biol Behav 1981; 6(4):283–290.

92. Kelly AJ. Practical tips on fostering. In: Harris PA, Gomarsall GM, Davidson HPB, Green RE, eds. Proceedings of the BEVA Specialist Days on Behaviour and Nutrition; 1999:39–41.

93. Houpt KA. Domestic animal behaviour for veterinarians and animal scientists, 2nd edn. Ames: Iowa State University Press; 1991.

94. Boyd LE. The natality, foal survivorship and mare–foal behavior of feral horses in Wyoming's Red Desert. Thesis, University of Wyoming, Laramie; 1980.

95. Porter RH, Duchamp G, Nowak R, Daels RF. Induction of maternal behavior in non-parturient adoptive mares. Physiol Behav 2002; 77(1):151–154.

96. Cameron EZ, Stafford KJ, Linklater WL, Veltman CJ. Suckling behaviour does not measure milk intake in horses. Anim Behav 1999; 57:673–678.

97. Monard AM, Duncan P, Fritz H, Feh C. Variations in the sex ratio and neonatal mortaity in a natural herd of horses. Behav Ecol Sociobiol 1997; 41(4):243–249.

98. Barron JK. The effect of maternal age and parity on the racing performance of Thoroughbred horses. Equine Vet J 1995; 27(1):73–75.

99. Martinet-Rosset W, Doreau M, Cloix J. [Activities of a herd of draught brood mares and their foals on pasture] [French]. Ann Zootech 1978; 27(1):33–45.

100. Duncan P, Harvey PH, Wells SM. On lactation and associated behaviour in a natural herd of horses. Anim Behav 1984; 32(1):255–263.

101. Calinescu E. [Behaviour of foals and mares in lactation] [Romanian]. Revista de Cresterea Animalelor 1982; 32(7):37–43.

102. Tsujii H. [Suckling behaviour of Kiso horses] [Japanese]. J Faculty Agric Shinshu Univ 1986; 23(2):57–64.

103. Smith-Funk ED, Crowell-Davis SL. Maternal behaviour of draft mares (Equus caballus) with mule foals (equus asinus x equus caballus). Appl Anim Behav Sci 1992; 33:93–119.

104. Rudman R, Keiper RR. The body condition of feral ponies on Assateague Island. Equine Vet J 1991; 23(6):453–456.

105. Apter RC, Householder DD. Weaning and weaning management of foals: a review and some recommendations. J Equine Vet Sci 1996; 16:428–435.

106. Kiley-Worthington M. The behaviour of horses — in relation to management and training. London: JA Allen; 1987.

107. Kaseda Y, Ogawa H, Khalil AM. Causes of natal dispersal and emigration and their effects on harem formation in Misaki feral horses. Equine Vet J 1997; 29(4):262–266.

108. Mal ME, McCall CA, Cummins KA, Newland MC. Influence of preweaning handling methods on

post-weaning learning ability and manageability of foals. Appl Anim Behav Sci 1994; 40:187–195.

109. Jezierski T, Jaworski Z, Gorecka A. Effects of handling on behaviour and heart rate in Konik horses: comparison of stable and forest reared youngstock. Appl Anim Behav Sci 1999; 62:1–11.

110. Crowell-Davis SL. Developmental behavior. Vet Clin North Am Equine Pract: Behav 1986; 573–590.

111. Hoffman RM, Kronfeld DS, Holland JL, Greiwe-Crandell KM. Preweaning diet and stall weaning method influences on stress response in foals. J Anim Sci 1995; 73:2922–2930.

112. Coleman RJ, Gary MS, Mathison GW, Burwash L. Growth and condition at weaning of extensively managed creep-fed foals. J Equine Vet Sci 1999; 19:45–50.

113. McCall CA, Potter DG, Kreider JL. Locomotor, vocal and other behavioural responses to varying methods of weaning foals. Appl Anim Behav Sci 1985; 14(1):27–35.

114. Nicol CJ, Wilson AD, Waters AJ, et al. Crib-biting in foals is associated with gastric ulceration and mucosal inflammation. In: Garner JP, Mench JA, Heekin SP, eds. Proceedings of the 35th International Congress of the ISAE. Davis, CA: The Center for Animal Welfare, UC; 2001.

115. Nicol CJ. Equine learning: progress and suggestions for future research. Appl Anim Behav Sci 2002; 78(2–4):193–208.

116. McCall CA, Potter GD, Kreider JL, Jenkins WL. Physiological responses in foals weaned by abrupt or gradual methods. J Equine Vet Sci 1987; 7:368–374.

117. Malinowski K, Hallquist NA, Helyar L, et al. Effect of separation protocols between mares and foals on plasma cortisol and cell-mediated immune response. J Equine Vet Sci 1990; 10:363.

118. Houpt KA, Hintz HF, Butler WR. A preliminary study of two methods of weaning foals. Appl Anim Behav Sci 1984; 12:177–181.

119. Heleski CR, Shelle AC, Nielsen BD, Zanella AJ. Influence of housing on weanling horse behavior and subsequent welfare. Appl Anim Behav Sci 2002; 78(2–4):297–308.

120. Pugh DG, Williams MA. Feeding foals from birth to weaning. Compend Contin Educ Pract Vet 1992; 14:526–532.

121. Waters AJ, Nicol CJ, French NP. Factors influencing the development of stereotypic and redirected behaviours in young horses: findings of a four year prospective epidemiological study. Equine Vet J 2002; 34(6):572–579.

122. Krzak WE, Gonyou HW, Lawrence LM. Wood chewing by stabled horses: diurnal pattern and effects of exercise. J Anim Sci 1991; 69:1053–1058.

123. Taylor TS, Matthews NS. Mammoth asses – selected behavioural considerations for the veterinarian. Appl Anim Behav Sci 1998; 60(2–3):283–289.

124. McCort WD. The behavior and social organization of feral asses (Equus asinus) on Ossabaw Island, Georgia. Unpublished doctoral dissertation, The Pennsylvania State University, State College, 1980.

125. Clayton HM, Lindsay FEF, Forbes AC, Hay LA. Some studies of comparative aspects of sexual behaviour in ponies and donkeys. Appl Anim Ethol 1981; 7:169–174.

126. Vandeplassche GM, Wesson JA, Ginther OJ. Behavioral, follicular and gonadotropin changes during the estrous cycle in donkeys. Theriogenology 1981; 16:239–249.

127. Henry M, McDonnell SM, Lodi LD, Gastal EL. Pasture mating behaviour of donkeys (Equus asinus) at natural and induced estrus. J Reprod Fertil 1991; 44:77–86.

128. McDonnell SM. Reproductive behavior of donkeys (Equus asinus). Appl Anim Behav Sci 1998; 60(2–3):277–282.

129. Juarbe-Diaz SV, Houpt KA, Kusunose R. Prevalence and characteristics of foal rejection in Arabian mares. Equine Vet J 1998; 30:424–428.

130. Matoock MS. Maternal behaviour in Arabian mares. PhD thesis, Cairo University, 1992.

131. McDonnell SM. Pharmacological aids to behaviour modification in horses. Equine Vet J Suppl 1998; 27:50–51 (abstr).

132. Christensson J. [The effect of progesterone on mild forms of nymphomania in mares] [Swedish]. Svensk Veterinartidning 1992; 44(3):111–115.

133. Paul JW, Rains JR, Lehman FD. The use and misuse of progestins in the mare. Equine Pract 1995; 17(3):21–22.

134. Budzynski M, Kameniak J, Soltys L, et al. [Evaluating reproductive traits in Malopolski mares in relation to excitability] [Polish]. Annales Universitatis Mariae Curie-Sklodowska. Sectio ee Zootechnia 1995; 13:97–102.

135. Feh C. Relationships and communication in socially natural horse herds. Havemeyer Workshop on Horse Behaviour and Welfare, Holar, Iceland, 2002:84–91.

136. McDonnell SM. Reproductive behavior of the stallion. Vet Clin North Am Equine Pract: Behav 1986; 2:535–556.

137. Withrow JM, Sargent GF, Scheffahn NS, Kesler DJ. Induction of male sex behaviour in pony mares with testosterone proprionate. Theriogenology 1983; 20(4):485–490.

138. Schumacher EMA, Blackshaw JK, Skelton KV. The behavioral outcome of anabolic steroid administration to female horses. Equine Pract 1987; 9(6):14–15.

139. Beaver BM, Amoss MS. Aggressive behaviour associated with naturally elevated serum testosterone in mares. Appl Anim Ethol 1982; 8:425–428.

140. Stabenfeldt GH, Hughes JP, Kennedy PC, et al. Clinical findings, pathological changes and endocrinological secretory patterns in mares with ovarian tumours. J Reprod Fert Suppl 1979; 27:277–285.

141. Meinecke B, Gips H. Steroid hormone secretory patterns in mares with granulosa cell tumours. J Vet Med A (Anim Physiol, Pathol Clinic Vet Med) 1987; 34(7):545–560.

142. Perino LJ, Dider PJ. Equine granulosa cell tumours. Equine Pract 1985; 7(4):14–17.

143. Milne FJ. Granulosa cell tumors in mares — a review of 78 cases. In: Proceedings of the 23rd Annual Convention of the American Association of Equine Practitioners, Vancouver, British Columbia; 1977,

133–143. Ontario Veterinary College, Guelph, Ontario, Canada; 1978.

144. Baumann LE, Sillerud CL, Spolar-Kilroy CR. Equine granulosa cell tumors: a review of fifteen cases. Minnesota Vet 1985; 25(1):52–54.

145. McDonnell SM, Garcia MC, Blanchard TL, Kenney RM. Evaluation of androgenized mares as an estrus detection aid. Theriogenology 1986; 26(2):261–266.

146. McDonnell SM, Hinrichs K, Cooper WL, Kenney RM. Use of an androgenized mare as an aid in the detection of estrus in mares. Theriogenology 1988; 30(3):547–553.

147. Dunn HO, Smiley D, Duncan JR, McEntee K. Two equine hermaphrodites with 64,XX/64,XY and 63,XO/64,XY chimerism. Cornell Vet 1981; 123–135.

148. Thursby-Pelham RHC. Uterus unicornis in mares. Vet Rec 1997; 141(5):132.

13

Training

Andrew McLean and Paul McGreevy

BACKGROUND

There are a number of reasons for training problems. Many of them are considered from an ethological perspective in Chapter 15. They also include inconsistencies in the terms that are used, what is understood by them and the way in which training techniques are applied. The current chapter explores what horses can learn from their interactions with humans and encourages readers to engage with what should be considered *equitation science*.

WHAT CAN BE LEARNED?

Behavior is the product of the interaction of an animal's genes and its environment. As with all mammals, genetics only *predispose* the horse to behave in certain ways – actual behavior on any occasion will be the result of a combination of that predisposition and learned behavior in the environment or context. Learning can emphasize or suppress genetic tendencies, so that all equine behavior can be modified by experience. For example, the sex drive of a stallion can be modified by learning to the extent that a well-trained stallion behaves obediently around mares. In general, horse riders and trainers give far too much credence to genetic predispositions and pay insufficient attention to the potential for learning. Rather than being destined to be that way, vicious stallions, 'crazy' horses, horses that pull, shy, kick, bite or whatever are products of their life experiences and training.

HORSES FOR COURSES

It is important to be mindful that the behavioral responses required of horses, even at the highest level of dressage, are not beyond their physical capabilities. While physical limitations due to conformation may affect the *quality* of the training outcome (see Ch. 7), dressage movements are essentially derived from natural movements innate to the species.

The sorts of conformation problems that limit performance in dressage and jumping generally involve the height ratio of the wither and the croup. If the wither is substantially lower than the croup, then horses generally have trouble collecting and carrying weight on the hindquarters with the extra weight of the rider, which is a critical component of dressage and jumping training. Such croup-high horses are frequently found in the breeds bred for speed, such as Arabians and Thoroughbreds, and incidentally in the plains zebra (*E. burchelli*). Conversely, wither-high horses, such as all of the draft breeds, have formed the genetic basis of the modern performance dressage and jumping horse (Fig. 13.1). Interestingly, as the speed and endurance phase of three-day-eventing has become progressively reduced due to welfare considerations and, correspondingly, the relative influence of dressage phase on overall performance has increased, the predominance of the Thoroughbred in that sport is now giving way

to the slower and less enduring but dressage-designed warmbloods (draft and Thoroughbred crossbreds).

TRADITIONAL DOGMA

It is appropriate here to challenge some of the central features of traditional equine educational dogma. Despite empirical data that demonstrate the phenomenal memories of equids[1,2] and the likelihood that horses do not need to be reminded how to execute their schooling tracks, trainers remain committed to regular schooling activities that usually comprise repetitive maneuvers involving 10-meter circles, 20-meter circles, serpentines and so on. If horses can indeed learn after a single trial only,[3] it could be argued that these exercises are of more importance to riders than to horses. At the same time many classical riding tutors maintain that through such drilling the horse develops the musculature required to maintain self-carriage (see Glossary) without having learned anything. This circumvention of the need for any understanding of learning theory is unfortunate because it contributes to the mystification of equestrian technique by denying the central role of negative reinforcement.

Horses are adept at habituation to riding-related stimuli such as the girth, saddle, bridle, boots, the sight and general movements of a person on their backs, as well as to environmental aspects of their

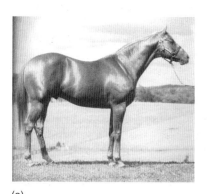
(a)

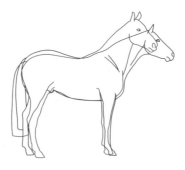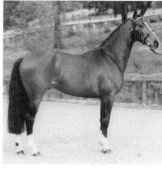
(b)

Figure 13.1 Examples of (a) a croup-high and (b) a wither-high horse. The central superimposed image illustrates the relative proportions (the dotted line representing the outline of the croup-high Thoroughbred). ((a) Thoroughbred stallion 'Rancher', photography by Neil McLeod; (b) warmblood stallion 'Rohirrim Tintagel Magic' owned by Victoria Kendall-Hawk, photography by Julie Wilson.)

habitat. Trainers must ensure that horses *do not* habituate to the training signals, an outcome which commonly shows up as hard mouths and laziness to the rider's leg signals. The schooling aspect of training sessions should make it possible to elicit maneuvers with increasingly subtle signals, providing that the subtle signal precedes and is contiguous with the reinforcement. With stimuli (rein, leg, whip-tap) using the pressure-release system, there is already an inherent subtle cue: the initial light increase in pressure. This precedes the immediate increase in pressure that results from a lack of response from the horse. The pressure is subsequently released immediately when the horse gives the desired response. The initial light increase is the mild cue that signals each intervention. Later on, through repetition of this protocol, the horse responds to extra cues, including the subtle changes of the rider's seat and position, through classical conditioning.

A recent industry survey (reported by Harris[4]) notes that 25% of the time owners spend with horses involves schooling (Fig. 13.2). Riders should be clear about the purpose of this activity. The benefits of schooling attributed to muscular development as opposed to neurological development may be overrated. The aim in the preparatory work for each schooling session should be to assess the progressive qualities of the horse's basic responses within each gait (immediacy of reaction, reaction to the light cue, rhythm, straightness, adjustability, suppleness and unconditional

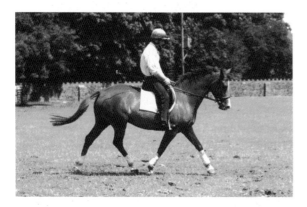

Figure 13.2 Horse being schooled. (Reproduced by permission of the University of Bristol, Dept of Clinical Veterinary Science.)

responses – does the horse give the same response wherever and whenever the rider signals?). Clearly, optimizing these outcomes will tend to improve the horse's dressage scores. Show-jumping and eventing, if executed correctly, also rely on the same principles, i.e. rhythm (self-maintained rhythm and speed), straightness (self-maintained line and body straightness), and contact (self-maintained leg and rein connections and outline). At any speed, the more correct the execution of turns and lines, the better the performance. Therefore instead of slavishly tracing circles in the manège, riders should aim to refine the horse's responses through a process of shaping (see Ch. 4). Having acknowledged the undoubted benefits of absolute obedience for many competitive disciplines, it is also worth remembering that horses who retain some innate responses may be much safer in novel and complex environments such as may be encountered during trail-riding.

SHIFTING THE MINDSET

The prevailing mindset throughout history has been to abandon, one way or the other, the less 'willing' equids because they have been regarded as having some moral (and even spiritual) involvement in the training process so that they are assumed to have 'decided' that they would not comply. These are the horses that, instead of learning what is required of them, learn to resist and escape and become the bolting, jibbing, balking, refusing, rearing, bucking and shying animals that are regularly described in books on so-called problem horses. These are the animals that change hands rapidly with the consequent addition of different commands and consequences that exacerbate the inconsistency of earlier training and increase the pressures to which they have already shown themselves to be particularly sensitive.

Learning theory provides principles and guidelines for training. While these are usually adhered to by good trainers, they are not proposed as the first principles in contemporary horse-training literature. It seems strange that throughout the world, the language of learning theory is almost never taught as a basic first principle in riding schools. We submit that these omissions precipitate confusion and therefore conflict in horses and ultimately contribute to welfare problems and wastage.

Training is most rapid and consistent and training-related stress is minimized when training practices exactly match an animal's mental abilities. This is evident in the results of great scientific animal trainers such as Marian Bailey, a student of Skinner, and those largely responsible for the tremendous advances in training cetaceans, pinnipeds and canids.

In the normal distribution curve that constitutes the components of what is termed 'trainability', the range of horses that are 'good', 'eager to please' and in fact easy to train in the ad hoc systems that comprise modern training, occupy a relatively small portion at the top of the trainability scale (Fig. 13.3). It would seem that this could be significantly increased by introducing a scientific approach to training and management and utilizing the principles of learning theory so that we can expedite training, reduce training-related stress and vastly improve horse–human interactions. This chapter aims to demystify the training of horses. Furthermore, by exploring best practice in horse training, it complements some of the techniques in behavior modification that appear elsewhere in this book (see Chs 1, 4 and 15).

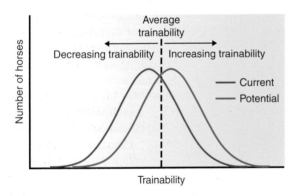

Figure 13.3 Theoretical normal distributions to show how the number of horses that cope with training may be increased by using more enlightened approaches including greater clarity of cues, better timing, greater consistency and more flexibility in educational approaches. (Courtesy of Peter Thomson.)

WELFARE AND WASTAGE

There are welfare implications in failing to identify adequately the mental abilities of all animals in the care of humans. Overestimating an animal's mental ability must be seen as a major contemporary welfare issue when it manifests as abuse, wastage, stress and conflict behaviors.

As horse trainers and handlers, our understanding of the horse's mental abilities is based largely on a centuries-old tradition of horsemanship. Horse-training textbooks (including pony club texts) throughout the world take their reference from traditional horse practice or from the 'great masters' of horsemanship who lived in the last 500 years. Such texts generally abound with words to describe horse behavior that imply reasoning abilities (Fig. 13.4). They generally assume that the horse 'understands' his training rather than simply responding through reinforcement. Training a horse within the traditional anthropomorphic framework has a number of potentially negative implications for horse welfare, as well as for the safety of riders and handlers.

Furthermore, the anthropomorphic view of the horse is not supported by scientific examinations which suggest that equids possess little or no higher mental abilities. Mindful of this, equine ethologists avoid interpreting responses as reflections of human emotions and values. They do not do this to demean horses but to recognize that there are often simpler and more plausible explanations for the responses.

Training does not always go according to plan. Some horses are predisposed genetically to trial undesirable responses rather than desirable ones. Some horses learn to evade stimuli most effectively when the stimuli are predictable by association, e.g. in a schooling context. Horses that have been subjected to inconsistent signals, such as the lack of release of pressure, or to the pain of bad schooling, often acquire the reputation of being difficult and are sold on to homes where more often than not the harshness of schooling is escalated. This contributes to disturbing slaughter statistics. For example, in a recent French study of more than 3000 non-racing horses, some 66.4% died aged between 2 and 7 years.[5] Unlike data

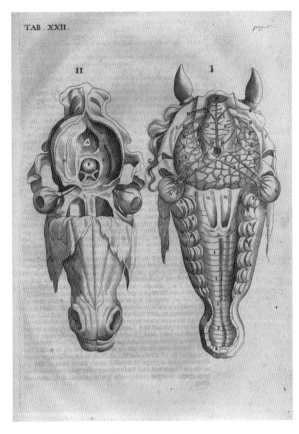

Figure 13.4 Etching of cranial dissection of the horse showing how 17th-century veterinary anatomists attributed to the horse a much larger brain than it truly has. (From *The Anatomy of an Horse*, by Andrew Snape, published by J Hindmarsh, Cornhill, 1686.)

from the racing industry,[6,7] this wastage was not attributed to orthopedic or respiratory disease so much as to inappropriate behavior. The welfare implications of this wastage suggest that veterinarians and equine scientists should become well versed in learning theory since it is the basis of good training, continuing education and behavior modification. The wrong approach to training can have consequences far worse than simple time-wasting.

The relevance of learning theory

Modern behavioral psychology has established learning theory as the cornerstone of elegant training programs in many laboratory and performance species, but this has yet to be incorporated in any significant way into contemporary equine training or into the education of equestrian coaches. Because horse training was well entrenched in its ways by the time Pavlov, Thorndike and Skinner came along, riders have not been altogether receptive to such wisdom.

The assumption that the horse is a willing partner and that the aim is largely to train the rider's biomechanics to merge into those of the horse is widely accepted in dressage circles. While it is not disputed that, after the consolidation of operant responses, this ideology plays a part in the later development of horse training, the overall approach neglects trial-and-error learning. Problems arise when equestrian methodologies focus on classical conditioning *before* or *instead* of the more deeply ingrained pressure-release responses through trial-and-error learning. This is because confusion (and therefore conflict) often arises in horses unless the basic responses have been installed thoroughly in the first place by trial-and-error learning through negative reinforcement. Training the horse by simple cue associations neither ensures controllability in all environmental contexts, nor provides the range of responses that is required for ultimate control in the Olympic equestrian disciplines of show-jumping, horse-trials or dressage. Furthermore the randomness in behavioral response that horses are able to exhibit when not under complete handler/rider control results in inconsistent stimulus–response relationships which frequently cause chronic stress.[12] It is assumed that the prevalence of such methodologies has arisen in the absence of a logical framework based on learning theory.

The cognitive revolution of the 1970s rejected behaviorism. Its legacy is the 'tendency to underestimate the power of Skinnerian conditioning to shape the behavioral competence of organisms into highly adaptive and discerning structures'.[8] This probably contributed to the resistance to the understanding of learning theory in those domains within animal training where it had not already been accepted. Indeed, many texts on equine behavior seem to imply subjective mental experiences in horses.[9–11] It would be a scientific error to assume the existence of abilities in the absence of data. Even if there are no data supporting the negative or affirmative case, assuming subjective mental experiences in animals would constitute an unacceptable rejection of the null hypothesis.[8] Moreover, all the published peer-reviewed data strongly indicate that horses lack insight into their instinctive behaviors. As we shall see in the discussion of equine mentality that follows, there are strong selective pressures for this lack of insight to occur.

HORSE WHISPERERS

It should be acknowledged that, when trainers are on the 'right track', they generally achieve desirable results. Throughout history, there have been riders who were adept at putting learning principles into practice, but who did not have the advantage of a theoretical basis. They were considered 'natural horsemen'. Biographies of gifted riders repeatedly suggest that they were at a loss to explain their talents. Unfortunately, this has led to the myth of horse whispering and the mistaken belief that training is more art than science. This set of beliefs has led to a consequent denial of the benefits of applying structured behavioral principles to horse training.

Although the equine industry is steeped in tradition, its stakeholders have demonstrated that they can nonetheless take heed of new information, especially when it is demonstrated convincingly. The new global wave of horsemanship, as expounded by the 'horse whisperers' and 'new age' trainers, is slowly raising awareness of alternative ways to view the horse and approach horse training. By approaching the so-called 'problem horse' with a different set of tools, these trainers have provided some enlightening solutions to problems that have presented difficulties for traditional equestrian ideology.

Sometimes the horse-whispering myth provides an irresistible superhuman kudos to the practitioner. But perhaps the greatest limitation of many horse-whispering systems is that training practices are once again locked into *method* without the illuminations and extrapolations provided by learning theory. Their techniques have arisen from the historical trials of practical horsemanship. Furthermore, the paranormal

mystique that surrounds horse whispering and the tremendous variety of techniques tend to confound any search for a unifying principle. Thus horse whispering is often applied without the sort of paradigm shift in thinking about the cause of the problems that we have seen in the behavior modification of other domestic species such as dogs. For this reason much of the current wave of 'new age' horse training remains within an anthropocentric and anthropomorphic framework. This is unfortunate because any assumption that the horse is motivated by anything other than its basic, instinctual drives adds an unnecessary layer of complexity to its training. Anthropomorphic explanations of how compliant horses 'understand' and 'oblige' us are unhelpful for at least two reasons: first, they mystify the training process for novice riders; and second, they imply that non-compliant horses are somehow malevolent. This explains why in one text of equine behavior modification, some horses have even been described as 'depraved'.[13]

Unfortunately, some of the 'modern' training systems are recycled in that they are just old horsemanship skills repackaged in a pseudoscientific wrapper. Predictably, these systems do not always follow the principles of the psychology of training as clearly as they should. Some retain familiar pitfalls such as: too many signals given concurrently; different signals for a single response; lengthy delays in reinforcement.

Finally, a note about the increase in the popularity of round pens that has resulted from the global interest in 'whispering' and relies on an understanding of the flight zone of an animal. A tame animal has a flight distance of zero. Animals are acutely aware of this zone of safety around them so that when it is breached, they move away. In a round pen situation the horse stops moving when the trainer retreats from the flight zone (Fig. 13.5). It seems that there is sometimes a perceived notion that creating an emotional crisis during round-pen training is actually desirable, probably because it forces the horse to offer a change in 'attitude' after which it accepts the human as 'leader'. The simplest explanation of this change is that the horse's running away in the round-pen does not increase the distance between it and the human, thus allowing the trainer to use

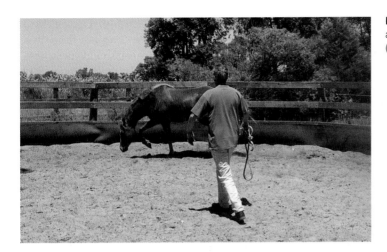

Figure 13.5 Round-pen work relies on an appreciation of the horse's flight zone. (Photograph courtesy of Portland Jones.)

actions and postures to reinforce slowing and shape the horse to approach. Similarly, the practice of lungeing (see Glossary) reactive horses before training can be seen as problematic as it is often little more than an opportunity for the horse to learn and practice flight-related behaviors.

We must exercise caution before advocating approaches to equine training that involve chasing horses and causing them to associate fear responses with any human interactions, because we now know that fear responses and associations are not as prone to extinction as other learned responses.[14] The horse may well learn to approach humans, but the means does not justify the end, because, if Le Doux's findings are to be given any credence, the experience of being chased can leave the horse with a more 'hair trigger' flight response. The danger is in the retention of flight-response associations, and its translocation to other interactions with humans.

THE PROBLEMS WITH CONTEMPORARY TRAINING

By tailoring training strategies to the species' mental ability, we can increase the efficiency of training and minimize misunderstandings in human–animal interactions. For example, when humans have expectations that animals 'understand' what is required, they often give inappropriate signals to the animals – such as delayed, inconsistent or meaningless reinforcements – that result in deleterious behavioral changes.[15] Wiepkema[12] indicates that unpredictability in the stimulus–response relationship causes conflict behaviors such as redirected, ambivalent and displacement behaviors. If these behaviors fail to reduce drive, the animal may learn that it is unable to improve its well-being. Not surprisingly, learned helplessness has been identified in domestic horses.[16,17] Although learned helplessness is a manifestation of compromised welfare,[18] it is often referred to as 'staleness' in equestrian texts.

Trainers are frequently at a loss to explain the origin of the seemingly 'naughty' or 'bad' behavior in their horses. Their dilemma arises from the fact that they believe the horse has a temperament problem or 'vice', rather than seeing that it has a training problem, an enlightened view that releases the horse from responsibility for the problem and puts it squarely at the feet of the trainer. Most likely the signals trained by pressure-release in the early training of the horse were either incompletely installed or have since deteriorated through lack of attention to their integrity.

EQUINE MENTALITY

Horses pass with flying colors the experimental tests of: their excellent memory;[2] their ability to learn through instrumental conditioning (sometimes rapidly);[10] their ability to discriminate; their powers of stimulus generalization; and how one learning experience can enhance their uptake of another.[10] However, empirical evidence suggests that they have little or no capacity for reasoning or insight.[15] From an anatomical perspective, Bermond[19] uses the argument from analogy to propose that animals without well-developed prefrontal cortices (including horses) would be unable to perform the mental abilities (such as reasoning) conferred by such brain features. Furthermore, he contends that reasoning has a maladaptive downside in that it allows animals (i.e. humans) to project and prolong their worst fears, and develop psychotic behaviors. He states that 'the prolongation of the emotional feeling (in humans) is a well known phenomenon and psychological defence mechanisms such as displacement, projection and suppression are, for example, unlikely to occur in the absence of this process'.[19]

Throughout evolution, grazing animals have been on the menu for predators. Being aware of such a plight would be maladaptive in terms of stress and interrupted foraging if an animal were slow, young, ill, lame, in foal, fearful of darkness or had a foal at foot. But horses never required higher mental abilities such as reasoning because, as Budiansky[20] points out, grass (unlike a mouse!) doesn't hide or require planning or ambush to catch it.

Reasoning is an expensive luxury and is most likely not selected for by the grazing niche. Brain tissue is many times more expensive to fuel than other tissues[21] and is subject to strong selective pressure.[22] The impoverished grazing niche that the horse has evolved to exploit adds an extra imperative for neural efficiency. Moreover the lack of higher mental abilities is adaptive for grazers such as equids, because it allows the formation of repetitive behavior patterns such as escape routines. The advantage of these 'habits' over more reflective mental processes lies in their speed of acquisition, and the immediacy and stability of reactions.[15]

Horse handlers frequently witness that horses have little or no insight into their own instinctive behavior. As humans we are astounded that an animal would maim or kill itself in the execution of pulling back from a tie-up post, thrash itself to bits in a trailer (float), or literally bolt towards solid obstacles, as sometimes seen in cross-country phases of horse trials competition. The riders in the latter instance frequently believe that these horses are simply 'keen'. Another sign of horses' apparent lack of insight is that they have little concept of 'form'. For example, many horse people have noticed that some horses show tremendous fear when confronted by changes in form of objects or even in conspecifics. If such horses have never seen a small white pony, they seem unable to extrapolate that it is a horse. Similarly, some horses (such as Topper in the case study in Ch. 11) seem unable to interpret correctly the form of their closest relative, the donkey, and react as if it were a potential predator.

HARD-WIRING AND HABITS

The horse is born with a neural template for all the different instinctive behaviors that it will require throughout its life. In a sense, the horse's brain has the neural architecture of a ready-made internalized structure of the external world. Here the neural pathways are predetermined – the animal is born with a motor-pattern to walk, trot, canter, flying-change, suckle, startle at certain shapes, be especially aware around water, caves and ditches and be pre-programmed for sex later in life. This has been referred to as hard-wiring. An obedient horse is one that offers desirable learned responses which, under the control of humans, override instincts such as to run, eat, socialize and copulate in the presence of eliciting stimuli.

In the early stages of learning, associations form in the brain as simple, fragile pathways and networks. The more a particular response is practiced as a consequence of its eliciting stimulus, the more that neural network develops. After a number of repetitions, a repetitive behavior pattern (a habit) forms. Learned responses in mammals modify instinctive drives, and thus can override or enhance their expression. For example, with enough practice, shying (Fig. 13.6) is shaped by learning in that it frequently develops into a faster and larger leap sideways and may even evolve into a rear and spin away.

Horses are highly motivated to seek freedom from confinement, pressure or effort. Panic and fearful responses are often the vehicles of their

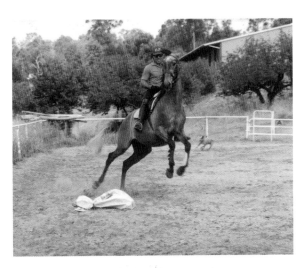

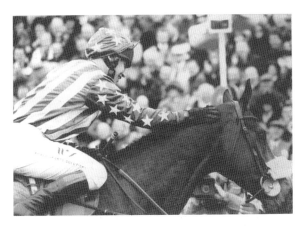

Figure 13.7 In many cases, patting may be irrelevant to horses. (Photograph courtesy of Sarah Brooks.)

Figure 13.6 Shying horses learn that evasive responses are effective means of reducing their exposure to aversive stimuli. (Photograph courtesy of Sandra Hannan.)

freedom and, when horses bolt, buck or rear, the freedom associated with the shedding of the predators from their backs is highly rewarding. It is therefore not difficult to understand why *expressing* the flight response is inherently reinforcing. Evolution has bequeathed to the horse automatically hard-wired patterns of behavior, such as bucking, because of their high survival value. It is not surprising that these patterns of behavior may be subject to one-trial learning, and that they themselves are modified by experience. So the horse can begin to adopt natural responses (that profit it) rather than the responses the rider wants. Such equine strategies prompt traditional horsefolk to label the horse as nasty or vengeful while in truth it is simply expressing a summary of its genetic predispositions and previous training.

INEFFECTIVE REWARDS

Patting the horse (Fig. 13.7) is an overrated reward endemic among equestrians. One of the dangers of patting the horse as a reward is that it can become the focus of our reinforcement system to the detriment of the release of pressure. Indeed some riders can be seen patting their horses while still pulling on the reins. Sometimes too the distinction between patting as a reward

and slapping the horse on the neck as some kind of punishment is a blurry one indeed.

Horses are not born with an innate understanding of patting; it is at best a secondary reinforcement. For it to be perceived as a reward, it would need to be associated consistently with a primary reinforcer (such as food) after an act (and just before the food). Scratching at the lower neck and withers, however, is a different story altogether (see Ch. 10). Feh and de Mazieres[23] propose that because grooming at this site lowers heart rate more than grooming of any other area of the body, it produces relaxation.

If we touch the horse and say, 'good boy' whenever we feel pleased with it, we run the risk of extinguishing associations with primary reinforcers (see the section on using reinforcers in Ch. 4, p. 96), and thus at best these things can come to mean 'I like you', but not 'well done!'. In animal training, failure to consolidate the attachment of rewards to responses will render such rewards as background noise.

CONFLICT BEHAVIORS – THE MANIFESTATION OF PROBLEMS

CONFLICT

In the natural habitat or indeed in many domestic contexts, horses are rarely frustrated for long because they are free to attend to the reduction of their basic drives. For example, in agonistic encounters they can compete and resolve disputes with other horses. When frightened, they can flee. If faced with hunger, they can search for and consume forage. Whichever way, the conflicts between competing drives will usually be resolved very rapidly.

Behavioral responses have evolved to lead to the reduction of the basic drives, including hunger, thirst, sexual desire, and freedom from predators, pain and discomfort. Throughout their lives horses learn to offer responses that result in the reduction of these drives. Domesticated horses learn during their early training that the pressure of the bit via the reins disappears when they stop or slow. They learn that the pressure of the rider's legs or spurs disappears when they go forward. However, when horses consistently cannot obtain their freedom from such pressures, chronic conflict may arise which is detrimental. Importantly, chronic conflict as a result of training manifests in situations where the horse receives constant pressure or pain; it tends not to arise directly as a

result of mild cues, although it does arise when random behaviors appear that are not under the stimulus control of those mild cues.[24] Such conflict leads to greater and greater amounts of tension and a frustrated flight response (Fig. 13.8).

A useful example of conflict in equitation arises when horses are trapped between the rider's 'go' and 'stop' signals. Unable to resolve the pain, they may resort to shying, spinning away, leaping, or bucking, depending on their genetic make-up. Shying may evolve progressively to rearing if a horse receives sufficient practice, motivation (pressures are not resolved) and reinforcement in the form of dislodging the rider. Bucking is a conflict response that arises from unclear installation of the 'go' signal when the reins are also pressuring the horse to stop to some extent. It is also made more likely when the leg signals are incompletely and inconsistently trained and when the horse has been poorly trained by benign cues (such as voice commands) that have no operant basis and the rider later has to resort to hitherto unused leg pressures. Most behavior problems in-hand and

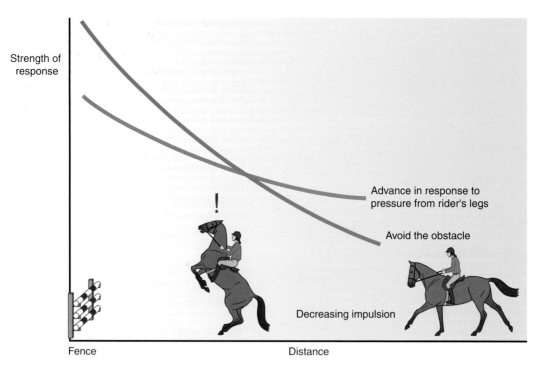

Figure 13.8 A horse that is reluctant to jump a fence may enter conflict if it fails to resolve the competing drives to avoid the fence and to respond to pressure from the rider's legs.

under-saddle can be resolved by retraining the pressure-release responses of 'go' and 'stop'. This entails training these responses so that they are immediate, occur from a light version of the pressure, and that speed, direction, and consistent leg and rein connections are retrained.

As we see in the case study at the end of this chapter, problems loading into a trailer (float) are similarly resolved when the horse is retrained so that the 'go' signal from anterior lead rein pressure and the 'stop' signal from posterior lead rein pressure are re-established.

In training situations, chronic states of stress and conflict increasingly emerge when the association between cues and outcomes is not sufficiently predictable for the horse. An example of this is when a stimulus does not always lead to the same response and a deteriorated state of pressure-release responses prevails. It is within this schema that most manifestations of the so-called 'problem horse' arise. Therefore conflict behaviors, including loading and traveling problems, tension in-hand and under-saddle, and many other problem behaviors may have their roots in the confusion or incomplete installation of one or more of the basic pressure-release responses that are derived from their interactions with humans.

The more horses experiment with conflict behaviors and associate them with positive outcomes, even on a variable schedule, the more they are likely to extinguish other learned responses.[24] They are driven by their hard-wired instincts to escalate tension when they experience conflict. This can have the effect of alarming or annoying the rider, with a resultant loss of relaxation in the horse. This is contraindicated because better learning performances are achieved by horses that are calm, probably due to reduced interference in the learning process.[25]

THE POTENTIAL CONTRADICTION OF CONTACT

The nature of the sport of dressage predisposes it to creating training-related conflict.[24] Dressage requires the horse to maintain a constant contact with the rider's hands (via the reins and bit), to be 'on the bit' (see Glossary), which entails the horse maintaining an arched neck, while simultaneously responding to signals from the reins (Fig. 13.9). Because the horse is highly motivated to seek release from pressure (especially in his sensitive mouth), the process of habituating the horse to the rein contact is often problematic within a traditional training regime. The problem is that the horse must habituate to the level of normal 'contact' *and* learn to differentiate this from 'stop'.[24] The contemporary framework for dressage training places less emphasis on maintaining a light contact than on other aspects of the

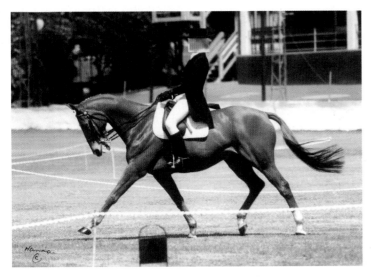

Figure 13.9 Horse being ridden with a 'strong' contact. (Photograph courtesy of Sandra Hannan.)

outline and locomotion of the horse. Thus, instead of training the horse to carry his head and neck freely on a light contact, it is not uncommon to find that the horse is heavy in the rider's hands and develops conflict behaviors. Furthermore, traditional dressage training obscures the signs of the onset of learned helplessness and offers few strategies to prevent it.[24]

Contact in the purist sense is simply the rider's feel of the horse's lips and tongue but not the premolar teeth or diastema so it therefore involves no pain, just a mild sensation. This contact should be targeted for the life of the horse in training. While seeking mild contact, which is implicit in the traditional notion of self-carriage, there will of course be times when the contact is escalated to produce a learned response, via operant conditioning, but the escalation is fleeting and is therefore unlikely to result in any learned helplessness. Sadly trainers and riders frequently prefer a much stronger pressure on the horse's mouth that includes pressure on other parts of the mouth and therefore is more likely to involve pain and learned helplessness.

Bloodlines of horses that tolerate the heavy rein (and spur) pressures and make it to the top in dressage, with few apparent side effects, are inadvertently selected for pain tolerance.[24] Such forbearance under saddle may come at the price of deterioration in the horse's behavioral repertoire. These changes may be easy to pinpoint (e.g. the horse may cease to turn or stop properly) or may be rather more obscure and general. For example, the horse may become generally sour and the manifestation of this may range from aggression during saddling to rearing or bolting. Since conflict typically manifests when the horse is least secure, he might develop 'panic' attacks away from home or may, for example, paw during traveling. We see a clear need for the empirical study of the relationship between training and stress responses.

THE SOLUTIONS

There is a series of ideas and strategies that practitioners can adopt to avoid and eliminate conflict

in horses. By clarifying thinking and simplifying the messages that are sent to horses, we can ensure that their responses become more predictable.

THE SCIENCE OF TRAINING

Although tradition has meant that learning theory has been overlooked by most equestrians, it is appropriate that readers acknowledge the extent to which scientists have developed ways of understanding the changes that occur in animals when they learn. Using the language of learning theory, some of the inconsistencies that confuse riders, and therefore ultimately horses, can be eliminated.

Trial-and-error (operant) conditioning or classical conditioning?

Most systems of horse training, especially traditions of classical dressage, focus on classical conditioning in the belief that this appeals to the horse's sensibilities. Indeed, there are numerous dressage discussion sites on the Internet devoted to classical conditioning.

While no mammalian habit is totally unconditional, many great riders have understood that the more habits are clear and consolidated, the less horses are at the mercy of their instincts. Stallions with good training of basics will work under-saddle in the presence of estrous mares, and throughout history the most reliable horses in the butchery of battle and across country are the well-trained ones – those with clear consistent and deeply entrenched responses.

When we consider the mechanisms of learning involved in training horses in-hand and under-saddle, it becomes clear that all trained responses in 'breaking-in' or, more correctly, foundation training are products both of trial-and-error (operant) conditioning and classical conditioning. Trial-and-error learning with both positive and negative reinforcement is the mechanism underlying the training of the basic responses in-hand (lead forward, stop, and so on) and under-saddle (go forward, stop, turn forequarters, turn hindquarters).

Trial-and-error learning in response to pressure from the reins or the legs of the rider allows greater controllability of outcome than could be achieved by classical conditioning.[24] For example, the greatest chance of stopping a bolting horse is with the reins, provided the 'stop' response is sufficiently trained through trial-and-error learning. This is because a horse that has been operantly conditioned to slow down or stop to bit pressures of variable aversiveness, is able to apply that learning even in face of the adrenalin-charged flight response. In contrast, a horse that has been trained only by classical conditioning to obey a previously neutral 'stop' cue is less likely to respond appropriately in the face of novel fearful stimuli.

Positive reinforcement

The fundamental reason why negative reinforcement is used so extensively in horse training is because of the enforceability of signals such as rein pressure, compared with the difficulty of positively reinforcing ('stop' and 'go') responses after they have been randomly produced (see Ch. 4).

Positive reinforcement does have a role in horse training, especially in the form of secondary reinforcement that takes the form of target and bridge training (clickers, clicker words, etc.). Because of its enormous value in rapidly reinforcing otherwise hard-to-reward behaviors, and behaviors offered by animals at a distance from the trainer, this approach should be incorporated into training, particularly of passage and piaffe.

Strategic timing of training sessions

McCall et al[26] examined the effect of the number of trials per training session on avoidance learning and found that, regardless of the total number of learning opportunities, moderate repetition of training activities is needed for efficient learning. However, learning occurs throughout life in parallel with any training regime. It is unlikely that the horse regards training or schooling sessions as opportunities to concentrate on important lessons. Instead, it is more likely that it is simply aware of an increased intensity of signaling from its rider, provided that it has not habituated to the signals.

The temporal distribution of training trials influences equine learning abilities. Experimentally this was demonstrated when ponies subjected to a single weekly training session (to clear a small hurdle in order to avoid a mild electric shock) achieved a high level of performance in fewer sessions than ponies trained twice weekly or daily.[27] This would seem to highlight the importance of giving horses breaks from intensive schooling so that they can better process information. Turn-out periods after intensive training are thought to allow maturation and consolidation of associations. However, from a neurological viewpoint, it is not clear exactly how or why this should occur. It would appear to involve the transformation of operant actions into habits and so may be connected with the maturation and consolidation of neural pathways.

One stimulus for one response

It is important to train a single response from a single and distinct signal, where possible. Pavlov coined the term 'overshadowing' to describe the diluting effect a stronger signal has over another if applied simultaneously.[28,29] Overshadowing is a common error in contemporary horse training. So in early training 'go' should *always* be elicited by both of the rider's legs, without the simultaneous application of other signals, such as a click of the tongue or a shuffle of the seat. The 'stop' signal should initially be trained only by pressure from both reins equally, and 'turn' with pressure from the rein on the side to which the turn is to be made. These things must be consolidated; it is inappropriate to use the seat for stop before the horse has a consolidated stop response from the reins. Similarly it is important that the horse leads proficiently from pressure on the head collar rather than simply 'following' (classical conditioning) the handler, as this affords greater control in all situations and prevents the horse from practicing and making a habit of undesirable behavior.

One response at a time

If the basic trial-and-error responses are not consolidated, then two or more signals should not be applied simultaneously. Moreover, it can be particularly destructive to the horse's learned responses if 'stop' and 'go' pressures are applied at the same time at any stage of its life. This is the most common cause of chronic conflict in performance horses. The elements of half-halts (see Glossary) should not be simultaneous but be fractionally separated in time. As the horse's learned responses become more consolidated over time, signals can be given closer together, because their effects have proceeded beyond operant action to become habit. However, even with potentially less-destructive combinations of responses, conflict can develop and training efficiency plummets. For example 'go' and 'turn', or 'go' and 'leg-yield' ('turn hindlegs') should also not be applied simultaneously, otherwise the integrity of the constituent responses becomes dulled.

FOUNDATION TRAINING UNDER-SADDLE

Importantly, there are three phases to the training of the basic responses both in-hand and under-saddle during 'breaking-in' or, more correctly, foundation training in horses:

- the mild cue, followed contiguously by
- an increase in pressure of the signal, and ending with
- release of the pressure at the onset of the desired behavior.

This scheme is negative reinforcement, and it induces a small amount of stress by design, so that the animal is propelled to trial various behaviors. Generally speaking, all attempts to reduce drive raise alertness. Subsequently when the horse trials the behavior deemed 'correct' by the trainer, the pressure must be released immediately.

In all pressure-release training, it is important to *increase* the pressure if there is no response; and to release the pressure *immediately* at the onset of the correct behavior. The release of pressure is the intrinsic reinforcer. Contiguous praise is largely redundant and may even be counter-productive if it has the potential to confuse the horse.

The rider's aim should be to reduce the stress by aiming to increase the subtlety of the signals once successful trials have taken place. This mechanism, pressure-release training, is the broad scheme by which all the basic locomotory responses are established in foundation training, and re-established in the elimination of problems. These locomotory responses cover the basic movements of the horse in the two dimensions (anterior/posterior; lateral forelegs/hindlegs). In-hand these are 'go', 'stop' and 'turn the hindlegs'. Under-saddle, 'go', 'stop', 'turn forelegs' and 'turn hindlegs' encompass all the possible movements of the horse in the two dimensions. Generally speaking it is not essential to train the turn of foreleg responses as part of in-hand training as there are no sharp turn requirements in that modality.

In under-saddle training the rider draws the reins toward his hips and when the horse stops/slows the rider releases that pressure. The rider squeezes the horse's sides with both his calves and when the horse goes forward, the squeezing stops. Similarly, a single rein trains the turn steps of the forelegs (Fig. 13.10a), and the single leg

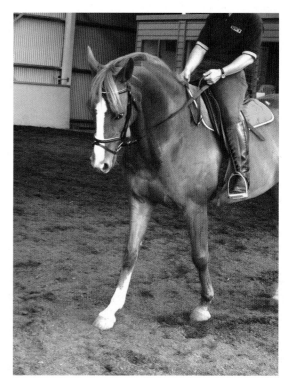

Figure 13.10a A single rein trains the turn steps of the forelegs.

application trains the turn steps of the hindlegs (Fig. 13.10b). The timing of this sequence of operant cues is critical. Problems right across the board in training – ranging from horses not leading into trailers to rearing under-saddle – result from the violation of this sequence, yet a description of it is a rarity in contemporary equine training texts.

FOUNDATION TRAINING IN-HAND

Training the horse in-hand is best begun with the trainer facing the horse, on the horse's nearside, holding the lead rein in the left hand 20 cm or so from the horse's chin. The horse should be wearing a thin rope halter so that the pressure is more readily perceived than with a thicker leather

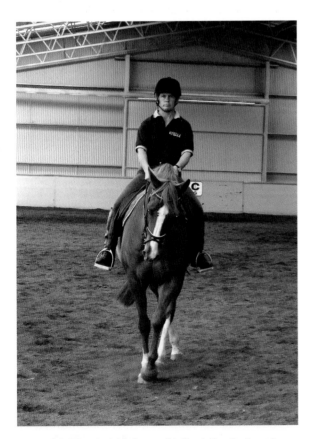

Figure 13.10b   A single leg application trains the turn steps of the hindlegs.

halter. If the horse has no leading response the entire lesson should be conducted in an enclosed yard. Generally the 'go' and 'stop' responses can be trained simultaneously through their various qualities because they arise in the training of each other.

During training in-hand, the handler pressures the lead-rein in the anterior direction for 'go', and in a posterior direction toward the horse's neck for 'stop'. For 'head down' the lead direction is vertically downwards, and for 'turning the hindlegs' the long whip is used for tapping the relevant hindquarter.

Go and stop

Forwards can be progressively shaped from a sideways move once this response has been established. When the horse can consistently achieve a step toward the trainer, further repetitions of increased pressure during the horse's delay will result in the response becoming immediate and light in the hand.

When the lead response is trained so that it is offered immediately from a light pressure, this will often result in the horse maintaining speed (rhythm) in its stride. However if the horse slows downs during leading, this is retrained by pressuring it more strongly during this loss of rhythm and releasing at the onset of the quicker stride. Next it can be trained to step forward in a straight line. This is achieved by stopping and repeating any drifting steps until the horse steps straight ahead. A consistent contact is trained by stopping the horse as soon as the contact becomes inconsistent. Longer steps are trained so that they also occur from a light contact, and finally these responses are tested and trained in different environments.

Similarly the stop is trained through increasing the pressure significantly during the time when the horse is not stopping/slowing, and releasing it as soon as locomotion has ceased. Increasing the pressure when the horse is slow to respond results in an obedient response. Rhythm in the stop response develops when the horse stops smoothly from a light contact. When the horse is being led forward, and it subsequently quickens of its own accord, an immediate downward transition will re-establish rhythm. A byproduct of successful training of rhythm in 'go' and 'stop' responses is that the horse will stay in the one place without being maintained by pressure. Conversely, retaining too strong a contact leads to habituation of the signal, which is detrimental to training. Vibrating the lead rein during the period of enforcement is sometimes more effective than pulling it, because it increases the aversiveness of the intervention.

Training a step backwards from the 'stop' pressure deepens the stop response. Drifting sideways during the 'stop' response can be corrected by increasing the lead pressure in the opposite direction during any drift. The 'stop' response should also be trained to be adjustable so that the stride can be shortened. The final quality to be trained is that the horse stops anywhere.

It is important to test that the pressures move the horse to go forward and stop, and this can be achieved when the handler is standing still (so as not to cue the horse) and pressuring the horse to go forward and stop. When this has been achieved, horses become relaxed and obedient.[24]

Sideways

The horse is first pressured to step sideways to its left to make a basic attempt at the desired response. As soon as the horse steps towards the trainer the pressure is released. The side step is done because pressuring the horse forward is sometimes difficult; it may simply not budge (75 kg vs 550 kg) or it may rear over.

It is also useful to train the horse to step sideways from pressure on its hock with the tapping of the light whip (Fig. 13.11). (It is important the whip is never used as a punishment as it will transform from a signaling device to one that triggers panic and precipitates conflict). At first even the slightest step is reinforced with the cessation of the tapping, but after some success, progressively larger steps across the midline are shaped. The response is trained through the cessation of the whip-tap until it is offered immediately after a light touch of the whip. During the early training of this response the horse will often

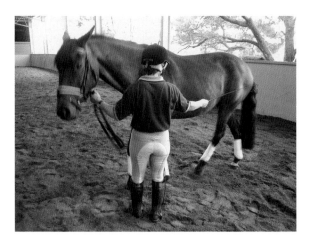

Figure 13.11 Train the horse to step sideways from pressure on his hock with the tapping of the light whip.

curl its neck. The aim should be to make it move smoothly, with a straight body and neck.

The tapping at the hock can progressively move up the sides of the leg and to the ribcage so that soon the handler's fingers or eventually a voice command such as 'Over!' can initiate the step across. The use of the whip on the flank at the outset is inadvisable since it tends to promote flinching and kicking-out because, typically, this area is extremely sensitive.

Lowering the head

It is also useful to train the horse to lower its head in response to pressure, because of the relaxing effect of this posture. Given the horse's apparent lack of higher mental abilities, it seems possible that posture can affect arousal and therefore responses by association. Therefore because a lowered head position is associated with activities that occur when horses are calm, such as grazing and drowsing, training the horse to lower its head results in a rapid and dramatic reduction in tension. Operant conditioning of head lowering is achieved by pressuring the horse's head directly downwards with the lead or reins until the horse lowers a little and releasing the pressure immediately (Fig. 13.12). Thus the horse consistently finds comfort, and calmness

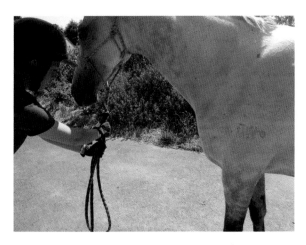

Figure 13.12 Head lowering is achieved by pressuring the horse's head directly downwards with the lead or reins until the horse lowers a little, and releasing the pressure immediately.

results. As with all responses, it is important to reinforce every good try according to the rules of shaping (see Ch. 4). Then progressively more immediate responses can be targeted, followed by the ability to lower all the way down to the ground in one smooth response.

Any lack of straightness in the neck is attended to using the rein to straighten the neck. The use of the rein in this way reduces the unhelpful effect of random neck movements laterally. Next, slightly faster downward movements of the horse's head are targeted, and then finally the horse is tested and trained in various other environments.

REFINEMENT UNDER-SADDLE AND IN-HAND

Refinement of the basics includes the conditioning of appropriate responses to signals of increasing lightness. The extent to which this can be achieved is often limited only by the handler's/ rider's ability to deliver more subtle signals. Unfortunately, as they struggle to balance, many riders inadvertently move around in the saddle too much to be consistent in the application of mild signals.

Assuming the horse has learned the basic responses, it can be trained to make these in response to increasingly subtle signals. Lightness in all the signals is extremely desirable for both in-hand training and under-saddle. This is why self-carriage is so critical and why it should occur from the beginning of training.[24] The horse's neck and head should be in the desired outline when it learns to go forward and stop. The rider should frequently release the reins to test that the horse is happy to carry its head in whichever position. If not, the horse will be leaning on the bit and the resultant pain will lead to some adverse behavior or learned helplessness.

Other features of refinement involve combining basic responses to build advanced movements and providing additional signals for these and indeed basic responses. For example, the half-pass involves the near simultaneous responses of 'go', 'turn forelegs' and 'turn hindlegs'. If such combinations do not arise from the lightest of pressure signals, then conflict behaviors are possible and the single constituent responses are subject to detraining.

It is tempting for novice trainers to use many cues at once when none is consolidated properly. They often use voice commands haphazardly together with leg or rein aids. In breaking-in or retraining the basics, trainers must train one stimulus for one response. Before adding other cues, trainers must be sure that the basics are well established and alternative behaviors are no longer trialled.[24] When the basic responses are consolidated and are under stimulus control (see Discrimination in Ch. 4), it is possible to add an extra signal to elicit a particular response. For example, a vocalized command may be added to the rein signal for the horse to stop.

RESOLUTION

Unwelcome behaviors (see Ch. 15) can be successfully modified by simply retraining the pressure-release regime of the problematic learned responses. One of the most important things to remember is that (re)training must progressively target consistent outcomes. The aim is to consolidate certain responses so that they become habits.

Retraining in-hand and under-saddle

With a young horse, or a horse in retraining, it is fundamental to (re)train the horse to go, stop, turn the forelegs and turn the hindlegs. But these responses must not be produced haphazardly with different outcomes each time or the horse will become confused. The targeting of consistent outcomes is achieved by progressively deleting random behaviors that arise from the handler's/rider's signals. However, because of the range of qualities of desirable behavior, the trainer must progressively train each separate quality of response. This involves ignoring undesirable qualities that can be successively targeted at a later point in the training process.

Shaping requires that the trainer initially reinforces every 'good try'. The horse may or may not trial all sorts of undesirable responses as a result of the maintained or increased pressure but it rapidly learns that the pressure is released only when it offers specific responses. Then the trainer can begin to target those specific responses so that the *same* response is reinforced. This brings the desired response under stimulus control.

Training of the basic responses in-hand and under-saddle involves gradually gaining complete control of the horse's locomotory responses. When this is achieved, random movements of the neck and head are deleted and horses universally show relaxation.

The order in which qualities are trained should reflect the problematic potential they offer. The first quality is simply to produce a basic attempt at the response. Then obedience is trained so that an immediate response arises from a light pressure signal.

The next quality to be targeted is the speed of the body and the subsequent rhythm of the leg responses. Then the exact direction of the horse is targeted so that any drift off the chosen line of the handler/rider is corrected. This results in the body and neck becoming straight, thus eliminating crookedness and drift.

Next the connection to the handler/rider is refined to be consistent. The penultimate quality to be targeted is to train adjustability in each response so that it can respond with increases in speed or stride length within each basic response. Finally, the horse is trained in various environments of increasing challenge potential so that it performs all the responses with all of the above qualities wherever and whenever required. The desired qualities of the basic responses should be shaped as follows:

1. basic attempt – an attempt or crude response
2. obedience – immediate and light
3. rhythm – self-maintained speed
4. straightness – self-maintained line, straight neck and body
5. contact – self-maintained leg and rein connections
6. engagement – adjustable within the gait
7. proof – performs response with above qualities whenever and wherever.

When the particular qualities of each response are trained and then consolidated, the horse will have no source of confusion in its training.[24] As we saw in the case study of police horse training (see Ch. 4), calmness is a feature of horses that have established consistent and predictable learned responses. The establishment of calmness is not always an easy or speedy task in retraining.

When the relationship between stimulus and response is variable, confusion is the result and conflict behavior involving tension is almost inevitable. Therefore it is important to progressively target responses of the same quality in each session, or progressively build on the quality during each session, and not to relax standards during training. Once modified, 'problem' behaviors can be managed by trainers through the frequent checking and refinement of the basic operant responses.

Sometimes, certain pressures applied with conventional equipment are insufficient to produce a response. This is particularly true when retraining a horse that has habituated to a pressure-release signal. For example, in leading the horse forwards, the horse may not be sufficiently motivated to step forward from lead pressure. Therefore the lead signal may require extra empowerment from an accompanying whip-tap on the shoulder. The horse must be able to lead reasonably well before you attempt this. Also, if you cannot touch your horse with the whip without him showing an excessive flight response, then habituate him to it by laying it on him then stroking him with it until he is relaxed.

It is important that strong lead pressure is *not* used in conjunction with the whip-tap, but instead mild pressure of the lead accompanies the whip-tap so that the whip-tap adds extra motivational power to the lead pressure. Such empowerment may be necessary in the case of leading a resisting horse into a float. Assisting the lead response with the whip-tap is inadvisable in early training of the lead forward response in a naïve horse because adding the whip-tap to a *novel* lead stimulus can result in overshadowing and therefore no learning of leading from the lead-rein.

SUMMARY OF KEY POINTS

- One of the abiding obstacles to effective training of ridden behavior is the rider's poor understanding of learning theory.
- Equine education is clouded by unhelpful terms such as 'natural' and 'unnatural' 'aids', and the use of anthropomorphic terminology in describing horse behavior as well as the implication that the horse has some moral culpability in its training.
- Contemporary horse training dogma provides many obstacles to effective equine learning such as training too many responses simultaneously and overshadowing of one signal over another.
- If novice riders used the principles of operant conditioning so that they did not apply conflicting signals as they learned to balance, many riding school horses would feel the immediate benefit.

CASE STUDY

Unexpectedly, a 12-year old half-bred gelding refused to load at the end of a show. The two-horse trailer being used that day was the vehicle in which he normally traveled. Despite an enormous variety of attempts to cajole him into loading he continued to back away from the ramp. He was eventually forced in with a combination of ropes and whips. Since then he seemed phobic of the trailer and required considerable coaxing even to feed near it. The owners felt that he may have worked out a way of avoiding going to shows.

Conferring subjective mental machinations on a horse that refuses to load into a trailer is an unconstructive approach. Even with the most difficult horses, trailer loading is a relatively simple process if it is considered a function of the leading response. When the horse is relatively unconditional in its leading responses, it will lead anywhere, including into the trailer.

The gelding was retrained to lead, using a thin rope halter. This provided maximum control of his 'stop' and 'go' responses. First he was tested in the qualities of the 'go' and 'stop' responses away from the trailer. Subsequent retraining also took place away from the aversive stimulus that the trailer represented.

The 'go' response was thoroughly trained as there was an inherent weakness in the normal leading stimulus supplied by the lead-rein pressure. Because the lead-rein pressure at the top of the gelding's head was not sufficiently aversive compared with the aversiveness of the stimuli he was expected to face, such as the trailer, his response to it needed to be deepened. This was achieved by *combining* the lead pressure with the incessant tapping with a long whip between the elbow and the shoulder.

At first the horse did not 'go' and 'stop' immediately from the respective pressures, so stronger pressure and quicker release at the onset of correct behavior were deployed. This also resulted in his becoming maximally responsive to a light pressure. The obedience of the 'stop' response was enhanced by training a step-back from the halt using pressure-release. When the gelding was obedient, the long whip was introduced to fortify the lead response that was already installed. This association was established because it was considered likely that it was going to be necessary when it was time to face the trailer. As the 'go' lead pressure was employed, he was tapped between the elbow and the shoulder (Fig. 13.13).

The leading response was deepened by making him step back using a light signal then immediately applying forward lead pressure coupled with mild tapping as above. Crucially, the trainer was careful not to cease the mild lead pressure and tapping until the horse stepped forward, no matter what resistance it offered.

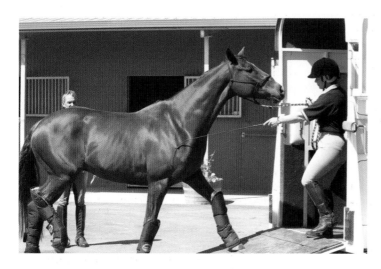

Figure 13.13 Horse being re-trained to lead and load.

Next the gelding was trained to move his hindquarters sideways from both sides. This was established to assist in straightening the horse if he trialed crookedness during loading onto the trailer. Facing the hindquarters of the horse, holding the lead with the hand that was closest to the horse, and holding the long whip with the other hand the trainer used the lead rein with the appropriate pressure to prevent him going forwards, rather than sideways with the hindlegs. Using the whip to tap the metatarsal region, the trainer increased the tapping intensity until the instant the horse stepped across. This was repeated until the response was reliable. The horse was then ready to be trained to load onto the trailer.

Facing the trailer for the first time, the gelding stopped and therefore failed his *basic attempt*. Although training him to load into the trailer was the ultimate goal, the proximate targets were simply to take steps forward towards the trailer. To train the horse to step forward towards the trailer, the trainer:

1.   Only ever tapped when he also had forward direction pressure on the rein (it fortified the lead response by *association*).
2.   Only ever tapped when the horse was not going forward (*never* when he was).
3.   Increased the intensity of the tapping, but not the lead pressure, when he felt there was no response within a reasonable period.

4.   Never had gaps of more than one second between taps.
5.   Softened both lead rein and ceased tapping the very second the horse moved his foot/feet forward.
6.   Used the 'stop' response to delete leaping onto the trailer; allowed him only to step to it.
7.   Immediately applied mild lead and whip-tap pressure if the horse rushed during backing out of the trailer and continued to do so until he stepped forward, no matter how far back he went.

Further repetitions and mild pressure of rein and whip-tap resulted in the horse developing a *rhythm* in his steps onto the trailer. Whenever he slowed or quickened, these inappropriate responses were dealt with progressively. With the focus on training *straightness*, it was important to step forward and back all over the trailer, especially the area of the roof overhang. (This is often a problem area where horses learn to balk). The gelding was trained to go forward and demonstrate he was willing to place his front feet anywhere in the trailer region. At this stage, wither scratching and voice praise associations were employed profusely to reinforce his learned responses. The horse no longer shows any evidence of reluctance to approach or enter the trailer.

REFERENCES

1. Voith VL. Pattern discrimination, learning set formation, memory retention, spatial and visual reversal learning by the horse. Thesis, Ohio State University, Columbus, 1975.
2. Wolff A, Hausberger M. Learning and memorisation of two different tasks: the effects of age, sex and sire. Appl Anim Behav Sci 1995; 46(3/4):137–143.
3. Mal ME, McCall CA, Newland C, Cummins KA. Evaluation of a one-trial learning apparatus to test learning ability in weanling horses. Appl Anim Behav Sci 1993; 35(4):305–311.
4. Harris PA. Review of equine feeding and stable management practices in the UK concentrating on the last decade of the 20th Century. The role of the horse in Europe. Equine Vet J Suppl 1999; 46–54.
5. Ödberg FO, Bouissou MF. The development of equestrianism from the baroque period to the present day and its consequences for the welfare of horses. The role of the horse in Europe. Equine Vet J Suppl 1999; 26–30.
6. Jeffcott LB, Rossdale PD, Freestone J, et al. An assessment of wastage in thoroughbred racing from conception to 4 years of age. Equine Vet J 1982; 14:1 85–198.
7. Bailey CJ. Wastage in the Australian Thoroughbred racing industry. Rural Industries Research and Development Corporation, Research Paper No. 98/52, 1998.
8. Dennett DC. Kinds of minds. London: Orion; 1996.
9. Williams M. Effect of artificial rearing on social behavior of foals. Equine Vet J 1974; 6:17–18.
10. Kiley-Worthington M. The behaviour of horses: in relation to management and training. London: JA Allen; 1987.
11. Rees L. The horse's mind. London: Stanley Paul; 1984.
12. Wiepkema R. Behavioural aspects of stress. In: Biology of stress in farm animals: an integrative approach. Wiepkema PR, van Adrichem PWM, eds. Dordrecht: Martinus Nijhoff; 1987.
13. Schramm U. The undisciplined horse. London: JA Allen; 1981.
14. Le Doux JE. Emotion, memory and the brain. Sci Am 1994 (June); 32–39.
15. McLean AN. Cognitive abilities — the result of selective pressures on food acquisition? Appl Anim Behav Sci 2001; 71(3):241–258.
16. Houpt KA. The intelligence of the Horse. Equine Pract 1979; 1:20–26.
17. McGreevy PD. How animals learn: basic insights. Ain't Misbehaving. The AT Reid refresher course for veterinarians. Proceedings 340, 11–15 June 2001. Published by the Post Graduate Foundation in Veterinary Science, University of Sydney; 2001:69–98.
18. Webster AJF. Animal welfare: a cool eye towards Eden. London: Blackwell Scientific; 1994.
19. Bermond B. The myth of animal suffering. In: Dol M, Kasanmoentalib S, Lijmbach S, Rivas E, van den Bos R, eds. Animal consciousness and animal ethics: perspectives from the Netherlands. Animals in Philosophy and Science. Assen, The Netherlands: Van Gorcum; 1997:125–143.
20. Budiansky S. The nature of horses — exploring equine evolution, intelligence and behavior. New York: Free Press; 1997.
21. Deacon TW. Fallacies of progression in theories of brain-size evolution. Int J Primatol 1990; 11:193–236.
22. Beilharz RG, Luxford BG, Wilkinson JL. Quantitative genetics and evolution: Is our understanding of genetics sufficient to explain evolution? J Anim Breed Genet 1993; 110:161–170.
23. Feh C, de Mazieres J. Grooming at a preferred site reduces heart rates in horses. Anim Behav 1993; 46:1191–1194.
24. McLean AN. The mental evolution of the horse and its consequences for training. PhD Thesis, Institute of Land and Food Resources, University of Melbourne, Victoria, 2003.
25. Nicol CJ. Equine learning: progress and suggestions for future research. Appl Anim Behav Sci 2002; 78(2/4):193–208.
26. McCall CA, Salters MA, Simpson SM. Relationship between number of conditioning trials per training session and avoidance learning in horses. Appl Anim Behav Sci 1993; 36(4):291–299.
27. Rubin L, Oppegard C, Hintz HF. The effect of varying the temporal distribution of conditioning trials on equine learning behaviour. J Anim Sci 1980; 50:1184–1187.
28. Hull CL. Principles of behavior. New Haven, CT: Appleton-Century, 1943.
29. Miller RM, Barnet RC, Grahame NJ. Assessment of the Rescorla–Wagner model. Psychol Bull 1995; 117(3):336–363.

14

Handling and transport

THE PRINCIPLES OF GOOD HANDLING

Horses are potentially dangerous because of their size, strength and speed. Using the responses that have evolved as part of their agonistic ethogram, they can kick, strike, bite and barge humans as readily as they do conspecifics. Additionally, they may deploy anti-predator strategies, such as charging, on humans.

Aggressive horses have usually learned that threats and attacks on humans are reinforcing because they effectively reduce the threat posed by the presence of humans. However, learning can be turned to our advantage, since for example, neonatal handling has a beneficial effect on the subsequent general tractability of foals.[1]

Naïve horses are usually frightened of being handled but are seldom actively aggressive, preferring to avoid contact. (This is central to early round-pen training.) They will be less distressed if they can be handled with educated conspecifics, preferably those with whom they have already had social interactions that have led to the more experienced animal emerging as the leader of the dyad.

The prior experience and temperament of a horse are significant for prospective handlers whether they be riders, trainers, farriers or veterinarians. However, even without a full history or the benefit of an owner to advise them, experienced personnel can predict the most likely response by studying the body language of horses. Regardless of the presence or absence of alarm bells in a horse's history and warning signs in its behavior, it pays to reduce risks when handling all

313

horses, e.g. by ensuring that during all procedures, equipment and personnel within a stable are kept to a minimum and that personnel remain on the same side of the horse as one another.

Tact and subtlety are the cardinal markers of good horsemanship. Young, naïve and fearful horses demand the greatest tact. Sudden movements by personnel should be avoided so that one can clearly identify which responses can be elicited and controlled by a steady approach. Correct handling procedures can lower reactivity levels in horses, and may facilitate learning in some circumstances.[2]

Since horse handling is commonly based on negative reinforcement (see Ch. 4), it is worth remembering that for as long as force is used it will continue to be needed. It is fundamental therefore that the application of pressure must be followed by release (see Ch. 13). Under ideal conditions this means that just as the pressures applied during the most desirable forms of equitation are minimal, the very least force should be used to lead and control a horse when one is on the ground. It is incumbent on the horse handler to use a minimum of force because each episode of handling represents a learning opportunity. The horse that has learned to struggle and been reinforced by being allowed to escape is more likely to offer the same behavior in future. Excessive force or the failure to release the pressure when the horse responds appropriately are likely to cause problems related to conflict and habituation.

It is always worth remembering how useful positive reinforcement can be in shaping desirable responses, especially when aversive stimuli have been used previously. For example, horses that are reluctant to load into a trailer (float) can first be trained to approach a target and then the target can be moved to various locations inside the vehicle.[3] The lessons learned this way rapidly generalize to novel conditions, such as different handlers and vehicles. A limited-hold procedure and the presence of a companion horse seem to facilitate training.

The use of the voice in horse handling has been both over-rated and under-rated. Horses respond to a handler's body language and voice. When both are consistent in all handling sessions, the horse's response becomes increasingly predictable. By using the same voice cues when training responses, a trainer can give a horse auditory cues that help to identify the required response (such cues become discriminative stimuli; see Ch. 4). If the human is conversing with the horse, there is the possibility that the horse may habituate to the noise and become reasonably calm if required to do little more than relax. However, the opportunities for associations between a verbal command and a certain response are diminished since the horse is challenged by the need to filter commands out of the conversation. In other words, discrimination becomes more difficult.

Since consistency is the cornerstone of all good training programs, the use of a routine is helpful in early training of basic manners. After these have been instilled, the horse can be taught to generalize the learning from these fundamental lessons to other contexts. Among other things, this should include being taught to lead from both sides.

For many vets the pleasure of equine work is somewhat offset by the reality that horses are often very fearful of such practitioners. With their ability to learn quickly from aversive events and their formidable memory, horses can remember individual veterinarians and demonstrate accurate recognition of their colleagues from a given clinic because of uniforms or even more generically because of odors (such as surgical spirit) frequently associated with members of the profession. The increased use of chemical restraint rather than physical restraint may reduce the fearfulness of the average equine patient. At the same time, owners can help by habituating horses to being handled in the way a veterinarian handles them. Following the model offered by puppy preschools, it is preferable to do this before rather than after a problem has developed.

The color of clothes worn for handling horse is immaterial when compared with the stimuli horses associate with certain clothing.[4] In the wake of reports that synthetic pheromones can modify behavior in other species,[5] it is worth considering ways in which odors may be used to calm horses. Perhaps the role of familiar odors helps to explain why horse-lore makes mention of the pacifying effects of rubbing one's hands on the chestnuts of a horse prior to 'befriending' it. On a more scientific basis, early reports of the effects of a synthetic 'equine appeasing pheromone' in reducing behavioral and cardiac indicators of fear during a fear-eliciting test (return to familiar conspecifics by parting a curtain)[6] are exciting and suggest that horses may be effectively calmed before novel husbandry and training experiences. By the same token it may be that angry and frustrated humans emit characteristic odors in their sweat that signal to horses the emotional states of their handlers.[7] The effects of different handlers on the behavior of horses are sparsely reported, but it has been proposed that by looking for excessive ear movements when horses are led around an obstacle course, one can detect inexperienced handlers.[8]

DONKEY HANDLING

The differences between the behavioural repertoires of donkeys and horses should be considered when handling donkeys and mules. Some of these differences are inherent; for example, donkeys tend to have different responses to fear-inducing stimuli, tending to freeze more readily than horses (a distinct advantage should they become stuck in barbed wire). Other differences are related to the amount of training and human contact experienced by the individual.

When faced with frustrating situations and forced to respond with aggression, donkeys tend to give fewer warning signs than horses. Additionally it should be borne in mind that because of their enhanced ability to balance, donkeys can easily cow-kick. Few donkeys have been taught not to lean when having their feet examined. This makes veterinary examinations of the hooves and farriery generally more difficult in donkeys than in horses and ponies. Despite their agility, restraint of most donkeys is straightforward if their head can be controlled. Unlike some other species, such as pigs, all equids follow the general rule of 'where the head goes, the body will follow'.

Generally, when compared with horses, donkeys tend to have experienced less close human contact because they are less likely to be ridden and, as a result, they tend to be less well trained. For instance, in the absence of any need, they are rarely taught stable manners. On the other hand, it appears that because fewer people are nervous of donkeys, they are likely to have been handled with more confidence (Jane French, personal communication 2002).

APPROACHING THE HORSE

Until we can, with certainty, unpick the relationship between horses and humans, we are likely to vacillate between explaining a horse's responses as those used with a predator or with a conspecific. If horses view humans as predators, the chances are that their fear responses will be rapidly extinguished if humans do nothing to justify their anxiety. Then it is possible that, during the gentling process, the representation of humans as a threat can be replaced by one of companionship.

The use of the voice can be helpful when approaching equids since it may alert and disarm them. Compared with human clothing, which changes regularly, voices can be a constant cue that assists horses to recognize their owners. As it happens, horse owners tend to use similar calls when calling horses (one of the more common ones being a drawn out 'come on'). While this can have helpful consequences in horses that are happy to be caught, since they respond by traveling towards the sound, it may alert others to the intentions of the approaching humans and prompt them to move away. In the case of horses that are being retrained to accept being caught, it is appropriate to abandon established cues completely so that new associations can be built.

When attempts are made to corner horses, the same principles of driving and blocking that are used in other herding species, such as cattle or sheep, apply. However, the speed and agility of horses means that this rarely works as a means of catching them. A horse in a confined space may attempt to escape either by scrambling over the fence or turning on approaching personnel to drive them away.

To avoid emerging from horses' blind spots (see Ch. 2), personnel should always approach them from the side. Convention is that horses are approached from the left, but this is something that can be revisited in horses that are being trained to extinguish fearful responses associated with handlers. By avoiding staring at horses one may be able to reduce the chances of this being misinterpreted as a prelude to predation or the challenge of a conspecific. Having said that, there is some evidence from a study of well-handled horses that eye contact does not necessarily affect a horse's latency to approach humans.[9] The speed with which humans move can certainly influence equine responses. For example, walking quickly past the point of balance at the animal's shoulder in the direction opposite to desired movement is an easy way to induce an animal to move forward.[10]

Generally it is helpful to approach an unfamiliar horse slowly in a non-menacing stance, with the body relaxed and slouching slightly. If a penned horse is facing away from the stable door or yard gate, handlers should make noises to encourage it to face them. This prevents handlers from being kicked as they approach the horse and is even considered by some to be an important sign that the horse is showing 'respect'. If horses ever regard humans as analogous to conspecifics, they could be excused for having problems reading our body language unless we are regarded as issuing constant (and often hollow) threats (because our ears are permanently pinned back).[11] Regardless of this, it remains unclear why horses would need to show 'respect' to other horses, and therefore submission or subordinance are perhaps more appropriate terms for displays of social deference. Having said that, most riders want their horses (whether they are companion or performance animals) to be compliant first and foremost, so interpretations of rank may be entirely irrelevant.

RESTRAINT

Once they have begun to exhibit a flight response, most horses that are restrained by the head will continue to struggle until the pressure around the head is released. Horses should be tied up with a secure halter (or headcollar) and rope and never by the reins or a lead attached to the bit. The rope

should be tied to a length of bailing twine, which is attached to a solid object. Because it is more readily broken than regular lead ropes and reins, bailing twine is used in combination with quick-release knots in case a struggle ensues. Many serious injuries have been inflicted on both horses and handlers when horses have thrown themselves to the ground in a bid for freedom (Fig. 14.1) or when rails have broken or posts have come out of the ground, so it is important that the bailing twine is weaker than the fixed object to which the horse is tied. The extent of flight responses among horses that are tied up means that the act of releasing horses can be very dangerous, even if they are secured only by quick-release knots. The danger is magnified when more than one horse is tied up and a wave of socially facilitated hysteria crashes over them.

Generally, it is best practice to tie horses at nose height so that normal head movement can be maximized within the limits set by the length of rope between the horse and the fence. This should be

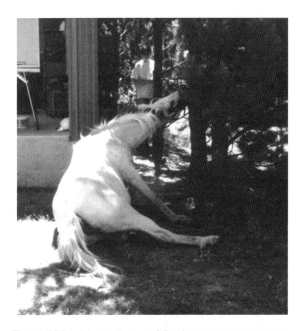

Figure 14.1 A horse that has fallen in an attempt to escape from physical restraint. (The horse was physically unharmed by this incident, but the possibility of it becoming an habitual puller as a result of panic could have been avoided if breakable twine had been used to secure it.) (Photograph courtesy of Claire Ruting.)

such that the horse can turn its head sufficiently to examine objects that would otherwise be in its blind spot, but cannot put a leg over the rope.

There is clear evidence that, as creatures of flight, horses value being able to remove themselves from the threat of discomfort. The danger of horses fighting against physical restraint by blindly paddling their limbs in pursuit of freedom means that hobbles and ropes should be avoided wherever possible. Even under conditions of best practice, rope-burns and even fractures are among the recognized sequelae of roping, strapping and hobbling techniques.

The various roping techniques developed by horsefolk who had no chemical agents with which to pacify horses during aversive interventions have been catalogued elsewhere.[12–14] While one cannot deny the inventiveness of the horse handlers who developed these approaches, the necessity that bred it may have passed. While it may be convenient to keep a horse still and safe for a given procedure, the crudity of these forms of physical restraint should be questioned in the light of current thinking about analgesia in companion animals. There is no justification for allowing animals to undergo pain.[15] Ethically one could argue that psychological threats are as aversive as pain itself. By the same token, there is no justification for allowing horses to fight against physical restraint when there is no evidence that they can predict that the episode will ever end.

If, during a handling procedure, a horse is not likely to learn good associations with personnel, there is a very strong argument for avoiding it learning anything. In practice, while emergencies may necessitate the use of physical restraint before veterinary assistance arrives, chemical agents are indicated more often than force. It is inevitable that some veterinary interventions with horses will be painful, so some level of physical restraint is usually needed to control equine patients, even if it is only to allow the administration of chemical restraint. Since horses show a peak in plasma beta-endorphin concentrations[16] (and so are likely to be least sensitive to noxious stimuli) in the early morning, it has been suggested that this may be the preferred time to undertake elective aversive procedures.[7]

The natural inclination of horses to run from trouble makes them difficult to deal with in the open. Although attempts are sometimes made to hold horses in a corner of a field or yard for interventions, horses are usually much safer in a stable, especially one with enough bedding on the floor to prevent them slipping. Anything that may get in the way during a struggle or a forced retreat by the handler, most notably water buckets, should be removed from the stable before any invasive handling or veterinary procedure. Stables with low ceilings are sometime helpful when handling horses that are inclined to rear or have learned to throw their heads up to avoid a twitch. Ceilings suitable for this application have no projections (such as jutting beams) from them that might damage a horse's head or neck. The presence of the ceiling prevents the horse from gaining momentum as it swings its head up. Though the horse might throw its head up once, it is likely that it feels the ceiling with its ears, and rarely bothers a second time. Rectal examinations may be safely carried out by working round the side of a door. Temporary stocks can be built by placing bales of straw around the horse's hindquarters.

EQUIPMENT FOR RESTRAINT

For most veterinary procedures all that is needed is a reliable attendant who holds the horse firmly with a halter and reinforces appropriate behavior by stroking the animal in anatomical areas associated with stress reduction, including the forehead, neck and withers. Cupping a hand over a horse's eye on the side on which it is being treated is often very helpful, especially for needle-shy horses (Fig. 14.2). Tying horses up for aversive procedures is inadvisable since their tendency to fight against such restraint usually precipitates an attempt to flee and ultimately increases fear and the likelihood of damage to equipment or, worse still, injury to themselves or personnel.

Physical restraint should not be used in ways that directly compromise horse welfare. When increased restraint is required, hobbles, a tail rope or service hobbles (see Fig. 12.5) may be used, but these should be seen as emergency measures rather than routine approaches. Horses may be controlled completely by being cast and tied with ropes, but this is rarely necessary since the same result can be achieved more readily by methods of general anesthesia. Occasionally it is suggested that a twitch or rope gag, often found useful when dealing with the hindquarters of a fearful horse, may work by distracting the animal. This is something of an understatement since, at least in the short term, the distraction is pain. However, the pain may be rapidly modified by endorphins.[17]

The twitch

A time-honored method of applying restraint in horses is to apply a constriction to the upper lip as a so-called twitch (Fig. 14.3). It has the merits of being simple, effective and easy to apply, and is comparatively safe for the horse and the operator.

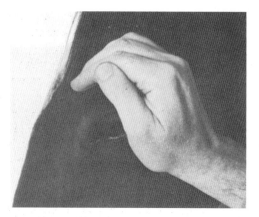

Figure 14.2 A hand cupped over the eye of a horse can reduce fearful responses to veterinary personnel. (Reproduced from Rose & Hodgson.[14])

For mildly painful, brief procedures, a twitch will give some added security. It certainly has a place in the protocol for nasogastric tubing of many horses since it seems to reduce their ability to flick the advancing tip out of the esophageal sphincter (Ken Sedgers, personal communication 2002). Twitches come in a variety of forms, from a simple loop of rope attached to a bull's nose ring, through to a pair of metal pliers called the humane twitch (because it may be associated with less tissue damage in the hands of a novice than a home-made twitch). As with any means of applying pressure, the narrower the element in touch with the horse the greater the chances of pain and even permanent damage. Twitches with soft, thick rope and light (i.e. plastic) handles are generally safest. Snaring as much of the upper lip as possible when applying a twitch seems to increase its effectiveness and reduce the chances of it slipping. The constriction should be loosened every 15 minutes or so to maintain perfusion of tissues distal to it. Additionally this is sound practice since the effectiveness of the twitch tends to wane after this period in many cases.

Twitching of the lip is an approach that should be adopted only when chemical restraint is not available and is best regarded as a last resort of restraint justified only by a bid to inject a psychotropic drug. In very difficult horses, the ear can be grasped transiently (Fig. 14.4) as a brief means of controlling the horse while a twitch is put on the upper lip. Twitching the ear should always be avoided as it may scar the skin, paralyze the ear or make the animal head shy.[7]

The central mechanism (thought to be mediated by beta-endorphins) by which the twitch is

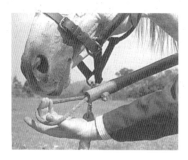
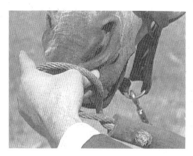
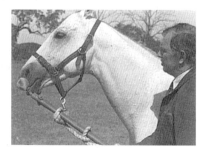

Figure 14.3 Application of a twitch. (Reproduced from Rose & Hodgson.[14])

believed to work is discussed briefly in Chapter 3. However, regardless of the pathways involved, there is little doubt that the twitch works because it hurts.[18] Horses undergo a transient increase in

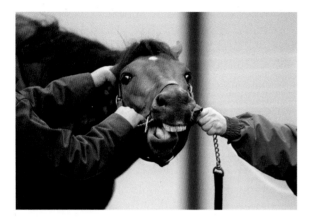

Figure 14.4 Grasping of the ear can have unwelcome long-term behavioral consequences and should therefore only be used with caution. (Photograph by Vince Caligiuri, reproduced by permission of the Sydney Morning Herald.)

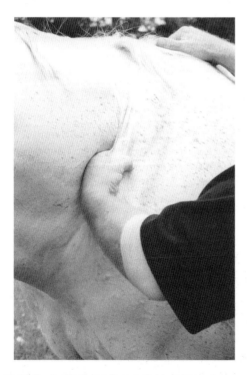

Figure 14.5 A skin twitch (or gaucho twitch) involves grasping and twisting a good handful of skin from the area cranial to the shoulder. (Photograph courtesy of Greg Hogan.)

heart rate when twitched.[11] Intriguingly, heart rate returns to baseline values more rapidly in the crib-biters than in normal horses.[19] Also crib-biters are reported to be less reactive to being twitched than normal horses, being more likely to remain calm.[19] This has prompted the proposal that twitching be used to detect covert stereo-typers,[20] but more empirical data are needed before the management or fate of horses should rest on responses to such a crude intervention.

Broadly speaking, the effects of a nose twitch can often be achieved by 'twitching' a generous fold of skin on the side of the neck (Fig. 14.5). Using this technique, handlers can often restrain fearful horses well enough to facilitate the administration of injectable forms of restraint.

War bridle (or rope gag)

A rope or chain passed over the poll and under the upper lip and then threaded through a loop at the side of the face to form a running noose (Fig. 14.6) acts in a similar way to a twitch when pulled tight. Many variations on this theme arise in the literature and are sometimes even advocated for problems in the ridden horse, even though they are simply vehicles for escalated force and should therefore be avoided. A piece of rubber tubing slipped over the portion of the rope that

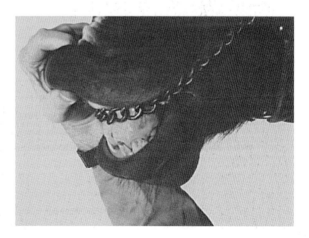

Figure 14.6 A war bridle. (Reproduced from Rose & Hodgson.[14])

presses on the under part of the lip reduces any risk of injury and does not seem to interfere with the effectiveness of the device. The appealing claims made for the efficacy of commercial versions of this device (e.g. Stableizer®) in calming horses even when ridden suggest that its function deserves scientific scrutiny.

Service hobbles

Service hobbles are designed to limit a mare's ability to kick the stallion during mating. They also offer some protection to veterinarians performing rectal or vaginal examinations (see Restraint of Hindlimbs, p. 321), though a physical barrier is more usual for this purpose. Various patterns of service hobbles have been described elsewhere in horse-management literature. All limit the motility of the hindlegs by attaching them by ropes to a band around the horse's neck and most are fitted with some form of quick-release device. Because they occasionally cause horses to fall (usually while struggling) they should be considered for use only in combination with deep, soft bedding materials.

RESTRAINT OF THE HEAD

Generally speaking, horses are not dealt with unless some harness is put on the head. If a horse darts forward, experienced handlers can hold their ground, with the benefit of a pair of strong gloves, and pull the horse's head towards them to arrest the horse's forward movement. An excitable, reactive or flighty horse is best controlled if the handler is standing caudal to the horse's head and cranial to its shoulder. With this approach, any horse can be controlled in an open space as its momentum can be thrown off course by a sharp tug on the lead rope. When applying this technique, one should keep in mind that the horse's rump will tend to swing out away from the handler, exposing it to the possibility of collision with objects to the side. Equally, the maneuver brings with it the risk of the horse being placed in an ideal position to rear, strike or bite the handler. The suggestion has been made that simply lowering the head may have a pacifying effect on horses

(see Ch. 13).[21] The use of a horse rug slung around the cranial pectoral region as a barrier to striking forelimbs has been proposed,[14] but the associated risk of the horse becoming entangled by the rug as a consequence of a flight response means that this approach has limited appeal.

A halter is designed to be placed on the horse from the near side. It should be tight enough to prevent the horse from removing it, and the nosepiece should not rest below the nasal bone. The noseband should be loose enough to allow the horse to open its mouth and chew. When designed to allow tightening around the head if the horse resists, this works especially well, in the right hands, within the pressure-release framework (see Ch. 13). However, it is often knotted to prevent it becoming dislodged should the horse struggle. This safety measure often does little to affect the halter's usefulness because few handlers seem to understand the importance of releasing pressure immediately to reinforce leading responses. As discussed in Chapter 7, it seems likely that there are left- and right-handed horses, so although horses generally lead better from the near side, this is simply because this is what they are accustomed to. By leading horses from both left and right, one can determine whether one side suits the horse better.

A headcollar is stronger than traditional rope halters but does not pull tight. Although the straps that comprise a head collar give alternative handgrips for the attendant, best practice is to attach a rope so that, if the horse throws its head up violently, control is not completely lost (since the attendant has a length of rope to pay out). Consistent pressure-release conditioning (as explained in Ch. 13) quickly teaches horses, by the application of exceptionally subtle downward tension on the lead rope, to lower their heads. Ropes should never be wrapped around the hand or fingers because serious injuries can occur. If the horse snatches its head back with such speed and force that the handler finds it impossible to let go, skin burns and even fractured bones may result.

If the mouth is not being examined, a bit and bridle may be used for restraint. When considering the effect of different pieces of tack, the broader the area in contact with the horse the less discomfort

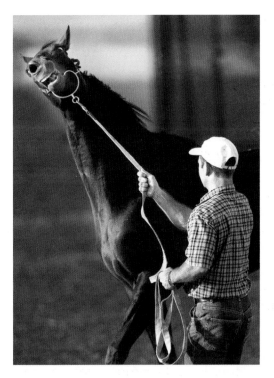

Figure 14.7 Despite the use of an anti-rearing bit, many horses in behavioral conflict will continue to rear. (Photograph by Vince Caligiuri, reproduced by permission of the Sydney Morning Herald.)

it causes and the less readily it can be used in the negative reinforcement paradigm. This is why horses can easily be trained to pull against harnesses, breast-plates and collars used on well-muscled areas, such as the shoulders and pectoral regions, but are reluctant to fight pressure from bits in the mouth (especially if they make contact only in small areas as is the case with the bladed and twisted bits). When used only occasionally, chains in the curb groove or in the mouth are likely to have a strong effect, especially in the short term. Anti-rearing bits usually have reasonably fine elements and therefore a more severe action than normal riding bits, such as a regular snaffle. Working on several parts of the mouth, these bits help to control particularly reactive animals such as naïve youngsters that may readily toss their heads (Fig. 14.7) and stand up on their hindlegs, but they must be used with sensitivity. Again, the

emphasis should be on using light pressure that is released as soon as the desired response has been made. They should never be used in attempts to punish a horse, e.g. by reefing on a lead rope.

RESTRAINT OF FORELIMBS

Roping techniques are mentioned in this book only for use in emergencies that arise in the absence of veterinary support. Interested readers can find detailed accounts of such techniques elsewhere.[22]

During a veterinary examination of a potentially fractious horse, movement and risk of being kicked can be decreased by restraining one of the forelimbs. An additional purpose of raising the forelimb arises when injecting it, e.g. for a peripheral nerve block. A forelimb can be lifted and the hoof brought up to the elbow and held there by a handler. When holding the forefoot of a horse in this way, handlers must avoid teaching the horse to lean, because this defeats the object of transiently disabling the horse. A light grip on the foot is desirable, but it is important to avoid giving the horse an opportunity to snatch the foot away, which often happens before a horse kicks out at the veterinarian. After due consideration of the hazardous responses it can evoke (especially in naïve horses), the use of a 'knee strap' placed around the forearm and just proximal to the fetlock may be considered to hold the leg off the ground. A soft surface underfoot, such as deep bedding, is a prerequisite for this approach because many horses fall before learning that stoicism is the preferred response when normal locomotory responses are compromised in this way. Generally speaking, however, chemical restraint is the preferred option.

RESTRAINT OF HINDLIMBS

Hindlimb hobbles are often used on mares during mating (see Fig. 12.5) or pregnancy testing. Each hindlimb is attached to a collar around the horse's neck so that the horse can move the legs forward but not backwards. The straps around the pasterns should be made of soft but strong material, such as leather, that is unlikely to burn the horse's skin. The collar must be of a sufficient width to prevent undue pressure being concentrated on a small region of the neck.

Farriers and horse breakers sometimes teach a horse to pick up a hindleg by a modification of the breeding hobbles. A strap is placed around the horse's hind pastern and a rope attached to the strap. The rope is then run through a padded collar placed around the horse's neck. The rope may be run back through the strap (if the horse's leg can be approached), and then pressure on the pulley system lifts the hindleg off the ground. For horses in a situation where the hindlegs cannot be handled (i.e. in the absence of veterinary support), a slip loop can be made in the end of the rope and placed on the ground. The horse is then walked over the rope so that the targeted hindhoof is located within the loop. The rope is then pulled so the loop tightens around the pastern. Once the rope is through the collar, it is shortened until the horse's leg is at the required position. Unfortunately, rope burns may arise at this point, so the use of a soft rope is critical. The rope is then secured so that the handler can approach and handle the hindlimb safely. Because it is akin to one method of casting a horse, it is unsurprising that, when undergoing this method, many unhandled horses throw themselves on the ground. For this reason the procedure should take place only in a safe paddock with a soft landing (e.g. a round yard containing deep sand). The extent to which the horse also undergoes learned helplessness in this situation is worth considering. With horses that have thrown themselves to the ground, it is said that holding the nostrils closed is an effective means of getting them to struggle to get to their feet. However, adding asphyxiation to the woes of a restrained horse may be ethically inhumane.

DONKEY RESTRAINT

Some donkeys tend to move towards negative stimuli,[23] and this may help to explain why they have been found useful in guarding other species, such as sheep, from predation by dogs.[24] Being less inclined to flee, donkeys are regarded as stoical, but this reflects a higher threshold to respond, not necessarily a higher threshold for pain or, for that matter, fear. This must be borne in mind when practitioners weigh up the apparent need for chemical restraints in donkeys.

While a horse's first response is to flee and, if it cannot, to rear and kick, donkeys more usually freeze and simply stand their ground when confronted by aversive stimuli. As a result they have attracted a reputation for being difficult to force into situations. Indeed, it is often the case that the more a handler tries to push them, the more forcefully they will move towards that person.[23] Since donkeys cannot easily be forced towards hazards undetected by riders, their resolve makes them safer than horses as riding animals in certain sorts of terrain. If donkeys become entangled in wire or rope, they do not thrash about like horses and so are far less likely to injure themselves, e.g. injuries from barbed wire are less frequent in donkeys. By the same token, when tied securely, to the point at which they accept that they cannot leave, donkeys usually accept most veterinary procedures.[23]

It is important to note that the twitch is far less effective on donkeys. It is said that it can do no more than distract them from aversive procedures and may do so only transiently before they lower their heads and attempt to drag their handlers away.[23] This is especially likely to be an effective and therefore learned evasion in mammoth breeds.[23]

In cases of lameness, the stoicism of donkeys may make them challenging patients when veterinarians use hoof testers to locate a seat of pain. Foot-care in donkeys presents other interesting challenges because they are so sure-footed and therefore dislike having their balance compromised. This is why they are more likely than horses to refuse to pick up a foot or, if they do oblige, to snatch it back or lean on the handler. One solution to leaning and snatching during foot-care is to capitalize on the tendency of donkeys to accept physical restraint, albeit after a struggle. So, using quick-release knots, one can tie the patient up short and use a sideline for a hindleg and an over-the-back rope or elbow strap for a foreleg.[23] Most importantly, before the foot-care procedure commences, the donkey should be allowed time to test its predicament and convince itself that it can stand on three legs. It should also be taught this lesson separately for each leg, since donkeys do not appear to automatically transfer to the remaining limbs acceptance of the tying up of one leg.[23]

CHEMICAL RESTRAINT

The innate inclinations of horses to react strenuously when control is applied is sometimes referred to as 'opposition reflex'. This explains in part the escalation of force that is required when horses are said to panic. The use of drugs to modify the behavior of horses is always preferable to the use of force. Just as pre-operative analgesia reduces the need for sustained post-operative analgesia,[25] so the reduction of fearfulness seems to reduce the need for sedation. The psychological state of the animal before administration of tranquilizers may markedly affect the degree of sedation achieved. Animals that are intractable and in a state of excitation are likely to need very high doses before becoming manageable, so for routine procedures such as clipping, owners are well advised to avoid a struggle of any sort before the administration of chemical restraining agents.

Chemical agents with a variety of pharmacological mechanisms make it possible to alter a horse's behavior by tranquilization, sedation or immobilization (see Ch. 3). The distinction between sedatives and tranquilizers is reasonably subtle and focuses on the extent to which an agent causes central nervous system (CNS) depression (what would be described in humans as clouding of consciousness). Tranquilizers, such as the benzodiazepines, dissipate anxiety without CNS depression. Meanwhile sedatives, such as phenobarbitone, induce a dose-dependent spectrum of CNS effects.[26] To complicate matters, the classification of various psychotropic drugs used in horses can also depend on dose, i.e. some tranquilizers, such as the alpha-2 agonists, can cause sedation. Generally, horses are not good subjects for those tranquilizers that cause muscle weakness or ataxia because these outcomes can evoke 'panic' responses.[27] By the same token, if sedatives are used to produce manageability, high doses should be avoided since these may result in ataxia, depressed response to stimulation and some respiratory depression. Tranquilization during transportation can be

dangerous with horses since some react adversely under novel circumstances.[28]

TRANSPORTATION OF HORSES

Factors that influence horse behavior and welfare during transportation include:

- preparation of the horse and vehicle
- the extent of social isolation
- sex of and familiarity with travelling companions
- experience of the driver
- travel duration
- hydration status
- ventilation and air quality
- temperature and humidity
- previous transport experience of the horse
- medications
- the horse's temperament and orientation
- the means of restraint.

Although research efforts have focused on road transport, much of the information derived from research into the road transport of horses is also applicable to transportation by sea and air.

For many handlers the most unwelcome behaviors arise in their horses during loading and occasionally unloading. Many horses refuse to load and thus add considerable stress to and delays in travel, while a few rush during unloading, sometimes injuring themselves or personnel. Both of these problems should be seen as problems with being led. The case study in Chapter 13 gives a detailed approach to a loading problem. As part of the therapy, the horse is trained to stand still in any spot on the ramp and floor of the vehicle. This rapidly resolves rushing in any direction and is the preferred approach for unloading problems.

Horses brace themselves against and in anticipation of the changes in momentum during road transport by adopting certain body postures (notably the base-wide stance). Efforts expended by horses as they continuously adjust their posture during transit reflect both muscular and emotional stress related to road conditions and the

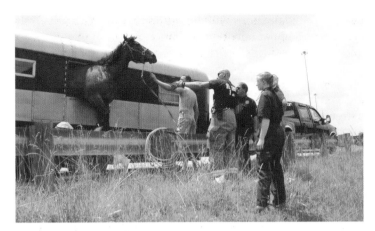

Figure 14.8 Horse that has tried to force its way out of a vehicle. (The horse made a complete recovery.) (Photograph courtesy of Michael Watiker.)

driver's behavior.[29] All of these effects are readily evaluated by monitoring heart rates during transport.[29] Horses have been shown to have higher heart rates in a moving vehicle than in a stationary vehicle[30,31] and, although heart rates decreased significantly during a road journey, they did not return to resting levels.[30,32] Transport stress may increase susceptibility to diseases, including an equine herpes virus 1[33] and salmonellosis infections.[34,35] Other common problems resulting from transportation include traumatic injuries, dehydration and pleuropneumonia. With adequate preparation and care, the incidence and severity of these disorders and their complications can be reduced. Previous experience largely determines the response of the horse to being transported, and it is worthwhile spending time accustoming the horse to the vehicle before transport is required. The calmer the horse remains during loading and transport, the less likely are injuries. Beyond that there is a need for vehicles of strong construction in case horses struggle (Fig. 14.8).

The longer a journey, the more one can expect to find increases in a horse's white blood cell count,[36] weight loss,[37,38] level of dehydration[39] and body temperature.[40] Body temperatures as high as 39.9 °C have been reported in horses after a 41-hour road trip.[41] Unsurprisingly, as the length of the road journey increases, the risk of horses developing shipping fever also increases.[42] A report describing six horses following a 9-hour flight noted elevated white blood cell counts, dehydration, and the loss of 4.1 ± 0.8% body weight that took 7 days to return to a pre-flight range.[43] So it is most likely as a result of the environmental conditions imposed on them during a 39-hour flight, that 7 of 112 horses developed pleuropneumonia (shipping fever) 1–2 days after arrival in one study.[44] Air temperature and humidity tend to peak when planes are stationary, e.g. during loading, unloading, refueling and delays. It is important to keep the latter to a minimum.[45] Frequent monitoring of rectal temperature is indicated in horses during transit because an elevated temperature is a familiar finding in dehydrated horses[40] and may also signal respiratory disease.[46]

The following discussion will focus on behavioral aspects of transportation and how research is providing data on best practice when horses are transported.

ORIENTATION

When facing forward during transport, horses may incur damage to the head, throat and neck as a result of being propelled forward by braking. Many owners report that traditional forward-facing transportation makes some horses lean back against the rear of the vehicle and sometimes even sit down. In contrast, horses facing backwards are thought to absorb deceleration with their haunches and are better able to maintain stability.[47] This explains why rear-facing horses have fewer side and total impacts and losses of balance.[48]

Several attempts have been made to determine the best orientation of the horse during transport.

Untethered horses in transit spend significantly more time facing the rear, and several horses have displayed strong individual preferences for orientation during travel.[49] Horses facing forward tend to move and vocalize more frequently and have higher heart rates than when facing the rear.[32] While Gibbs & Friend[50] found no significant preference for facing forwards or backwards, they noted a slight preference for traveling at about 45° to the direction of travel. Some studies have failed to find significant differences in heart rate and plasma cortisol concentrations between horses facing forward and backward during transport.[30,48] While this suggests that the imposition of forward-facing travel is not distressing, it does not rule out the possibility that it is tiring and increases the likelihood of injury.[51]

When a horse with an orthopedic injury must be transported, it should travel with the injured leg to the rear of the vehicle to protect it from the effects of deceleration. So a horse with an injured hindleg should travel facing forwards, and one with an injured foreleg should travel facing the rear. The head should be able to move freely to enable the horse to remain balanced while shifting weight off the injured leg. Horse slings, either commercial or homemade, should be used only in vehicles strong enough to support the weight of the horse in such a manner.[52]

As horses attempt to balance during changes in speed and direction, they tend to move their heads and feet rapidly. Leg wounds can occur through loss of balance when the vehicle brakes, while traveling around corners, and on uneven surfaces. The most common injuries are to the pastern and coronet.[53] The risk of injury can be minimized by the use of protection such as a padded headstall or a poll guard (head bumper in the USA) and protective leg bandages, thoughtful driving and generous tie ropes.[53] Bandaging the tail can protect it from damage resulting from repeated contact with the tailgate or wall.

HEAD POSITION

Equine pleuropneumonia can result from contamination of the lower respiratory tract by normal pharyngeal microflora and has been closely associated with transport. In enclosed containers the respiratory system is often further challenged by increased humidity, ammonia concentrations[54] and numbers of airborne microorganisms,[55] while in especially dry conditions the mucociliary clearance capacity may be further reduced by desiccation. Depression of cellular immunity may also occur due to stress-induced elevations of cortisol levels.[55]

Horses have evolved to spend long periods with their heads to the ground. Maintained elevation of the head facilitates the introduction of normal pharyngeal flora into the lower respiratory tract and hinders their removal by forcing the mucociliary transport system to work against gravity. When transported horses have their heads restrained, restricted head movement can compromise their ability to both balance and avoid respiratory disease.[56] Valuable horses traveling individually in stalls are commonly cross-tied for road transport to stabilize them, but this is not recommended for long-term transportation because it involves elevation of the head. When compared with transportation loose in small groups, cross-tying causes white blood cell counts, neutrophil:lymphocyte ratios and glucose and cortisol concentrations all to become significantly elevated.[57]

While frequent breaks when traveling help prevent fatigue and dehydration, allowing horses to lower their heads for brief intervals (30 minutes every 6 hours) is ineffective in preventing the accumulation of bacteria and mucus in the respiratory tract.[58] In one study,[58] at least 8 hours was required to clear the secretions that accumulated after maintaining an elevated head position for 24 hours.

Permitting the head enough freedom to allow the cranial trachea to be below the caudal trachea is the most effective way of preventing accumulations of mucus and bacteria and assisting the mucociliary transport system.[59] In a horse that is tied, one method of facilitating this head position and indeed horizontal and vertical head movement is to use a 'log and rope tie'. This involves passing a lead rope through a loop fixed to the inside of the vehicle and weighting the other end with a block that the horse cannot pull back through the loop.[53] Other appropriate measures include lowering hay and food containers, and soaking hay to minimize the inhalation of spores and bacteria.[60] It has also been suggested that allowing horses to face away from the direction of travel means that they are more likely to relax and hold their heads down.[51]

PREVENTING DEHYDRATION

Dehydration is associated with transport because voluntary intake of water during transit is low and, in any case, water is rarely offered during transport. While up to 5% dehydration may pass undetected, even 2–3% dehydration can affect the performance of competition horses.[53] Dehydration has also been implicated in the onset of acute laminitis and colonic impaction after extended road travel.[53] Horses are sometimes given electrolyte solutions via nasogastric tube to prevent gastrointestinal impaction. Familiarity with and frequency of transport are regarded as important risk factors in colic. Horses that travel one to six times per year have a higher risk of colic than those not transported.[53] Interestingly, more than six trips per year are associated with reduced risk of colic.[53] It is suggested that this reflects the effect of habituation and correspondingly reduced distress that facilitates adequate drinking and general hydration.[53]

Breaks in journeys are recommended every 4–6 hours. They offer the opportunity to give the horse some exercise, to offer it water and even to give it electrolyte solutions via nasogastric tube if a veterinarian is present. Horses can tolerate 6–8 liters of electrolyte-enriched water by nasogastric tube every 15 minutes, for up to 2 hours if required.[53]

Studies in hot weather have shown that the provision of water during transport in summer can have favorable effects on several physiological parameters of hydration and distress.[61] Compared with watered horses, unwatered horses showed greater weight loss, higher plasma cortisol concentrations and elevated respiratory and heart rates. Their plasma concentrations of sodium, chloride and total protein, and their plasma osmolality greatly exceeded normal reference ranges, indicating severe dehydration.[61]

While the provision of water to group-transported horses (viz. slaughter horses, see below) reduces the incidence of dehydration,[62] it is not straightforward because high-ranking horses may prevent others from gaining access to the water. Furthermore, there is a risk of water spillage that would make the flooring more slippery and compromise the horses' ability to maintain their balance. Providing water on both sides of vehicles and ensuring that bedding is sufficiently absorbent may help to resolve these problems.

RESTRAINT OF HORSES DURING AIR TRANSIT

The differences between road and air transport are few. In level flight, horses being transported in enclosed containers (Fig. 14.9) regularly doze and rest and their heart rates are close to resting levels.[45]

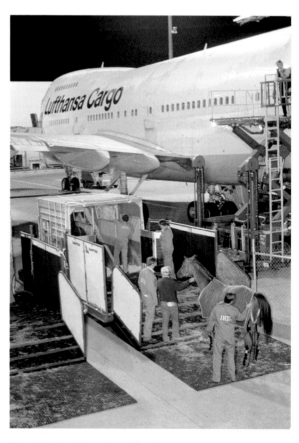

Figure 14.9 Horse being loaded into an enclosed container for transportation by air. (Photograph courtesy of International Racehorse Transport.)

Horses seem distressed by movement only during cargo handling, take-off and landing.[63] Agitation at these times can include regular changes in body postures to maintain balance and agonistic responses, such as aggression and appeasement.[45] Aggression may indicate distress as a result of certain environmental stressors[64,65] and is accompanied by increases in heart rate. Fortunately these episodes do not seem to be frequent or long enough to raise significant welfare concerns.[45] They are not accompanied by any changes in hematological or blood biochemical values that would be suggestive of any detrimental effects.[63]

Persistent pawing and stamping may be features of some horses' response to air travel.[66] It is interesting that this behavior prior to a race is seen as one of several characteristics of poor performance in racehorses.[8] Although rare, the occasional possibility of a horse becoming truly panicked in mid-air merits consideration and forward planning. Even if it may result in the horse being disqualified from competition on arrival, the use of tranquilizers in an airborne horses is preferable to manual restraint.[55] With the availability of potent equine psychopharmaceuticals, it is rarely necessary nowadays to euthanase horses in emergency situations.[55]

TRANSPORT OF HORSES FOR SLAUGHTER

The welfare of slaughter horses is of concern because inadequate head-room, high stocking rates, poor ventilation, dehydration and long travel times are common. Additionally, the pre-transport condition of slaughter animals is often suboptimal,[67] which compromises their ability to cope with transit stressors. It is suggested that even when governments attempt to regulate the conditions under which horses are transported and slaughtered, such rules are often flouted.[68] Horses destined for the abattoir are most commonly transported by truck, unrestrained and in groups. A study comparing two densities of horse groups in transit found that more horses fell and more were injured in the higher-density group.[69] This reflects the fact that it was more difficult for fallen horses to get to their feet in the higher-density group.[69]

Horses traveling loose in small groups exhibit less physiological distress than those tied up,[56,57] but economies of scale dictate that sufficient individual space is rarely given to horses bound for slaughter.

Fighting during transportation is a major cause of injuries.[67] Many of the injuries incurred during transport occur through aggression between freshly mixed animals. This may explain why the condition of established bands of feral horses after transport is often better than that of domestic horses from a variety of origins, such as arise in groups of horses traveling from saleyards to slaughterhouses. Clearly, one of the easiest means of avoiding such injuries is to avoid mixing horses. Where this is not possible, it is appropriate to separate stallions and particularly aggressive animals from the main group.

SUMMARY OF KEY POINTS

- Regardless of whether or not they realize it, good handlers of horses are students of equine behavior.
- By keeping horses as calm as possible, the type of restraint required for current and future handling can be kept to a minimum.
- Horses rarely forget aversive procedures.
- Horses should never be punished for showing flight responses.
- Donkeys respond differently to horses during restraint and veterinary procedures.
- Numerous factors associated with transport can compromise health and welfare.
- Prevention of dehydration is a priority in transported horses.

REFERENCES

1. Simpson BS. Neonatal foal handling. Appl Anim Behav Sci 2002; 78(2–4):309–323.
2. Nicol CJ. Equine learning: progress and suggestions for future research. Appl Anim Behav Sci 2002; 78(2–4):193–208.
3. Ferguson DL, Rosales-Ruiz J. Loading the problem loader: the effects of target training and shaping on trailer-loading behavior of horses. J Appl Behav Anal 2001; 34(4):409–423.
4. McGreevy PD. Why does my horse …? London: Souvenir Press; 1996.
5. Mills DS, Mills CB. Evaluation of a novel method for delivering a synthetic analogue of feline facial pheromone to control urine spraying by cats. Vet Rec 2001; 149(7):197–199.

6. Gaultier E, Pageat P. Effect of a synthetic equine appeasing pheromone in a fear-eliciting test. In: Dehasse J, Biosca-Marce E, eds. Proceedings of the 8th ESVCE meeting on Veterinary Behavioural Medicine, Granada, Spain, 2 October 2002. Paris: Publibook; 2002:59–64.

7. Saslow CA. Understanding the perceptual world of horses. Appl Anim Behav Sci 2002; 78(2–4):209–224.

8. Hutson G. Watching racehorses: a guide to betting on behaviour. Melbourne: Clifton Press; 2002.

9. Seaman SC, Davidson HPB, Waran NK. How reliable is temperament assessment in the domestic horse (Equus caballus)?. Appl Anim Behav Sci 2002; 78(2–4):175–191.

10. Grandin T. Behavioural principles of livestock and handling. Professional Animal Scientist 1989 (December); American Registry of Professional Animal Scientists.

11. Morris D. Horsewatching. London: Jonathan Cape; 1988.

12. Fraser AF. The behaviour of the horse. London: CAB International; 1992.

13. Waring GH. Horse behavior: the behavioral traits and adaptations of domestic and wild horses including ponies. Park Ridge, NJ: Noyes; 1983.

14. Rose RJ, Hodgson DR. Manual of equine practice. London: WB Saunders; 1993.

15. Ladd LA. Pain behaviour in animals. Ain't Misbehaving. The AT Reid refresher course for veterinarians. Proceedings 340. Published by the Post Graduate Foundation in Veterinary Science, University of Sydney; 2001:69–98.

16. Hamra JG, Kamerling SG, Wolfsheimer KJ, Bagwell CA. Diurnal variation in plasma ir-beta-endorphin levels and experimental pain thresholds in the horse. Life Sci 1993; 53:121–129.

17. Lagerweij E, Nelis PC, Wiegant VM, van Ree JM. The twitch in horses: a variant of acupuncture. Science 1984; 225(4667):1172–1174.

18. Webster AJF. Animal welfare: a cool eye towards Eden. London: Blackwell Science; 1994.

19. Minero M, Canali E, Ferrante V, et al. Heart rate and behavioural responses of crib-biting horses to two acute stressors. Vet Rec 1999; 145(15):430–433.

20. Marsden DM. A new perspective on stereotypic behaviour problems. In Practice 2002 (Nov/Dec):558–569.

21. McLean AN, McLean MM. Horse training the McLean way – the science behind the art. Victoria, Australia: Australian Equine Behaviour Centre; 2002.

22. Kerrigan RH, Hunt ER. Practical horse sense and safety. Maitland, Australia: Equine Educational; 1992.

23. Taylor TS, Matthews NS. Mammoth asses – selected behavioural considerations for the veterinarian. Appl Anim Behav Sci 1998; 60(2–3):283–289.

24. Smith ME, Linnell JDC, Odden J, Swenson JE. Review of methods to reduce livestock depredation, I: Guardian animals [review]. Acta Agric Scand A Anim Sci 2000; 50(4):279–290.

25. Shafford HL, Lascelles BDX, Hellyer PW. Preemptive analgesia: managing pain before it begins. Vet Med 2001; 96(6):478–480.

26. Steffey EP. Drugs acting on the central nervous system. In: Adams HR, ed. Veterinary pharmacology and therapeutics, 8th edn. Ames: Iowa State University Press; 2001:153–171.

27. Hall LW, Clarke KW. Veterinary anaesthesia, 8th edn. London: Baillière Tindall; 1983.

28. Lumb WV, Jones EW. Veterinary anesthesia, 2nd edn. Philadelphia: Lea & Febiger; 1984.

29. Giovagnoli G, Marinucci MT, Bolla A, Borghese A. Transport stress in horses: an electromyographic study on balance preservation. Livestock Production Science 2002; 73(2–3):247–254.

30. Smith BL, Jones JH, Carlson GP, Pascoe JR. Effect of body direction on heart rate in trailered horses. Am J Vet Res 1994b; 55(7):1007–1011.

31. Waran NK, Cuddeford D. Effects of loading and transport on the heart rate and behaviour of horses. Appl Anim Behav Sci 1995; 43:71–81.

32. Waran NK, Robertson V, Cuddeford D, et al. Effects of transporting horses facing either forwards or backwards on their behaviour and heart rate. Vet Rec 1996; 139(1):7–11.

33. van Maanen C, Willink DL, Smeenk LAJ, et al. An equine herpes virus 1 (EHV1) abortion storm at a riding school. Vet Q 2000; 22(2):83–87.

34. McClintock SA, Begg, AP. Suspected salmonellosis in seven broodmares after transportation. Aust Vet J 1990; 67(7):265–267.

35. Owen RR, Fullerton J, Barnum DA. Effects of transportation, surgery, and antibiotic therapy in ponies infected with Salmonella. Am J Vet Res 1983; 44(1):46–50.

36. Yamauchi T, Oikawa M, Hiraga A. Effects of transit stress on white blood cells count in the peripheral blood in thoroughbred racehorses. Bull Equine Inst 1993;30:30–32.

37. Foss MA, Lindner A. Effects of trailer transport duration on body weight and blood biochemical variables of horses. Pferdeheilk 1996; 4:435–437.

38. Mars LA, Kiesling HE, Ross TT, et al. Water acceptance and intake in horses under shipping stress. J Equine Vet Sci 1992; 12:17–20.

39. Van den Berg JS, Guthrie AJ, Meintjes RA, et al. Water intake and electrolyte intake and output in conditioned thoroughbred horses transported by road. Equine Vet J 1998; 30:316–323.

40. Friend TH, Martin MT, Householder DD, Bushong DM. Stress responses of horses during a long period of transport on a commercial truck. J Am Vet Med Assoc 1998; 212:838–844.

41. Oikawa M, Takagi S, Anzai R, et al. Pathology of equine respiratory diseases occurring in association with transport. J Comp Pathol 1995; 113: 29–43.

42. Oikawa M, Kusunose R. Some epidemiological aspects of equine respiratory disease associated with transport. J Equine Sci 1995; 6:25–29.

43. Marlin DJ, Schroter RC, White SL, et al. Recovery from transport and acclimatisation of competition horses in a hot humid environment. Equine Vet J 2001; 33:371–379.

44. Leadon DR, Daykin J, Backhouse W, et al. Environmental, hematological and blood biochemical changes in equine transit stress. Proc Am Assoc Equine Pract 1990; 36:485–490.

45. Stewart M, Foster TM, Waas JR. The effects of air transport on the behaviour and heart rate of horses. Appl Anim Behav Sci 2003; 80(2):143–160.

46. Leadon DP. Transport stress. In: Hodgson DR, ed. The athletic horse: principles and practice of equine sports medicine. Philadelphia: Saunders; 1994:371–378.

47. Cregier SE. Reducing equine hauling stress: a review. J Equine Vet Sci 1982; 2(6):187–198.

48. Clark DK, Friend TH, Dellmeier G. The effect of orientation during trailer transport on heart rate, cortisol and balance in horses. Appl Anim Behav Sci 1993; 38(3/4):179–189.

49. Smith BL, Jones JH, Carlson GP, Pascoe JR. Body position and direction preferences in horses during road transport. Equine Vet J 1994a; 26(5):374–377.

50. Gibbs AE. Friend TH. Horse preference for orientation during transport and the effect of orientation on balancing ability. Appl Anim Behav Sci 1999; 63(1):1–9.

51. Cregier SE. Transporting the horse. In: McBane S, ed. Behaviour problems in the horse. Newton Abbot, Devon: David & Charles; 1994:123–132.

52. Deboer S. Transporting horses with severe leg or body injuries. Equine Vet Data 1989; 10(15):260–261.

53. Mansmann RA, Woodie B. Equine Transportation problems and some preventatives. J Equine Vet Sci 1995; 15(4):141–144.

54. Katayama Y, Oikawa M, Yoshihara T, et al. Clinico-pathological effects of atmospheric ammonia exposure on horses. J Equine Sci 1995; 6(3):99–104.

55. Leadon DP. Transport stress and the equine athlete. Equine Vet Educ 1995; 7(5):253–255.

56. Stull CL, Rodiek AV. Physiological responses of horses to 24 hours of transportation using a commercial van during summer conditions. J Anim Sci 2000; 78(6):1458–1466.

57. Stull CL, Rodiek AV. Effects of cross-tying horses during 24 h of road transport. Equine Vet J 2002; 34(6):550–555.

58. Raidal SL, Love DN, Bailey GD. Inflammation and increased numbers of bacteria in the lower respiratory tract of horses within 6–12 hours of confinement with the head elevated. Aust Vet J 1995; 72:45–50.

59. Racklyeft DJ, Love DN. Influence of head posture on the respiratory tract of healthy horses. Aust Vet J 1990; 67:402–405.

60. Jeffcott L. Recommendations for horses going to the 1996 Atlanta Olympic games. The Equine Athlete 1996; 9(3):19–25.

61. Friend TH. Dehydration, stress, and water consumption of horses during long-distance commercial transport. J Anim Sci 2000; 78(10):2568–2580.

62. Gibbs AE, Friend TH. Effect of animal density and trough placement on drinking behavior and dehydration in slaughter horses. J Equine Vet Sci 2000; 20(10):643–650.

63. Thornton J. Effect of the microclimate on horses during international air transportation in an enclosed container. Aust Vet J 2000; 78(7):472–477.

64. McCall CA, Potter GD, Kreider JL. Locomotor, vocal and other behavioural responses to varying methods of weaning foals. Appl Anim Behav Sci 1985; 14:27–35.

65. Scheepens CJM, Hessing MJC, Laarakker E, et al. Influences of intermittent daily draught on the behaviour of weaned pigs. Appl Anim Behav Sci 1991; 31:69–82.

66. Judge NG. Transport in horses. Aust Vet J 1969; 45:465–469.

67. Reece VP, Friend TH, Stull CH, et al. Equine slaughter transport – update on research and regulations. Animal Welfare Forum: Equine Welfare, J Am Vet Med Assoc 2000; 216(8):1253–1258.

68. Endenburg N. Perceptions and attitudes towards horses in European societies. The role of the horse in Europe. Equine Vet J Suppl 1999; 28:38–41.

69. Collins MN, Friend TH, Jousan FD, Chen SC. Effects of density on displacement, falls, injuries and orientation during horse transportation. Appl Anim Behav Sci 2000; 67(3):169–179.

15

Miscellaneous unwelcome behaviors, their causes and resolution

INTRODUCTION

Physical causes of unwelcome behavioral responses should always be ruled out before any purely behavioral therapy is adopted. Such impediments should be eliminated because beyond their effects on horse welfare and development of annoying habits, they are likely to compromise athletic output (Fig. 15.1). For example, it has been proposed that undiagnosed pelvic or vertebral lesions could be important contributors to poor performance in horses.[1] While occasional disorders such as 'cold-back syndrome' and the relationship between dental problems and behavior under saddle have yet to be thoroughly explored, the treatment of most physical disorders that reduce performance is considered in detail in the veterinary literature.

Since most problem behaviors that emerge in stables or at pasture are considered elsewhere in this book, the current discussion will focus on handling problems and problems with the ridden horse. In combination with Chapters 1, 4 and 13, this chapter aims to help veterinarians and equine scientists in their creation, from first principles, of humane and effective therapies for unwelcome behaviors. The current chapter indicates the basic approaches to therapy that can be tailored for each affected horse, defines some of the more common problems and offers a framework for understanding the origins of these problems.

Unfortunately, as discussed in Chapter 13, there is a lack of scientific data in these realms. This may reflect the importance we place upon the performance of the horse under-saddle and the

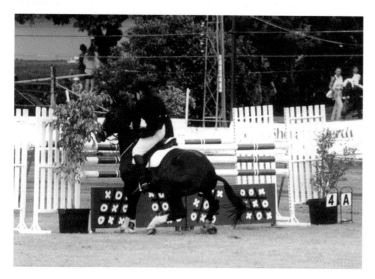

Figure 15.1 A horse making a so-called dirty stop (getting very close to a fence before refusing). Horses refusing fences may have learned that they are physically unable to clear the top rail or that landing is a painful consequence of taking off. (Photograph courtesy of Sandra Hannan.)

consequent development of riding instruction that tends to focus on outcomes rather than mechanisms. Since the ideals of equestrian technique combine art and science, students of equitation encounter measurable variables such as rhythm, tempo and outline alongside many more ethereal ones such as impulsion and harmony.[2] This mixture and the dearth of mechanistic substance frustrate attempts to express equestrian technique in empirical terms[3] and account for some of the confusion and conflict that arises in many human–horse dyads. With time, the application of science to the plethora of undesirable behaviors that horses trial and learn to adopt will undoubtedly reduce the ill-considered demands for quick fixes and ultimately decrease the wastage in the industry.

MECHANICAL APPROACHES

Most naïve horses respond to humans as they would to any predator. They behave in ways that help them avoid pressure, physical or psychological, by moving away bodily or posturally. These basic evasive responses can be modified successfully to produce a highly responsive equine performer or unsuccessfully to produce a problem horse.

When trainers encounter horses that rapidly enter conflict and as a result do not comply, they often experiment with increased pressure to overcome resistance. Mechanical restraints and stimulants may be used to magnify the pressure that riders can apply. Because of the perceived need to force horses into an 'outline' and make them work 'on the bit' (see Glossary), the tendency is to use stronger bits as the first approach to solving the problem. This accounts for the multiplicity of bits on the market. As with any device, it is true to say that if there are many of them available, the chances are that none of them provides all the answers. Furthermore, enlightened trainers recognize that where aversive stimuli have failed to elicit the desired response and have begun to cause behavioral conflict, the application of more force is contraindicated. They rarely reach for such gadgets.

Frustrated trainers often try bits that apply pressure to different parts of the mouth or to the same area of the mouth but with greater severity (Fig. 15.2). Even though they can and sometimes do sever the tongue,[4] saw chain bits (so-called mule bits and correction bits) are readily available to riders who are having problems getting horses to respond to milder bits. If changing or increasing mouth pressure is unsuccessful, an alternative or additional means of making the horse adopt

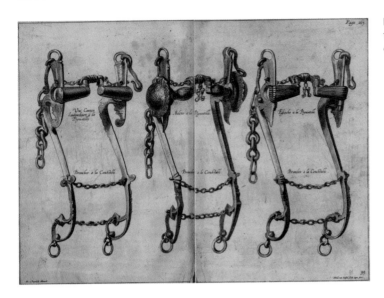

Figure 15.2 Etching of 18th-century bits. At times it seems that more effort has gone into designing bits than addressing poor equitation.

the desired shape is to apply pressure to the other parts of the head, so training devices such as curb chains, gags, hackamores, bosals, draw reins, balancing reins and chambons may be employed. Unfortunately the tendency is to develop a reliance on these extra pulleys, rather than use them solely for retraining as the name might imply. Martingales and tie-downs are similar in that they apply pressure to prevent evasive raising of the head and are rarely dispensed with.

If the horse fails to show sufficient forward movement or impulsion, trainers direct their attention to the flanks where they can increase the pressure and more effectively drive the horse forward or simply away from the rider's leg using whips and spurs. Although, for some, these stimulants are distasteful, they are not necessarily contraindicated since they can be used with subtlety and employed transiently to empower the rider's leg signals.

BEHAVIOR MODIFICATION

Behavior therapy can help overcome undesirable equine responses that may have an innate component but are largely learned. The temptation may be to treat such traits in isolation. However, an holistic approach has tremendous merit since

better results tend to occur if the human–horse relationship is nurtured when the rider is both on the ground and in the saddle. At the same time punishment is regarded by many owners as unenlightened, since it presupposes that horses know the difference between good and bad behavior. So, it is increasingly inappropriate for veterinarians to advocate punishment as a response to undesirable behavior in the horse. It undermines the human–horse bond and carries the risk of injury, which may place any practitioner who advises it in a legally liable position.

Examples of acceptable techniques used for behavior modification include habituation and counter-conditioning (see Chs 4 and 13). Habituation is the key to overcoming fear-related responses such as traffic shyness but it can be expedited with counter–conditioning, an approach that relies heavily on the shaping of alternative responses through operant conditioning. At its most elegant, equine operant conditioning takes the form of positive reinforcement and subtle negative reinforcement. Consistent use of negative reinforcement is the key to retraining the basics, but is notably more likely to work in horses that have not habituated to pressure. Meanwhile, clicker training employs positive secondary reinforcement that is particularly useful for refinement of responses, once negative reinforcement has established the basics.

Horses with innate or learned evasion responses may have the rewarding outcomes of these responses removed by a process of extinction. Furthermore they can be trained to associate the aversive stimuli with positive outcomes in the same way that laboratory primates can be trained to voluntarily present their forelimbs for intravenous injections. (A case study that required a pony to learn to cope with hypodermic injections appears at the end of this chapter. It followed the injection desensitization training technique developed by ethologists at Pennsylvania State University.[5]) A far less humane approach to fearful horses is to flood them by exposing them to an overwhelming amount of the fear-eliciting stimulus in the hope that their responses are exhausted. For example, so-called 'tarping', a method of breaking by flooding, involves evoking learned helplessness by casting the horse, covering it with a tarpaulin and beating it until it no longer resists.

Practitioners are strongly encouraged to become extremely conversant with learning theory (see Ch. 4) before counseling owners on the application of these techniques. All of the undesirable responses in the current chapter can be remedied by behavior modification. But a prerequisite is correct identification of the motivation for a given response. Readers are urged to consider the ethological content of this entire volume when determining causal factors. Beyond that the success of behavioral therapy depends on the consistency of administration and compliance of owners, who must be counseled that the latency for desirable outcomes depends largely on the number of times the horse has trialed and learned from the unwelcome response. With a thorough knowledge of learning theory, practitioners can customize behavior modification programs, modify advice in the light of initial responses and counsel owners when proximate results surprise the uninitiated. So, for example, when as a result of an extinction protocol, undesirable responses become more frequent, the accomplished student of learning theory can explain that this is a manifestation of the frustration effect (see p. 105 in Ch. 4) and that it is transient.

HANDLING PROBLEMS

As discussed in the previous chapter, physical restraint of horses during painful procedures is often possible but rarely preferable to chemical restraint since it tends to escalate the aversiveness of the procedure and is therefore ultimately likely to compromise the horse–human bond and make the horse less compliant for future procedures. So many handling problems are the legacy of previous (often unintentional) abuse. Others can have proximate causes in physical pathologies, so practitioners should always check first (with an examination and a thorough case history) for the involvement of these anomalies before embarking on any course of behavior therapy. By way of an example, a horse that is reluctant to step backwards must be checked for wobbler syndrome.

Horses fearful of clippers may have had a cutting injury or mild heat damage during clipping. Head shyness can be the manifestation of partial blindness, dental anomalies and, occasionally, spinose ear ticks.[6] Girthing and saddling problems may be related to thoracic and spinal lesions. Horses that are eager to rub their heads against handlers may have lice or, very occasionally, flying insects or spinose ear ticks that make them generally itchy and sometimes irritable. In a similar vein, when acute in onset, hypersensitivity to being touched may be attributed to strychnine poisoning and even lightning strike.[6]

Assuming that painful pathologies have been ruled out, the role of learning is of tremendous significance in emergent handling problems. Horses showing fear of veterinarians may simply remember them as the immediate precursors of pain or of unpleasant physical restraint prior to painful interventions. Similarly, those showing fear of farriers (Fig. 15.3) may have received a nailing injury in the past. The horse's ability to form general relationships between certain activities and pain should not be overlooked. For example, painful lesions (e.g. subclinical orthopedic disorders that are exacerbated by riding) may make a horse generally reluctant to work and, by a process of backward chaining (see Ch. 4), difficult to catch.

As with all behavior problems, it is the responsibility of handlers and therapists alike to establish that the horse is not only capable of an appropriate response but that it is also free from pain. Furthermore, the horse must know what is being asked of it, i.e. it must have learned the cue. Only when these prerequisites are in place can the horse be helped to unlearn the inappropriate associations (Table 15.1). Techniques in behavioral therapy can be used in combination so the suggestions that appear in Table 15.1 should not be considered the complete or sole approach.

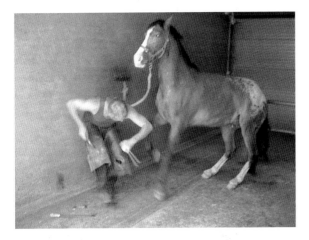

Figure 15.3 A horse attempting to escape from a farrier. (Photograph courtesy of Sandro Nocentini.)

PROBLEMS WITH THE RIDDEN HORSE

Horses can demonstrate various unwelcome behaviors under-saddle, often in combination. For the sake of simplicity, inappropriate responses are considered separately.

INAPPROPRIATE OBSTACLE AVOIDANCE

It is appropriate for horses to avoid hazards that may jeopardize their safety, but such innate

Table 15.1 Common handling problems, their interpretation and suggested approaches to therapy that can be employed after any primary physical causes have been removed

Problem	Interpretation	Approaches to therapy
Barging (trampling)	Agonistic response to displace personnel	Avoidance learning or shaping of lateral movement in response to being touched on the flank
Biting and bite threats	Aggression to deter approaching personnel	Total refurbishment of the human–horse bond.[a] For example, experienced personnel may make great strides with such horses in a round-pen
Claustrophobia	Innate fear of enclosed spaces such as stalls, stables and trailers (floats) Learned fear of aversive and coercive human responses	Clicker training to approach, stand beside and enter enclosures[c] Reinstall leading cues[d]
Difficult to bridle	Learned evasion of discomfort from bit, crown-piece and brow band	Partially dismantle bridle and apply in parts to identify the most aversive element Counter-conditioning[b] Clicker training to stand quietly in usual area used for bridling[c] Shape tolerance of key elements of the bridling process
Difficult to saddle-up	Learned evasion Response to past pain	Counter-conditioning[b] Clicker training to stand while being saddled[c]
Difficult to shoe	Learned evasion from fear	Extinction of fear responses by habituation and counter-conditioning Clicker training of appropriate responses, such as approaching farriers and their equipment[c]

(contd.)

Table 15.1 *(Contd.)*

Problem	Interpretation	Approaches to therapy
Dislike of grooming	Innate ticklishness Learned evasion	Habituation Counter-conditioning[b]
Fear of being clipped	Learned evasion and sometimes learned aggression	Counter-conditioning.[b] Clicker training to approach and stand beside clippers[c]
Fear of veterinarians	Innate aversion to pain and learned evasion of associated stimuli	Extinction of fear responses by habituation and counter-conditioning.[b] This should involve the owner in the first instance and then the practitioner Clicker training of appropriate responses, such as approaching veterinarians and their equipment[c]
Hard to catch	Learned evasion	Clicker training of appropriate responses such as approaching personnel[c] Extinguish associations with being removed from group. Therefore habituate the horses to being caught but not necessarily brought in from the paddock or ridden
Head rubbing	Innate response to irritants Learned association with gratification from rubbing against personnel	Extinguish gratification. Offer visual cues (such as a body brush) that allow the horse to discriminate times when rubbing against a more appropriate object (such as a brush) is worth trying, i.e. is 'permissible'
Head shyness	Learned evasion, e.g. of being twitched or being struck around the head	Clicker training of appropriate responses such as approaching personnel, especially their hands and hand-held equipment[c]
Kicking and kick-threats	Aggression to displace personnel	Extinguish fear and then undertake total refurbishment of the human–horse bond
Pulling	Motivation to ignore or override pressure from headcollar or halter (headstall) Habituation to pressure from headcollar or halter	Reinstall leading cues[d]
Pushing	Agonistic response to intimidate personnel	Reinstall leading cues[d]
Rearing	Learned evasion Habituation to pressure from headcollar or halter Aggression	Reinstall leading cues[d]
Refusal to back	Learned evasion	Reinstall leading cues[d]
Refusal to leave company	Lack of training Excessive bonding usually with one particular field-mate	Consider restructuring social group Reinstall leading cues[d] Counter-conditioning to develop positive associations with temporary isolation[b]
Refusal to load	Learned evasion ± claustrophobia	Reinstall leading cues[d] Clicker training of appropriate responses, such as approaching and entering vehicle[c]
Refusal to stand while being mounted	Learned evasion of bit pressure and anticipation of kinetic behavior	Reinstall leading cues[d] Clicker training of appropriate response[c] Shape the horse to stand quietly for increasing periods before moving forward
Striking	Aggression	Refurbishment of the human–horse bond

[a]Refurbishment of horse–human bond is also discussed in the case study in Chapter 11, on page 261.
[b]Counter-conditioning is explained on page 91 (see Ch. 4) and also in the case study at the end of the current chapter, on page 344.
[c]Clicker training is explained on page 100 (see Ch. 4).
[d]Reinstallation of leading cues is explained in Chapter 13 and highlighted in the case study in that chapter on page 309.

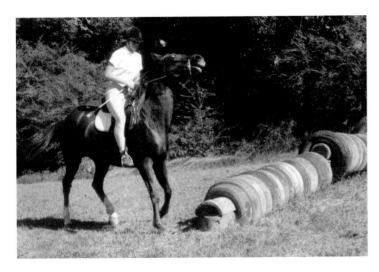

Figure 15.4 A horse avoiding obstacle despite (or perhaps even as a result of) the efforts of a novice rider. (Photograph courtesy of Mellisa Offord.)

self-preservation responses sometimes inconvenience riders (Fig. 15.4). Examples include avoidance of ground hazards, manifested as running out and refusal of fences, ditches and water jumps, while avoidance of lateral confinement may prompt a horse to refuse to enter starting stalls. Unfortunately, the original causes of these responses may be obscured and the subsequent application of aversive stimuli may simply confirm to the horse the need to avoid such obstacles because they become associated with pain. Shying behavior is most rapidly learned and incorporated into the horse's behavioral repertoire when it permits complete escape. As the horse escalates its shying behavior, the reinforcement from escape is compounded by the incremental loss of control by the rider.[2] Additionally, riders who predict the responses may inadvertently apply pressure that may increase the horses' motivation to find freedom.[2] Re-training the 'go' response in such horses (see Ch. 13) is the preferred remedial course of action.

The importance of rhythm and direction in basic training is explained when one considers horses that learn to refuse jumps. Habitual losses of rhythm and tempo or directional line often lead to stalling while approaching fences.[2] When horses learn to stall in the jumping effort, outright refusal is generally their next step.

HYPER-REACTIVITY RESPONSES

While innate obstacle avoidance responses may paradoxically help to ensure the safety of riders (e.g. by prompting the horse to steer around a hazard unseen by its rider), other innate self-preservation action patterns of horses, especially those that keep them safe from predators, are sometimes triggered too readily or are performed with speed that riders are unable to predict. These are chiefly flight responses motivated by a need to get away from the stimulus, rejoin a group of conspecifics or return to the home range. Depending on the human observer, horses that readily offer theses responses are variously described as sharp, keen, fizzy or flighty.[7]

There are several common examples of hyper-reactivity in the ridden horse. As discussed above, shying is an avoidance response that sends horses leaping laterally or backwards away from auditory, olfactory or visual stimuli. Many horses in unfamiliar surroundings offer this response innately but some adopt it as their default response to novelty. Traffic shyness is a particularly important example. The most successful approach to this dangerous problem involves a process of habituation, but the challenge for trainers is to present a comprehensive range of diverse stimuli (A model for habituation

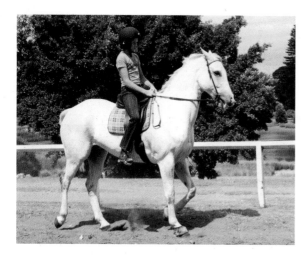

Figure 15.5 A jogging horse. Jogging is a choppy trot that wastes energy and often indicates the need for better training of clear transitions.

Table 15.2 Selected examples and descriptions of agonistic responses to conflict

Response	Description
Bucking	Response used to fight conspecifics and dislodge predators
Rearing	Response used to fight conspecifics and predators
Balking, bolting home, napping and jibbing	Motivation to return to home range or social group is greater than motivation to respond to rider's signals
Rushing fences	Although the behavioral mechanism is unclear, horses choosing to travel too rapidly toward fences are thought to be making a perverse attempt to reduce the aversiveness of the stimulus by running towards it
Falling out through the shoulder	Failure to turn appropriately on command

of former racehorses appears in the case study in Ch. 4.).

Jogging, on the other hand, is largely learned and manifests as a horse that is unresponsive to signals to walk (Fig. 15.5). This undesirable gait is often accompanied by persistently repeated extension of the neck to pull the reins through the rider's hands in horses that have learned to 'pull'. These horses demonstrate a clear need for reinstallation of the 'stop' cue. Similar unresponsiveness takes an extreme form in horses that bolt, i.e. that gallop with no response to rein pressure. These animals may learn to ignore bit pressure whenever they wish to remove themselves from a perceived threat or return to their home range or social group.

AGONISTIC RESPONSES TO CONFLICT

When faced with discomfort or a threat, most horses move away. If horses cannot escape from such a stimulus, they enter behavioral conflict and increase their kinetic effort in a bid to relieve the pressure (Table 15.2). Some horses develop seemingly irrational phobias by becoming sensitized to associated stimuli and anticipating the escalation of bit or leg pressure that riders use to make them 'behave'. The therapeutic approach to conflict is discussed in detail in Chapter 13.

EVIDENCE OF PAIN AND IRRITATION

When a horse fails to respond as requested by the rider, the innate human tendency is to repeat the cue with greater force in a bid to increase the animal's motivation to relieve the pressure. However, it is important that somatic causes of a horse's disinclination to respond are eliminated before more aversive stimuli are applied. There is a strong argument for the use of analgesics as a diagnostic probe when horses fail to respond appropriately, especially if this departure is sudden.

Pain is recognized as an important contributor to unwelcome behavioral responses.[8] Occasionally horses may learn to relieve pressures caused by riders by removing the riders themselves, e.g. by bucking (Fig. 15.6), rolling or even rubbing the riders against fixed objects. Grunting and groaning are expiratory noises associated with tenesmus and abdominal guarding. As such they reflect low-grade discomfort in the very general region of the horse's forequarters. Far more profound an indication of thoracic and lumbar pain is seen in 'cold-back' syndrome during girthing and mounting. This often includes responses to being saddled, mounted and especially to being girthed that vary from aggression to recumbency.

Horses commonly learn to reduce the discomfort of the bit by manipulating it to lie in relatively insensitive parts of the mouth. Common names for these evasions include raking, boring, getting the tongue over the bit and seizing the bit between the teeth (Fig. 15.7). Mouth pain is usually associated with heavy-handed riding or inappropriate equipment. For example, pinching between the commissures of the lip and the second premolar is thought to occur as a result of the action of some jointed bits. Some maintain that in the event of a horse fighting the bit, comfort in this part of the mouth can be maximized by the creation of a 'bit seat' or 'cheek seat', i.e. the removal of an appreciable portion of the second premolar.[9] While one study reported improved athletic performance in most horses after the creation of bit seats,[9] an abiding question is whether a simple change of bits (e.g. to an unjointed design) would be just as effective.

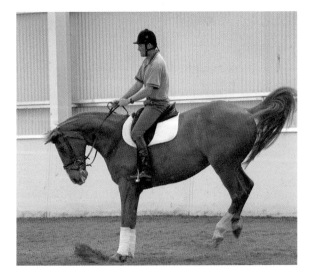

Figure 15.6 A horse bucking under-saddle. (Photograph courtesy of Andrew McLean.)

EVIDENCE OF POOR PHYSICAL ABILITY

While some horses do not comply because they associate the responses desired by riders with musculoskeletal discomfort, others are insufficiently athletic because of poor conformation or lack of fitness (Table 15.3). Clearly, as with those resulting from pain, these cases are unresponsive to behavior therapy.

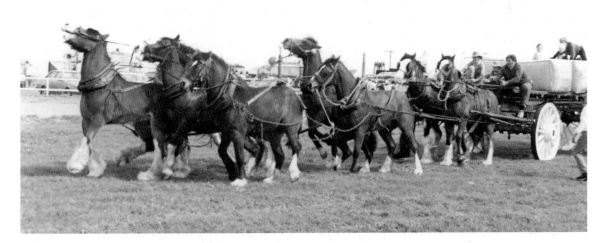

Figure 15.7 A draft team in which several horses can be seen evading the bit. (Photograph courtesy of Les Holmes.)

Table 15.3 Selected examples of inadequate performance under-saddle that reflect poor physical ability

Response	Description
Fatigue	Lack of energy as distinct from lack of willingness to respond
Problems in transition	Congenital propensity, e.g. to disunite at the canter (see Glossary)
Tripping, toe-dragging, stumbling and clumsiness	Poor locomotion due to fatigue, conformation or excessive hoof growth
Forging, clicking and over-reaching	Inappropriate farriery, conformation problems and inattentive equitation
Brushing, speedy cutting and dishing	Inappropriate farriery and conformation problems
Hitting fences	Failure to elevate limbs, especially the leading foreleg while jumping

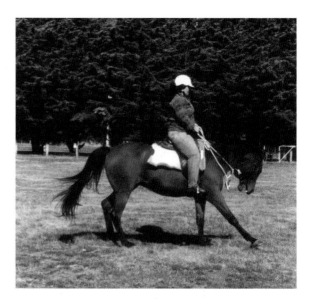

Figure 15.8 A hard-mouthed horse. (With kind permission of Elvira Currie.)

EVIDENCE OF LEARNED HELPLESSNESS

Horses may learn that they are unable to help themselves when responses they use to relieve pain or discomfort or threats (or their precursors) are unsuccessful. By a process of habituation, such horses often become unresponsive to the stimuli, but it is unclear whether they all do so with a concurrent reduction in physiological distress.

Horses that exhibit general reluctance to work and resistance to signals from the rider are described as 'stale' or 'sour'. Specifically they may be referred to as being hard-mouthed (Fig. 15.8) or lazy and sluggish, whereas, more correctly, they should be considered to have habituated to rein pressure or leg pressure, respectively. It is difficult but not impossible to re-educate these horses (see Ch. 13).

CAUSES OF UNWELCOME RESPONSES IN THE RIDDEN HORSE

Two broad sections are proposed here: unwelcome behavioral responses caused directly by humans, and those attributable more to the horse than the rider. However, it is accepted that while the dichotomy is not absolute, the responsibility for equine behavior problems ultimately lies with humans, since we have undertaken the domestication and exploitation of equids. Because humans are so directly involved in the first group, it is likely that interventions such as behavior therapy are more likely to work in these cases.

HUMAN CAUSES OF UNWELCOME BEHAVIORAL RESPONSES

Some unwelcome responses disappear if management deficiencies are corrected or if the rider becomes more skilled or is replaced by a more talented equestrian. Horses learn to evade discomfort in both appropriate and inappropriate ways. Sometimes, for example in rodeos, horses are required to produce exaggerated agonistic responses as part of their work. Indeed Schonholtz[10] points out that some horses are purpose-bred for a heightened anti-predator response (e.g. one line of buckers accounted for 30 horses used at the US National Rodeo Finals in 1996). While this is claimed by some to be evidence for the increasingly humane treatment of rodeo animals, it may simply indicate that hypersensitive horses can be bred. This means that selected animals are less likely to habituate to being ridden with a bucking strap in place because they continue to find the procedure aversive. So purpose breeding seems an unconvincing justification for the use of selected rodeo animals on welfare grounds.

While schooling in the form of operant conditioning can make a horse respond desirably, it can also evoke resistance, conflict and learned helplessness when administered crudely, inconsistently or too rapidly.[11] Avoidance and resolution of problems in the ridden horse have already been explained in Chapter 13.

Poor riding technique

The importance of rider position is always stressed in riding manuals, with good reason (see Fig. 7.20). Without this pre-requisite, riders attempt to maintain or resume a centered position and usually have a significant effect on the horse's movement and balance in the short term (Fig. 15.9). In the long term, a rider's lack of balance allows the horse to practice unrequested responses. The more opportunities the horse has to trial responses that are not under stimulus

control, the greater it perceives its freedom from the control of the rider. This allows an escalating series of random behaviors to be trialed and possibly reinforced. For these reasons, novice riders should never be paired with uneducated horses.

Poor application of learning theory

Although horses are adaptable and therefore tolerant of poor handling and training, this does not obviate the need to use tact and sensitivity when applying aversive stimuli. Punishment and inappropriate negative reinforcement are prevalent because few riders appreciate the importance of learning theory (Table 15.4).

Unrealistic expectations

As the commercial value of a horse is often related to its ability to compete, many owners seek to push their horses to the limits of their performance. When the expectations of the owners are not met, this may account for some abiding dissatisfaction and the application of interventions that can elicit conflict. Coercion is ineffective and inhumane when the real problem is ignorance of the true limitations of the horse's

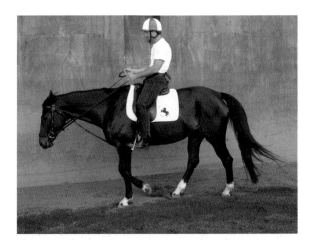

Figure 15.9 An inexperienced rider showing lack of balance, with the hands uneven and the legs placed too far forward. Typically these characteristics predispose the rider to being 'left behind' the horse whenever it moves forward with unexpected speed, an outcome that prompts many novices to compensate by using the reins to balance. (Photograph courtesy of Sandro Nocentini.)

Table 15.4   Common rider faults that demonstrate poor application of learning theory and may serve to confuse horses

Rider fault	Example
Nagging	Repeated application of aversive stimuli regardless of response
Poor timing	Application of signals *after* the response has been offered
Inconsistency	Failure to relieve pressure to reinforce every desirable response
Failure to reinforce	Ignorance of the need to relieve pressure
Inappropriate punishment	Punishment for fear responses
Poor balance	Inability of the rider to balance without signaling to the horse
Pursuit of style at the expense of other appropriate goals	Prioritizing desirable outline over self-carriage

ability. For example, although the majority of Thoroughbreds are physiologically suited to fast work, one study demonstrated that only 10% win prize money to offset the purchase and ongoing expenses.[12] Such horses may be viewed as under-achievers and may even attract more use of the whip than those that run fast enough to meet their owners' expectations.

Hyper-reactivity

While reactivity is selected-for in some high-performance breeds, especially those used for racing, it is unwelcome in the breeding stock of others such as those used for draft purposes. Motivation to respond to pressure may be reduced in the more stoic animals that are commonly labeled sluggish. Perversely the so-called warmbloods may be so tolerant of bit pressures that they can perform in dressage competitions while subjected to bit pressures that hotbloods cannot ignore.

Hyper-reactivity may arise from inappropriate matching of horses with the work required of them. For example, some horses cannot be used in traffic because they are intolerant of large objects moving in their peripheral vision. Additionally, most traffic-shy horses learn to anticipate aversive stimuli from riders (including rein and leg pressures) when traffic is encountered. This means that instead of habituating to traffic as most horses do, they recognize the rider's alarm and become especially responsive to traffic-related stimuli; in other words, they become sensitized (see Ch. 4). As discussed with shying, even in the absence of anticipation, inadvertently applying pressure may increase the horses' motivation to find freedom (Fig. 15.10).[2]

Beyond mismatching horses for work, two general causes of hyper-reactivity are management and schooling. We know that the frequency of unwanted behavior during training is increased by stabling.[13] By feeding horses inappropriately and housing them without regard for their need for conspecific company and spontaneous exercise and play, humans increase the likelihood of

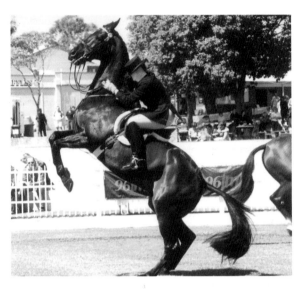

Figure 15.10 A rearing horse under-saddle. (Photograph courtesy of Sandra Hannan.)

explosive displays of locomotory behaviors. So, the influence of intensive management should always be considered when a horse presents with training problems. For example, because shying appears more likely in stabled horses it is appropriate to consider the effects of post-inhibitory rebound[14] and the role of over-feeding high-energy foods as contributors to hyper-reactivity in the wake of confinement. As far as the role of schooling is concerned, it is worth remembering that some riders train their horses to be acutely sensitive to leg pressure. This is appropriate only if the horses are never ridden by novices who may trigger responses inadvertently, e.g. by using their legs to balance.

Failure to consider social needs

Most equestrian pursuits require riders to thwart the horse's innate need to have constant conspecific company. Inattention to this need or inadequate training of the horse to cope without it can lead to undesirable responses under-saddle. Separation-related distress may cause bolting, while aggression to conspecifics while under-saddle may mean that a horse cannot be ridden in company. The inadequate provision of space between horses that are strangers or occasionally even affiliates can cause horses to show aggression to conspecifics while being worked. This is unwelcome since it can cause injuries to both horses and riders. The more obedient a horse is under-saddle the less likely are these responses, so retraining the 'go' and 'stop' responses is clearly indicated. Due consideration should also be given to the social environment to which the horse is exposed at home and the relevance of this at exercise.

HORSE-RELATED CAUSES OF UNWELCOME BEHAVIORAL RESPONSES

If horses continue to perform poorly, despite demonstrable improvements in management or technique, they may have innate or acquired physical anomalies that make them unsuitable for ridden work. This is not meant to suggest that the horses are at fault, since most of these problems can ultimately be attributed to human intervention or omission.

Pain

The application of pressure in sensitive areas is an implicit feature of traditional equitation, which relies on negative reinforcement. While humans routinely inflict discomfort on ridden horses intentionally with rein and leg pressure via bits and spurs, they may also do so unintentionally as a result of poor management or oversight (Table 15.5).

Physical inability

Some horses will never be able to excel in some fields (Table 15.6). Their inability should be identified rather than misinterpreted as disobedience or the absence of a 'will to please'.

Because they had become associated with previous adverse experiences, raised voices and forceful restraint readily conveyed to this pony the message that any veterinary intervention was

Table 15.5 Selected examples of management factors that contribute to unintentional pain in ridden horses

Problem area	Example
Tack	Saddles can pinch the dorsal lumbar musculature
Hoof care	Inappropriate hoof trimming can contribute to bruising of the foot
Malnutrition	Overfeeding can increase the risk of rhabdomyolysis
Dental anomalies	Sharp spurs and hooks in the molar and premolar teeth may make jaw movement uncomfortable and therefore make the horse less likely to relax its jaw when ridden
Cranial discomfort	Trigeminal pain may cause head-shaking with frenzied flexion and extension of the poll
Musculoskeletal pathologies	Navicular pain may make the horse resistant to work on hard surfaces
Exercise surfaces	Certain exercise surfaces may cause unnecessary pain

Table 15.6 Examples of some of the ways in which horses are predisposed to poor performance

Problem area	Example
Anomalies in perception	Partial blindness can lead to generalized wariness
Conformation	Inadequate height or hindquarter strength can disadvantage a horse intended for jumping or dressage, respectively
Physiology	Inherently low thresholds for dehydration and fatigue
Gait anomalies	A familial tendency to trot may disadvantage some Standardbreds when asked to pace

going to be unpleasant and that the person doing it was to be avoided and feared. Clearly, the use of force and punishment was inappropriate.

This case was approached in two phases. The first was to counter the mare's fear of injections, and the second focused on her fear of the clippers. The overall goal was to make the experience of both more positive than negative.

SUMMARY OF KEY POINTS

- Equine behavior therapy relies on:
  - consideration of the ethological relevance of unwelcome behaviors
  - elimination of pain and discomfort as proximate causes
  - the application of learning theory to resolve learned responses.
- The reasons for failure of behavioral modification include:
  - inconsistent application of learning theory
  - a lack of reconciliation of the task required of the horse and its physical ability to oblige.
- Riders often experiment with increased force before seeking professional help.
- Persistent application of traditional techniques that have contributed to the emergence of unwelcome behaviors makes the problems themselves more persistent.
- Clinical examinations are essential to rule out non-behavioral causes of undesirable behaviors.
- Consideration of the motivation for undesirable responses in ethological terms helps to identify the causal factors.
- In all cases, the key to behavior therapy is sound application of learning theory.
- Clients should be counseled not to expect quick fixes, especially with long-standing problems.

CASE STUDY

A 5-year-old riding pony mare had developed a reputation for being impossible to inject. A veterinarian who was persuaded to inject her with a sedative prior to being clipped while she was restrained within a float had his spleen ruptured in the frenzied flight response that ensued when the mare appreciated she was going to be injected.

Injections

Using the technique established by Professor Sue McDonnell[5] for achieving compliance with any intervention, the mare had to learn three basic lessons. These were that the intervention:

- does not really hurt that much
- could lead to rewards, if tolerated
- could not be stopped with regular flight or fight responses.

The first step was to ensure that the restraint of the mare was not causing genuine discomfort or fear, so she was handled in a large corral in which she could move without crashing into anything if she withdrew at speed during the procedure. To avoid their conveying anxiety to the mare, it was important that personnel working with her were not tense or fearful. Many horses have learned that flinching or retreating on the part of personnel is a portent of their departure, which reinforces agonistic responses.

For injection shyness, it was important to ensure that the injections themselves were as painless as possible by using a small-gauge needle and a quick but gentle injection technique. Successive tolerable approximations of the procedure were patiently repeated. Initially, each improvement in compliance was rewarded with a primary reinforcer (see Shaping in Ch. 4). In this mare's case, carrots were demonstrably reinforcing, so they were used in the shaping process. Any adverse reactions were not punished. If she moved away, the mare was trained to find that this did nothing to help her avoid the procedure. Personnel stayed with her as much as possible, and calmly waited for her to stop recoiling.

The mare eventually learned to tolerate injections and even appeared to enjoy most normal non-painful veterinary or management procedures.

Clipping

Counter-conditioning was used to train the mare to associate the sound of the clippers with the arrival of her evening meal. The clippers were switched on every evening until the mare and her stable-mates were all responding to the sound of the clippers alone by demonstrating typical restlessness that one finds at feed times, e.g. when buckets are rattled. The next step was to introduce the sight of the clippers in combination with their sound. The mare had all meals presented only after the clippers had been switched on in her stable.

The final steps involved counter-conditioning the fear of the clippers making contact. With the attraction of the food, the mare was encouraged to move toward the clippers. When she did so they were switched off. In this way she was given some operant control of her fear. This was a form of negative reinforcement since the response was made more likely by the removal of the aversive stimulus. She was then target trained with food to move towards the clippers so that they developed associations with rewards.

The seasonality of clipping meant that the clippers would normally have been shelved for many months before being re-used. This was considered counter-productive since spontaneous recovery of the fearful response was a possibility. So, throughout the summer months, the mare continued to have the clippers presented and still has to approach them before they are switched off and she is fed. Now, when she has to be clipped, she can be clipped without any forceful restraint and, indeed, without any sweating.

REFERENCES

1. Haussler KK, Stover SM, Willits NH. Pathologic changes in the lumbosacral vertebrae and pelvis in Thoroughbred racehorses. Am J Vet Res 1999; 60(2):143–153.
2. McGreevy PD, McLean A. Development and resolution of behavioural problems with the ridden horse. In: Behavioural biology of the horse. Cambridge: Cambridge University Press; In press.
3. Roberts T. Equestrian technique. London: JA Allen; 1992.
4. Rollin BE. Equine welfare and emerging social ethics. Animal Welfare Forum: Equine Welfare. J Am Vet Med Assoc 2000; 216(8):1234–1237.
5. McDonnell SM. How to rehabilitate horses with injection shyness (or any procedure non-compliance). Annual Meeting AAEP, San Antonio, Texas, November 26–28, 2000.
6. Waring GH. Horse behavior: the behavioral traits and adaptations of domestic and wild horses including ponies. Park Ridge, NJ: Noyes; 1983.
7. Mills DS. Personality and individual differences in the horse, their significance, use and measurement. Equine Vet J Suppl 1998; 27:10–13.
8. Casey R. Recognising the importance of pain in the diagnosis of equine behaviour problems. In: Harris PA, Gomarsall GM, Davidson HPB, Green RE, eds. Proceedings of the BEVA Specialist Days on Behaviour and Nutrition; 1999:25–28.
9. Wilewski KA, Rubin L. Bit seats: a dental procedure for enhancing performance of show horses. Equine Pract 1999; 21(4):16–20.
10. Schonholtz CM. Animals in rodeo – a closer look. Animal Welfare Forum: Equine Welfare. J Am Vet Med Assoc 2000; 216(8):1246–1249.
11. McLean AN, McLean MM. Horse training the McLean way – the science behind the art. Victoria, Australia: Australian Equine Behaviour Centre; 2002.
12. More SJ. A longitudinal study of racing Thoroughbreds: performance during the first years of racing. Aust Vet J 1999; 77:105–112.
13. Rivera E, Benjamin S, Nielsen B, et al. Behavioral and physiological responses of horses to initial training: the comparison between pastured versus stalled horses. Appl Anim Behav Sci 2002; 78(2–4):235–252.
14. Houpt K, Houpt TR, Johnson JL, et al. The effect of exercise deprivation on the behaviour and physiology of straight-stall confined pregnant mares. Anim Welfare 2001; 10(3):257–267.

Further reading

Budiansky S. The nature of horses – exploring equine evolution, intelligence and behaviour. New York: The Free Press; 1997.

Houpt KA. Domestic animal behaviour for veterinarians and animal scientists, 3rd edn. UK: Manson Publishing; 1998.

Kiley-Worthington M. The behaviour of horses: in relation to management and training. London: JA Allen; 1987.

McDonnell S. A practical field guide to horse behavior – The equid ethogram. Lexington, Kentucky: The Blood Horse Inc; 2003.

McGreevy PD. Why does my horse … ? London: Souvenir Press; 1996.

McLean A. The truth about horses. Melbourne: Penguin; 2003.

Mills DS, Nankervis KJ. Equine behaviour: principles and practice. Oxford: Blackwell Science Publication; 1999.

Rees L. The horse's mind. London: Stanley Paul; 1984.

Waring GH. Horse behavior: the behavioral traits and adaptions of domestic and wild horses including ponies, 2nd edn. New York: Noyes Publications Williams Andrews Publishing; 2003.

Readers who are interested in learning more about equine behaviour may wish to join the international Equine Behaviour Forum (EBF). Founded in 1978 and based in the UK, the EBF is an entirely voluntary, non-profit-making group for people interested in equine (not only horse) behavior. Its membership comprises vets, scientists as well as professional and amateur horsepeople. The EBF produces the journal *Equine Behaviour* which is a platform for both scientific and 'amateur' content. *Equine Behaviour* is written and illustrated mainly by its members and includes letter, articles, views and experiences, book reviews, requests for and offers of help and advice. To find out more, visit www.gla.ac.uk/external/EBF

Glossary

Glossary of colloquialisms, ethological and equestrian terms

While it is clear that the use of unscientific terms has flourished in equestrian circles, the extent to which 'horsey' folk can agree on the meanings of these terms has been called into question.[1] The following glossary of terms is an attempt to demystify some of the terms that may confound novice practitioners on either side of the Atlantic.

Aerophagia: Pathological and excessive swallowing of air.

Agonistic behavior: Any behavior associated with threat, attack or defense. It includes related aspects of behavior, including passivity and escape as well as aggression.

Aid: Any of the signals used by riders to give instructions to horses. *See also* Artificial aids *and* Natural aids.

Air above the ground: A group of advanced maneuvers in which the horse rears up in a controlled fashion onto its hindlegs, with its forelegs curled under its chest and then either holds this pose, or jumps into the air off its hindlegs. *See also* Ballotade, Capriole, Courbette, Croupade, Levade *and* Mezair.

Allogrooming: Grooming action directed from one herdmate to another and most commonly followed by mutual grooming (i.e. in which allogrooming is reciprocated).

Alter: To castrate (or geld) a horse.

Anorexia: Abnormal reduction of ingestive behavior, e.g. in depressed and toxic clinical states.

Appetitive: In the broadest sense, appetitive behavior represents the first phase of a series of behaviors that leads to the consummatory phase involving the actual behavior and the refractory period.

Artificial aids: Equipment used to alter a horse's behavior under-saddle or in-hand, e.g. whips, spurs and martingales (q.v.).

Asking with the rein: Mild cues sent by the rider through the rein.

Aversion therapy: Treatment of an unwelcome behavior by associating it with an aversive stimulus such as an electric shock.

Aversive: Describes a stimulus that elicits avoidance or withdrawal.

Balanced seat: The position of the mounted rider that requires the minimum of muscular effort to remain in the saddle and which interferes least with the horse's movements and equilibrium. (*See also* Independent seat).

Balk (or baulk): Refuse to move forward.

Ballotade: An air-above-the-ground in which the horse half rears, then jumps forward with its hindlegs tucked underneath it.

Barn: *See* Yard.

Bars: Area of gum between the teeth in which the bit lies (also called diastema).

Behind the bit: An evasive posture that thwarts the development of impulsion, in which the horse persistently draws its nose in, allowing the rein to go slack.

Biological fitness: The ability of an animal to survive and reproduce, a concept referring to one genotype's ability to succeed relative to another's.

Bitless bridle: Any of a variety of bridles designed without bits so that pressure is exerted on the nose, poll or curb groove instead of the mouth.

Blind bucker: A horse that bucks indiscriminately, sometimes heading toward obstacles, when ridden.

Blow up: (a) When a ridden horse either breaks from the pace at which it is meant to be traveling or misbehaves generally. (b) (US To start bucking.)

Bolting: (a) Eating too rapidly. (b) Breaking out of control or trying to run away.

Bosal: The braided rawhide or rope noseband of a bosal hackamore.

Break: The basic training of a young horse to obey commands, and accept direction and control, for whatever purpose it may be required.

Breaking: The transition seen in trotters or pacers that leave their gait and start to gallop.

Bridle lameness: An appearance of lameness that arises when a horse is unable to free itself of bit pressure because of one or both reins being too tight and resulting in an irregular rhythm and a crooked longitudinal axis of the body.

Bronco: An unbroken or imperfectly broken feral horse.

Bronco-buster: A person who breaks and trains broncos (horses used for bucking competitions in rodeos).

Bucking: Leaping forwards and dorsally with speed while arching the back and descending with the forelegs rigid and the head held low.

Camp-drafting: A uniquely Australian rodeo contest in which a rider separates a bullock from a group of cattle and drives it at the gallop around a course marked with upright poles.

Canter: A rotary three time gait in which the hooves strike the ground in the following order: near hind, near fore and off hind together, off fore (leading leg); or off hind, off fore and near hind together, near fore (leading leg).

Capriole: An air-above-the-ground maneuver (often considered the ultimate of all high-school and classical training) in which the horse half rears with the hocks drawn under, then jumps forward and high into the air, at the same time kicking out the hindlegs with the soles of the feet turned upwards, before landing collectedly on all four legs.

Cast: A horse's having fallen or laid down close to a wall or fence so that it cannot get up without assistance.

Causal factors: Interpretation of external change or internal state that form inputs to a decision-making center of an animal's brain.

Cavalletti: A series of small jumps used in the basic training of a riding horse with the intention of encouraging lengthened strides, improved balance and loosened up and strengthened muscles.

Circadian rhythm: A rhythm in behavior, metabolism or some other activity that recurs about every 24 hours.

Cold-back: (US Cinch bound) Resentment or instability sometimes to the extent of collapse when the girth is tightened or a horse is mounted.

Collection: Shortening the pace by the application of light tension from the rider's hands and steady pressure with the legs to make the horse flex its neck and bring its hocks underneath it.

Combinations: In show-jumping, an obstacle consisting of two or more separate jumps that are numbered and judged as one obstacle.

Conformation: Features of the external morphology (i.e. relative musculoskeletal dimensions) of a horse that interest breeders and exhibitors, not least because they can affect its performance.[2]

Conspecific: Animals belonging to the same species.

Consummatory act: An act that reduces the levels of causal factors so that the activity is terminated.

Contact: A steady (and preferably light) tension in the rein(s).[3]

Coping: The short-term or long-term ability to have control of mental and bodily stability, an absence of which leads to reduced fitness and stress.

Coprophagia/coprophagy: Eating feces, a behavior that is regarded as abnormal except in foals.

Core area: The area of heaviest regular use within an animal's home range.

Corn/concentrates: (US Sweet feed) Dried, crushed or pelleted food.

Courbette: Rearing to an almost upright position, and then leaping forwards several times on the hindlegs alone.

Creep-feeding: Providing youngstock with concentrates or supplements via a feeding apparatus that denies access to older animals, including the dam, by having a small entrance.

Crib-biting: (US Cribbing) Holding onto a fixed object with the incisor teeth, arching the neck and leaning backwards with or without engulfing air with a characteristic grunting noise.

Croupade: Rearing and then jumping vertically with forelegs and hindlegs well flexed under the body, to land again on the hind feet.

Cryptorchid: A horse with at least one testicle in an abdominal position.

Curb bit: A type of bit consisting of two metal cheekpieces and a mouthpiece with a central indented section (called the port) used in conjunction with a snaffle bit and a curb chain in a double bridle.

Curb chain: A chain that lies in the curb groove of the horse's jaw when fitted to a curb or pelham bit and acts by applying pressure to this part of the horse's head in concert with regular bits in its mouth.

Cut: To geld or castrate a colt or stallion.

Cutting horse: A horse trained, and often bred, for separating selected cattle from a herd.

Depression: General state of behavioral atony, features of which can include sagged posture and unresponsiveness.

Diagonal: Refers to the forefoot's moving in unison with the contralateral hindfoot.

Direct flexion: A description of a horse that is correctly 'on the bit' (q.v.). For a horse to be showing direct flexion it must:

first, be straight (i.e. not laterally crooked); second, be extending its hocks cranially; and finally, be relaxed in the jaw.[4]

Displacement activity: An activity performed in a situation apparently different from the context in which it would normally occur. This term is often of reasonably limited use because it is dependent on the observer's ability to correctly determine the relevance of the behavior to the current context.

Disunited canter: This undesirable broken gait, more often seen in horses with a tendency to pace, occurs when the hindquarters lose coordination with the forequarters, and the horse leads with one leg in front and the diagonally opposite one behind.[5]

Diurnal rhythm: A rhythm in behavior, metabolism or some other activity that occurs on a daily basis or during daylight).

Double: In show-jumping, a combination obstacle consisting of two separate jumps.

Double bridle: A bridle comprising two bits, a curb and a snaffle, which are attached by means of two cheekpieces and may be operated independently.

Double-gaited: A term applied to a horse that can both trot and pace with reasonable speed.

Ecological niche: The environment that a species occupies in nature and usually in which it performs best.

Eliminative behavior: Patterns of behavior connected with the evacuation of feces and urine.

Engaging the hocks: The horse's bringing his hindfeet underneath his body so that proportionally more weight is placed on the hindlegs.

Epimiletic behavior: The provision of care and attention such as nursing behaviors.

Ethogram: A detailed description of the behavioral features of a particular species.

Ethology: The observation and description of behavior that leads to improved understanding of its mechanism, function, development and evolution.

Evading the bit: Oral behaviors and neck postures that enable horses to reduce the discomfort caused by bits or the extent to which riders can apply pressure.

Exploration: Any activity that offers the individual the potential to acquire new information about itself or its environment.

Extension: A vigorous forward movement involving straightened limbs that allow the horse to cover as much ground as possible with each stride.

Fall: In jumping, when the shoulders and quarters on the same side touch the ground. A rider is considered to have fallen when there is separation between him and his horse that necessitates his remounting.

FEI: The Fédération Equestre Internationale (International Equestrian Federation), body governing the international equestrian sports of show-jumping, three-day eventing, dressage and driving.

Feral: Horses that have escaped from domestication and become free-ranging, or their progeny.

Flehmen: Elevation of the upper lip to introduce odors, especially volatile fatty acids into the vomeronasal organ.

Flexion: Of the neck, when a horse bends ventrally at the poll, preferably while retaining a relaxed jaw. Of the body, when the longitudinal axis of the body bends dorsoventrally. Lateral flexion describes bending to the left or right at the atlanto-occipital joint.

Flight distance: The radius of space around an animal within which intrusion provokes a flight reaction.

Foraging: Behaviors that increase an animal's likelihood of encountering and acquiring food.

Forehand: Those parts of the horse that lie in front of the rider, i.e. the head, neck, shoulders, withers and forelegs.

Fraser Darling effect: The stimulation of reproductive activity by the presence and activity of conspecifics in addition to the mating pair.

Frustration: The process thought to occur when animals are thwarted from performing highly motivated behaviors.

Gee: The driving term that signals a turn to the right.

Geophagia/geophagy: Ingestion of soil.

Good mouth: *See* Soft mouth.

Green: (a) An inexperienced horse which has undergone foundation training but is not fully trained. (b) A trotter or pacer that has yet to undergo a time trial.

Group effect: A change in the behavior of a number of animals brought about by common participation.

Habituation: The waning of a response to a repeated stimulus as a result of frequent exposure (not simple fatigue).

Half-halt: A sequential application of rein and leg pressure intended to warn the ridden horse that it is about to be given a new command.

Half-pass: A lateral movement in which the horse moves both forward and sideways, bent toward the direction of movement. Half-pass may be performed at walk, trot and canter.

Hard-mouthed: (US Cold-jawed, tough-mouthed) Term used to describe the 'toughening of the bars of the mouth where the bit rests and the deadening of nerves because of the continued pressure of the bit' – more correctly this describes habituation to rein pressure.

Haute école: 'High school', classically the highest form of specialized training of the dressage horse.

Haw: The driving term that signals a turn to the left.

Head-pressing: Postural disorder usually linked to cerebral disease and characterized by apparent head stabilization through contact of the forehead with a vertical surface.

Hitch: (a) To fasten a horse, e.g. when hitched to a rail. (b) A connection between a vehicle and a horse.(c) A defect in gait noted in the hindlegs, which seem to skip at the trot.

Hollow: Extension of the vertebral column, considered undesirable in equitation.

Home range: Area that free-ranging animals use regularly. Though known intimately by its users, the home range may or may not be defended; those portions of it that are defended are called territories.

Impulsion: The response of an eager horse as it surges forward as soon as the rider signals. True impulsion, in which the horse conveys itself calmly and maintains a light rein pressure, is quite distinct from states of general excitement in which the horse pulls at the bit and requires forceful restraint to be controlled.

Independent seat: A rider's ability to maintain a firm, balanced position on a horse's back, without relying on the reins or stirrups. *See also* Balanced seat.

Ingestive behavior: Behavior concerned with the selection and intake of food, milk and water.

In-hand: In a routine of 'schooling in hand', the trainer works from the ground rather than from the saddle, standing beside the horse and controlling it with rein, voice, and schooling whip.

Initiator: The first individual in a social group to react in a way that elicits a new group activity.

Inside/outside: Terms used to identify sides of the horse as it is being schooled but that require some qualification to designate whether one is referring to the relative position in the arena, to the curvature of the path, or to the bend of the horse.

Intention movements: The preparatory activity that an animal may go through when switching from one suite of behaviors to another.

Jog: A short-paced trot.

Leaning on the bit: A sign of habituation to bit pressure which manifests with the horse persistently pulling on the rein(s) as though relying on the rider to support the weight of its head.

Leg yield: Lateral movement of a horse in response to pressure from the rider's leg, used as a schooling activity before training more complex lateral maneuvers such as a half-pass.

Levade: A controlled half rearing position, with the forelegs tucked well in toward the chest, the vertebral column inclined between 30° and 45° above the horizontal, and the hindlegs in a crouching position with deeply bent hocks.

Lightness: The bringing into action by the rider and the use by the horse of only those muscles necessary for the intended movement. Activity in any other muscle groups can create resistance and thus detract from the lightness.

Lignophagia/ lignophagy: Wood-eating, which may include bark-chewing.

Long-reining: Driving the horse without any vehicle or load. Used to train the horse to move forward without being led, to respond to bit pressures, to habituate it to distractions and to classically condition it to respond to vocal cues.

Loosebox: Stall or stable in which the horse is free to move about, as distinct from a tie-stall in which the horse is tied.

Lope: The western version of a very slow canter, this is a smooth, slow gait in which the head is carried low.

Lugging: *See* Pulling.

Lunge (also Longe): Exercising a horse on the end of a long lead or rope attached to a lungeing cavesson (q.v.), usually in a circle.

Lungeing cavesson: Head-collar with a strong, cushioned noseband used for exercising and training horses.

Manege (menage): *See* School.

Martingale: A device that is attached to the girth and passes between the horse's forelegs to help keep a horse's head in the 'correct' position by attaching to the noseband (standing martingale) or to the reins (running martingale) or directly to the bit.

Mezair: A series of levades (q.v.) is joined together by the horse rocking smoothly forward on the forelegs to touch the ground between each levade.

Monorchid: A horse with a single descended testicle.

Motivation: The process within the brain that controls the occurrence and performance of behaviors and physiological changes.

Motivational state: A combination of the levels of all causal factors.

Mouthing: (US: Champing) The horse's playing with the bit, a response that is encouraged in bitting a young horse by using a bit with 'keys' attached to the mouthpiece, which facilitates saliva flow and keeps the mouth moist.

Napping: When a horse fails to respond appropriately to the rider's signals, as in refusing to go forward or to pass a certain point.

Natural aids: The body, hands, legs, weight, and voice, as used in controlling a horse.

Neck rein: To guide or steer a horse by pressure of the rein on the neck.

Need: A deficiency in an animal that can be remedied by obtaining a particular resource or responding to a particular environment or bodily stimulus.

Numnah: (US Saddle blanket) A pad placed under the saddle to prevent undue pressure on the horse's dorsum.

Observational learning: Learning that occurs when one animal observes another and acquires a behavior without its own direct experience.

Off the bit: A lack of at least one of the three prerequisites for direct flexion (q.v.).

On the bit: Neck and poll flexion that involves the nasal planum being within 6° of the vertical, a posture intended to improve the extent to which the horse responds willingly to the signals transmitted by the rider through the reins. To most people, 'on the bit' means that the horse is going along with his nose nicely tucked in, moving smoothly from one place to another. However, a vertical nose does not necessarily mean that the horse is 'on the bit', although many observers may be fooled by it.[4] A perhaps more elegant term to describe being 'on the bit' is 'direct flexion' (q.v.).

On the forehand: An undesirable form of locomotion that effectively involves the horse leaning forward and therefore carrying an inappropriate proportion of its weight on its forequarter, a posture that runs counter to impulsion (q.v.), collection (q.v.) and self-carriage (q.v.).

Open bridle: Bridle without blinds or blinkers covering the eyes.

Outline: (US Shape, frame) An aspect of the horse's posture that refers particularly to the curvature of the vertebral column and the degree of flexion of the neck and poll. According to the ideals of equitation the nasal planum should be no more than 12° from the vertical at the walk and 6° from the vertical at other gaits and never behind the vertical, a fault which results in loss of self-carriage (q.v.) and lightness.

Over-crowding: A degree of crowding which reduces the biological fitness (q.v.) of individuals in the group.

Oxer: (US Hog's back) a spread obstacle in show-jumping with three sets of poles: the first close to the ground, the second at the highest point of the obstacle and the third slightly lower than the second.

Pace: A two time lateral gait in which the hindleg and the foreleg on the same side move forward together.

Pain: An extremely aversive sensation.

Parabola: The arc made by a jumping horse from the point of take-off to the point of landing.

Parallel bars: A spread fence used in both show-jumping and cross-country courses, comprising two sets of posts and rails.

Passada: A change of rein through a small half-volte performed in full-pass with haunches well in but moving on a somewhat larger circle than they do in a half-pirouette.

Passage: An haute école maneuver in which the horse shows an elevated, collected trot and appears to dance forward from one diagonal pair of legs to the other, elegantly pointing the feet to the ground during the movement of suspension when the legs are fully flexed at the top of each unsupported phase.

Pecking order: A hierarchy in which each individual is able to threaten, displace or attack individuals lower than itself.

Pelham bit: A bit with a single mouthpiece designed to produce the combined effects of the snaffle bit and the curb bit.

Piaffe: A very elevated, cadenced, collected trot, similar to a passage performed with minimal forward progression.

Pica: The searching-for and ingestion of inappropriate substrates that may be toxic and cause obstruction.

Pig-rooting: Lowering the head often as a prelude to bucking.

Pirouette: A turn within the horse's body length, on the center, the forehand or the haunches.

Pivot: A dressage maneuver in which the horse spins on its hindquarters, holding one hindleg more or less in place and side-stepping with the contralateral hindfoot.

Posting trot: *See* Rising trot.

Pulling: (US Lugging) Evasive behavior by ridden or driven horses leaning on the reins or bearing to the left or right without being prompted.

Punishment: A decrease in the likelihood of a response due to the presentation of an aversive stimulus or, in the case of negative punishment, the removal of a reinforcing stimulus.

Quidding: Dysphagia.

Rack: The most spectacular movement of five gaited horses, this is a very fast even lateral gait in which each foot strikes the ground separately in quick succession.

Redirected behavior: The direction of an activity away from the primary target and toward another less appropriate substrate, a term to be used only with care because it implies that the observer knows what the primary target is.

Red ribbon: A strip of red material tied round the tail-head of a horse, especially when hunting, to indicate that it has been known to kick conspecifics in company.

Rein back: To make a horse step backwards while being driven or ridden.

Reinforcer: An environmental change that increases the likelihood that an animal will make a particular response, i.e. a reward (positive reinforcer) or removal of a punishment (negative reinforcer).

Renvers: A dressage movement on two tracks in which the horse moves at an angle of not more than 30° along the long side of the arena with its hindlegs on the outer and its forelegs on the inner track, looking in the direction in which it is going and being bent slightly round the rider's inside leg.

Rig: (US Ridgeling): *See* Monorchid *and* Cryptorchid.

Rising trot: (US Posting trot) The rising and descending of the rider with the rhythm of the trot.

Ritual behavior: An originally variable sequence of actions that may have lost some of its original meaning, become almost rigid in sequence, and developed a role in communication.

Saddle blanket: *See* Numnah.

School (a) An enclosed area, either covered or open in which a horse may be trained or exercised. (b) To train a horse for whatever purpose it may be required.

Self-carriage: The characteristic way in which a well-trained horse deports itself with lightness of the forehand and reliance on the hindquarters for propulsion.

Sensitization: The increasing of a response to a repeated stimulus.

Shoulder-in: One of the lateral movements in which the shoulder is brought in from the track of the inside hindleg so that the forelegs travel on a separate, parallel but overlapping track and the horse's longitudinal axis is bent away from the direction of movement.

Slow gait: One of the gaits of the five-gaited breeds characterized by a prancing action in which each foot in turn is raised and then held momentarily in mid-air before descending.

Social facilitation: When a behavior is initiated or increased in frequency by the stimulus of another animal performing that behavior.

Soft condition: Easily fatigued.

Soft mouth: Sensitive mouth, responsive to bit pressure.

Spanish walk/trot: Extended gaits (usually trained in-hand) in which the forelegs are momentarily held out horizontally forward from the shoulder at each stride, the feet are brought to the ground without the knees bending and the head is held high to transfer weight onto the hindlegs.

Spooky: Nervous.

Spread fence: Any obstacle (such as an oxer, parallel bars, triple bar or water jump) in show-jumping and cross-country events that is wide as opposed to simply high.

Spur: A pointed device strapped on to the heel of a rider's boot and used to urge the horse forwards or laterally.

Yard: (US Barn) Accommodation for a group of horses.

Star gazer: A horse that moves in-hand or under-saddle with its head elevated in an awkward position.

Stereotypy: A repeated, relatively invariant sequence of movements that has no obvious function.

Straight fence: Any obstacle (such as gate, post and rails or planks) in show-jumping and cross-country courses that has all its component parts in the same vertical plane.

Stress: All extra-individual events capable of evoking a broad spectrum of intra-individual responses mediated by a complex filter labeled 'individual differences'.

Stride: The set of changes occurring during a single complete locomotory cycle, which includes the stance phase and the swing phase of a limb, from the one landing of a particular foot to the next.

Territory: The area an animal defends by demarcation or by fighting.

Tonic immobility: A behavioral state of a few seconds or longer during which an animal makes no movement

as a result of a pathological condition or an environmental event.

Transition: (a) The change from one gait type to another. (b) The changeover of support within a specific gait from one member of a diagonal pair of legs to the other.

Travers: A dressage movement on two tracks in which the horse moves at an angle of not more than 30° along the long side of the arena with its forelegs on the outer track and the hindlegs on the inner track, looking in the direction in which it is going and bent slightly round the rider's inside leg.

Turn on the forehand: A movement in which the horse steps in one spot with its forehand while describing concentric circles with its hindlegs. Usually executed with the same rhythm as the walk, turns on the forehand are commonly of 90°, 180° or 360°.

Turn on the haunches: A change of direction in which the hindlegs remain in one spot and the forequarters describe an arc. Unlike the lateral movement prompted by neck reining, a turn on the haunches is usually executed at the rhythm of the walk.

Twitch: A device used on a horse's upper lip that is tightened by twisting or pinching to pacify the horse for short periods by causing the release of endorphins.

Unlevel: A euphemism for abnormal action caused by either clinical lameness or a physical abnormality that changes the action of the horse.

Volte: (a) The smallest circle a horse is able to execute on either one or two tracks, the radius being equal to the length of the horse. (b) In dressage, a full turn on the haunches.

Walk: A four-beat gait of four time in which the hooves strike the ground in the following sequence: near hind, near fore, off hind, off fore.

Water jump: In show-jumping, a spread obstacle consisting of a sunken trough of water (with a minimum width of 4.2 meters and a length of up to 4.8 meters) with the option of small brush fence placed on the take-off side.

Wind-sucking: In Australia, the stereotypic gripping of a fixed object with the teeth while pulling back and engulfing air into the cranial esophagus. In the UK, engulfing air into the cranial esophagus without holding on to any fixed object.

REFERENCES

1. Mills DS. Personality and individual differences in the horse, their significance, use and measurement. Equine Vet J Suppl 1998; 27:10–13.
2. Loch S. The classical rider: being at one with your horse. North Pomfret: Trafalgar Square; 1977.
3. Sivewright M. Thinking riding, book 2: In good form. London: JA Allen; 1984.
4. Wallace J. The less-than-perfect-horse. London: Methuen; 1993.
5. Wynmalen H. Equitation. London: Country Life; 1947.

Index

Note: Page entries in **bold** refer to tables, those in *italics* refer to figures. All entries in the index refer to horses and equine behavior unless otherwise stated and hence entries under these headings have been kept to a minimum.